GOWNED AND GLOVED ORTHOPAEDICS

GOWNED AND GLOVED ORTHOPAEDICS:

INTRODUCTION TO COMMON PROCEDURES

Neil P. Sheth, MD

Instructor
Department of Orthopaedic Surgery
Hospital of the University of Pennsylvania
Philadelphia, Pennsylvania

Jess H. Lonner, MD

Director of Knee Replacement Surgery
Booth Bartolozzi Balderston Orthopaedics
Pennsylvania Hospital;
Medical Director
Philadelphia Center for Minimally Invasive Knee Surgery
Philadelphia, Pennsylvania

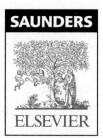

SAUNDERS

ELSEVIER

SAUNDERS
ELSEVIER

1600 John F. Kennedy Boulevard
Suite 1800
Philadelphia, PA 19103-2899

GOWNED AND GLOVED ORTHOPAEDICS:
INTRODUCTION TO COMMON PROCEDURES   ISBN: 978-1-4160-4820-6
Copyright © 2009 by Saunders, an imprint of Elsevier Inc.

Notice

Knowledge and best practice in this field are constantly changing. As new research and experience broaden our knowledge, changes in practice, treatment and drug therapy may become necessary or appropriate. Readers are advised to check the most current information provided (i) on procedures featured or (ii) by the manufacturer of each product to be administered, to verify the recommended dose or formula, the method and duration of administration, and contraindications. It is the responsibility of the practitioner, relying on their own experience and knowledge of the patient, to make diagnoses, to determine dosages and the best treatment for each individual patient, and to take all appropriate safety precautions. To the fullest extent of the law, neither the Publisher nor the Editors assume any liability for any injury and/or damage to persons or property arising out or related to any use of the material contained in this book.

The Publisher

Library of Congress Cataloging-in-Publication Data

Gowned and gloved orthopaedics : introduction to common procedures /
[edited by] Neil P. Sheth, Jess H. Lonner. — 1st ed.
     p. ; cm. — (Gowned and gloved)
     Includes bibliographical references and index.
     ISBN 978-1-4160-4820-6
   1. Orthopedics—Textbooks.   I. Sheth, Neil P.   II. Lonner, Jess H.   III. Series.
     [DNLM: 1. Orthopedic Procedures—methods. WE 190 G723 2009]
RD731.G69 2009
617.4'7—dc22

                                                    2008011021

Acquisitions Editor: James Merritt
Developmental Editor: Andrea Vosburgh
Publishing Services Manager: Joan Sinclair
Design Direction: Gene Harris

Printed in China

Last digit is the print number: 9 8 7 6 5 4 3 2 1

To the medical students who inspired the concept behind this text.

To my mentors, many of whom were involved with this project—thank you for your direction and guidance throughout the years and for getting me to this point in my career.

Most important, to my family and friends—thank you for your unconditional support of my academic endeavors.

NPS

To the students and residents who are considering a career in orthopaedic surgery—you are our future. I hope this book piques your interest and moves you to make a difference in this great specialty.

To the surgeons and residents who motivated, inspired, and taught me when I was learning the trade.

Most important, to my greatest joys—my wife, Ami, and our sons, Carson and Jared.

JHL

CONTRIBUTORS

JOSEPH A. ABBOUD, MD
Clinical Assistant Professor
Department of Orthopaedic Surgery
The University of Pennsylvania Health System
Philadelphia, Pennsylvania

JAIMO AHN, MD, PHD
Instructor
Department of Orthopaedic Surgery
Hospital of the University of Pennsylvania
Philadelphia, Pennsylvania

NIRAV H. AMIN, BS
Medical Student
Drexel University College of Medicine
Philadelphia, Pennsylvania

JOSHUA D. AUERBACH, MD
Instructor
Department of Orthopaedic Surgery
Hospital of the University of Pennsylvania
Philadelphia, Pennsylvania

KEITH D. BALDWIN, MD, MSPT, MPH
Instructor
Department of Orthopaedic Surgery
Hospital of the University of Pennsylvania
Philadelphia, Pennsylvania

PEDRO BEREDJIKLIAN, MD
Associate Professor
Department of Orthopaedic Surgery
University of Pennsylvania School of
   Medicine
Philadelphia, Pennsylvania

KAREN J. BOSELLI, MD
Instructor
Department of Orthopaedic Surgery
Hospital of the University of Pennsylvania
Philadelphia, Pennsylvania

ANDREA L. BOWERS, MD
Instructor
Department of Orthopaedic Surgery
Hospital of the University of Pennsylvania
Philadelphia, Pennsylvania

DAVID J. BOZENTKA, MD
Associate Professor
Department of Orthopaedic Surgery
University of Pennsylvania School of Medicine;
Chief
Department of Orthopaedic Surgery
Penn Presbyterian Medical Center
Philadelphia, Pennsylvania

KINGSLEY R. CHIN, MD
Assistant Professor of Orthopaedics
Department of Orthopaedic Surgery
Hospital of the University of Pennsylvania
Philadelphia, Pennsylvania

GREGORY K. DEIRMENGIAN, MD
Instructor
Department of Orthopaedic Surgery
Hospital of the University of Pennsylvania
Philadelphia, Pennsylvania

DEREK DOMBROSKI, MD
Instructor
Department of Orthopaedic Surgery
Hospital of the University of Pennsylvania
Philadelphia, Pennsylvania

DEREK J. DONEGAN, MD
Instructor
Department of Orthopaedic Surgery
Hospital of the University of Pennsylvania
Philadelphia, Pennsylvania

JOHN L. ESTERHAI, MD
Professor
Department of Orthopaedic Surgery
University of Pennsylvania School of Medicine;
Chief of Orthopedics
Department of Surgery
Veterans Affairs Medical Center
Philadelphia, Pennsylvania

JOHN M. FLYNN, MD
Associate Professor
Department of Orthopaedic Surgery
University of Pennsylvania School of Medicine;
Associate Chief
Department of Pediatric Orthopaedics
The Children's Hospital of Philadelphia
Philadelphia, Pennsylvania

THEODORE J. GANLEY, MD

Assistant Professor
Department of Orthopaedic Surgery
University of Pennsylvania School of Medicine;
Orthopaedic Director of Sports Medicine
Department of Pediatric Orthopaedic Surgery
The Children's Hospital of Philadelphia
Philadelphia, Pennsylvania

JONATHAN P. GARINO, MD

Associate Professor
Department of Orthopaedic Surgery
University of Pennsylvania School of Medicine;
Director
Adult Reconstructive Service
Penn Presbyterian Medical Center
Philadelphia, Pennsylvania

ALBERT O. GEE, MD

Instructor
Department of Orthopaedic Surgery
Hospital of the University of Pennsylvania
Philadelphia, Pennsylvania

DAVID L. GLASER, MD

Assistant Professor
Department of Orthopaedic Surgery
University of Pennsylvania School of Medicine;
Chief
Shoulder and Elbow Service
Penn Presbyterian Medical Center
Philadelphia, Pennsylvania

R. BRUCE HEPPENSTALL, MD, BSC, MA (HON.)

Professor and Vice Chair for Clinical Affairs
Department of Orthopaedic Surgery
University of Pennsylvania School of Medicine;
Department of Orthopaedic Surgery
Hospital of the University of Pennsylvania;
Department of Orthopaedic Surgery
Pennsylvania Hospital
Philadelphia, Pennsylvania

B. DAVID HORN, MD

Assistant Professor
Department of Orthopaedic Surgery
University of Pennsylvania School of Medicine;
Assistant Surgeon
Department of Orthopaedic Surgery
The Children's Hospital of Philadelphia
Philadelphia, Pennsylvania

G. RUSSELL HUFFMAN, MD, MPH

Assistant Professor
Department of Orthopaedic Surgery
University of Pennsylvania Sports Medicine Center
Philadelphia, Pennsylvania

CRAIG L. ISRAELITE, MD

Assistant Professor
Department of Orthopaedic Surgery
University of Pennsylvania School of Medicine
Philadelphia, Pennsylvania

KRISTOFER J. JONES, MD

Instructor
Department of Orthopaedic Surgery
Weill Cornell Medical College
Hospital for Special Surgery
New York, New York

JULIA A. KENNISTON, MD

Instructor
Department of Orthopaedic Surgery
Hospital of the University of Pennsylvania
Philadelphia, Pennsylvania

SAFDAR N. KHAN, MD

Orthopaedic Resident
Department of Orthopaedic Surgery
University of California at Davis
Sacramento, California

ERIC O. KLINEBERG, MD

Assistant Professor
Department of Orthopaedic Surgery
University of California at Davis;
Assistant Professor
Department of Orthopaedic Surgery
University of California at Davis Medical Center
Sacramento, California

ANDREW F. KUNTZ, MD

Instructor
Department of Orthopaedic Surgery
Hospital of the University of Pennsylvania
Philadelphia, Pennsylvania

J. TODD R. LAWRENCE, MD, PHD

Instructor
Department of Orthopaedic Surgery
Hospital of the University of Pennsylvania
Philadelphia, Pennsylvania

JESS H. LONNER, MD
Director of Knee Replacement Surgery
Booth Bartolozzi Balderston Orthopaedics
Pennsylvania Hospital;
Medical Director
Philadelphia Center for Minimally Invasive Knee
　Surgery
Philadelphia, Pennsylvania

JONAS L. MATZON, MD
Instructor
Department of Orthopaedic Surgery
Hospital of the University of Pennsylvania
Philadelphia, Pennsylvania

SAMIR MEHTA, MD
Assistant Professor
Department of Orthopaedic Surgery
University of Pennsylvania School of Medicine;
Chief, Orthopaedic Trauma Service
Department of Orthopaedic Surgery
Hospital of the University of Pennsylvania
Philadelphia, Pennsylvania

J. STUART MELVIN, MD
Instructor
Department of Orthopaedic Surgery
Hospital of the University of Pennsylvania
Philadelphia, Pennsylvania

SAMEER NAGDA, MD
Attending Orthopaedic Surgeon
Anderson Orthopaedic Clinic
Arlington, Virginia

CHARLES L. NELSON, MD
Associate Professor
Department of Orthopaedic Surgery
University of Pennsylvania School of Medicine
Philadelphia, Pennsylvania

ENYI OKEREKE, PharmD, MD
Associate Professor
Chief, Foot and Ankle Division
Department of Orthopaedic Surgery
University of Pennsylvania School of Medicine
Philadelphia, Pennsylvania

NIRAV K. PANDYA, MD
Instructor
Department of Orthopaedic Surgery
Hospital of the University of Pennsylvania
Philadelphia, Pennsylvania

DAVID I. PEDOWITZ, MD, MS
Instructor
Department of Orthopaedic Surgery
Hospital of the University of Pennsylvania
Philadelphia, Pennsylvania

STEPHAN G. PILL, MD, MSPT
Instructor
Department of Orthopaedic Surgery
Hospital of the University of Pennsylvania
Philadelphia, Pennsylvania

MATTHEW L. RAMSEY, MD
Associate Professor
Department of Orthopaedic Surgery
Thomas Jefferson University;
Shoulder and Elbow Service
Rothman Institute
Philadelphia, Pennsylvania

SUDHEER REDDY, MD
Instructor
Department of Orthopaedic Surgery
Hospital of the University of Pennsylvania
Philadelphia, Pennsylvania

ERIC T. RICCHETTI, MD
Instructor
Department of Orthopaedic Surgery
Hospital of the University of Pennsylvania
Philadelphia, Pennsylvania

SCOTT A. RUSHTON, MD
Assistant Clinical Professor
Department of Orthopaedic Surgery
University of Pennsylvania School of Medicine;
Director
Pennsylvania Hospital Spinal Reconstructive Fellowship
Pennsylvania Hospital
Philadelphia, Pennsylvania;
Medical Director
Center for Spinal Disorders
Lankenau Hospital
Wynnewood, Pennsylvania

WUDBHAV N. SANKAR, MD
Instructor
Department of Orthopaedic Surgery
Hospital of the University of Pennsylvania
Philadelphia, Pennsylvania

BRIAN J. SENNETT, MD
Assistant Professor
Department of Orthopaedic Surgery
Penn Sports Medicine Center
Philadelphia, Pennsylvania

NEIL P. SHETH, MD
Instructor
Department of Orthopaedic Surgery
Hospital of the University of Pennsylvania
Philadelphia, Pennsylvania

DAVID R. STEINBERG, MD
Associate Professor
Department of Orthopaedic Surgery
University of Pennsylvania School of Medicine;
Director, Hand and Upper Extremity Fellowship
Department of Orthopaedic Surgery
Chief, Hand Surgery
Veterans Affairs Medical Center
Philadelphia, Pennsylvania

WILLIAM TALLY, MD
Orthopaedic Spine Fellow
Pennsylvania Hospital
Philadelphia, Pennsylvania

JESSE T. TORBERT, MD, MS
Instructor
Department of Orthopaedic Surgery
Hospital of the University of Pennsylvania
Philadelphia, Pennsylvania

KEITH L. WAPNER, MD
Clinical Professor
Department of Orthopaedic Surgery
University of Pennsylvania School of Medicine;
Adjunct Professor
Department of Orthopaedic Surgery
Drexel University College of Medicine;
Director, Orthopaedic Foot and Ankle Fellowship
Department of Orthopaedic Surgery
Pennsylvania Hospital
Philadelphia, Pennsylvania

BRENT B. WIESEL, MD
Instructor
Georgetown University School of Medicine
Attending Surgeon
Department of Orthopaedic Surgery
Georgetown University Hospital
Washington, DC

Over the past decade, the field of orthopaedic surgery has become increasingly competitive from the perspective of a medical student. There are approximately 550 orthopaedic residency positions that are available for more than 1,500 student candidates.

Most medical students interested in pursuing a career in orthopaedic surgery will rotate through at least one orthopaedic sub-internship during their fourth year of school. Every year, students ask about the appropriate resources that they should use to prepare for these rotations, and often they are directed toward an anatomy atlas and a fracture handbook. However, most students spend nearly 90% of the day in the operating room, and their education is predominantly based on passive learning or occasional attending/resident formal teaching. On a busy service, teaching may not be the primary goal or it is done on the fly in the operating room.

The *Gowned and Gloved* series is designed to provide medical students, junior residents, and other members of the surgical healthcare team a resource to enable them to be more proactive about their intraoperative learning. This text offers a roadmap for the most common orthopaedic operative procedures. Each chapter presents a patient case, an algorithmic approach to patient evaluation, the pertinent applied surgical anatomy, and the sequence of steps used to treat the given pathoanatomy.

While referring to this text, please recognize that each individual attending surgeon will prefer his or her own variations or modifications of what is described. This text is geared toward providing readers a foundation on which to build their knowledge base for the surgical treatment of common orthopaedic problems. We hope that this publication assists you in optimally preparing for the operating room as you start your career in the exciting field of orthopaedic surgery.

NEIL P. SHETH, MD
JESS H. LONNER, MD

ACKNOWLEDGMENTS

We would like to thank the professional and enthusiastic staff at Elsevier, but particularly Jim Merritt and Andrea Vosburgh, who were with us from the start and put in countless hours to see this book through to completion.

Ultimately, this book never would have been possible without the commitment of the attending surgeons and residents who contributed chapters for this project. We are indebted to each of you for your participation.

In his outstanding oratory *Aequinimitas*, delivered to the graduating class of the University of Pennsylvania in 1898, Sir William Osler stated, "The first essential of a physician is to have his nerves well in hand." The quote is particularly appropriate to medical students and junior residents entering the operating room to observe and assist with operations that they have never seen or infrequently encountered. Certainly we all remember those experiences and the anxiety that these procedures provoked when, as junior members of the orthopaedic hierarchy, we were asked to observe or assist in these surgeries. How fitting that Neil Sheth and Jess Lonner have edited such an outstanding volume of surgical procedures that can be studied and learned in a straightforward and approachable manner. This text will provide much surgical knowledge to those early in their careers and will tremendously increase their understanding and appreciation for the procedures at which they will be assisting.

Orthopaedic surgery has evolved into a specialty driven by technology and rapidly improving surgical techniques. As one example, the advent of less invasive surgery that began with arthroscopic procedures has now spread to all areas of orthopaedic surgery. This text clearly explains the rationale for various surgical exposures and covers all anatomic areas as well as the fields of pediatrics, trauma, joint replacement, spine, and sports medicine. The procedures are well illustrated and precisely and succinctly demonstrated. The medical student or resident reviewing the surgical procedure that he or she will be scrubbing in on will effectively and quickly become familiar with the surgical approaches and the associated anatomy. There existed a real need for this text to provide this information in such a comprehensive yet user-friendly manner.

This text will be a great asset to the orthopaedic library of surgical techniques, but it will also be helpful as a guide to all levels of residents and even faculty members. With the subspecialization in orthopaedic surgery today, a text that covers a wide array of surgical approaches is necessary to educate all of us. Much credit goes to Dr. Sheth and Dr. Lonner for assembling a diverse group of authors, combining faculty, residents, and fellows, leading to this fine text. It is a needed addition that will be a great learning tool for both those in training and those doing the training.

THOMAS P. SCULCO, MD
Professor and Chair, Department of
  Orthopaedic Surgery
Weill Cornell Medical College;
Surgeon-in-Chief
Hospital for Special Surgery
New York, New York

CONTENTS

Basic Surgical Principles for Orthopaedic Procedures

Neil P. Sheth   and   Jess H. Lonner

This text is a compilation of surgical techniques used to treat the most common trauma-based or disease-based pathologies in orthopaedic surgery. The following guidelines are applicable to all orthopaedic surgical procedures and are presented here to avoid redundancy in the following chapters. Please keep these principles in mind as you read each section.

I. Each surgical patient should be properly identified in the holding area (by name, date of birth, or medical record number). The correct operative site should be marked and confirmed prior to transporting the patient to the operating room. Once in the operating room, the patient is once again identified with the operating room staff, and the site of surgery is confirmed in reference to the documented operative consent form in the chart. This is termed a "pause for safety" or "time-out," and it must be performed prior to starting any surgical procedure.

II. Make sure that the patient does not have a latex allergy prior to entering the operating room. If there is a documented allergy, it is imperative that all equipment used during the case, including Foley catheters, gloves, and tubing, be latex free.

III. Many longer cases or those with anticipated blood loss require the placement of a Foley catheter using sterile technique. It is typically removed on postoperative day 1 but may be left in place in specific instances.

IV. All patients should receive preoperative intravenous antibiotics approximately 30 to 60 minutes prior to the start of a case. Typically, 1 gram of cefazolin (Ancef), a first-generation cephalosporin, is the antibiotic of choice. The dose and choice of antibiotics can be adjusted according to weight and comorbidities. In patients with a penicillin allergy, IV vancomycin or clindamycin may be used as a substitute.

V. Prior to intubation, make sure that blood products are available for the patient if needed (e.g., bilateral total knee arthroplasty). In addition, it is important to check preoperative laboratory results, making sure that the patient is not coagulopathic and at an increased risk of bleeding or has a metabolic abnormality (e.g., hyperkalemia) that was not addressed preoperatively.

VI. Many cases involving the extremity use a tourniquet for minimizing blood loss during the operation. Procedures around the hip or the shoulder (e.g., total hip arthroplasty) are too proximal to allow for the use of a tourniquet. Typically, the tourniquet is set to 250 mm Hg and 350 mm Hg for the upper and lower extremities, respectively. The tourniquet is placed as high up on the extremity as possible to avoid interference with the sterile operative field. A typical formula used to determine the tourniquet setting is 100 mm Hg above the systolic blood pressure.

VII. An elastic Esmarch bandage or elevation of the extremity for 5 minutes can be used for limb exsanguination prior to tourniquet inflation. The tourniquet should not be inflated for longer than 120 minutes due to a risk of compartment syndrome or limb ischemia. If the tourniquet is needed for a longer period, it should be deflated for 10 minutes at the 120-minute time point, and then reinflated for up to an additional 120 minutes.

VIII. Before positioning, prepping, and draping the patient, ensure that the scrub technician is ready with the back table, all equipment is present, and the overhead operating room lights are in position.

IX. Both the upper and lower extremities are typically held in position for prepping with the use of a candy cane device (see images in individual chapters). Other devices may also be used to hold the limb steady while prepping. Some surgeons prefer to have the limb held by a person.

X. There are several prepping options available; however, many institutions use a Betadine scrub followed by a Betadine prep solution to sterilize the operative site. It is important to allow the Betadine to dry because it is bacteriostatic only when it has adequately dried. Other options include chlorhexidine-based or alcohol-based solutions, especially for patients with a Betadine or iodine allergy.

XI. Another important prepping principle is to prep the desired area from clean to dirty. In other words, start prepping over the proposed incision site and extend the prep area towards the periphery (i.e., the groin, axilla, or distal portion of the extremity).

XII. Several types of drapes exist and most draping techniques are attending and case-specific. In general, it is important to drape out as wide an area as possible to be prepared for extensile exposures to treat potential intraoperative complications. Inherent to proper draping is adequate patient positioning. Positioning of the patient on the operating room table is crucial to maintaining a stable position during the case and allowing sufficient surgical *exposure*.

XIII. In general, a nonsterile 1010 or 1015 drape is placed circumferentially around the proximal portion of the operative extremity. Once the limb has been adequately prepped, a down sheet is placed under the operative extremity to provide a barrier between the patient and the sterile field. A series of impervious drapes, including stockinettes, U-drapes, extremity drapes, and site-specific drapes (e.g., shoulder drape), are then used to secure a sterile surgical field. Many attending surgeons are very particular about draping and the order in which specific drapes are used. It is best to learn how to appropriately drape a patient from the attending or senior resident on your service.

XIV. Many attendings use an adhesive iodine-based drape called Ioban, which is placed directly on the skin of the surgical site. It is used to add an additional layer of sterility and also seals off the space between the operative area and the surrounding drapes.

XV. At the conclusion of a case, several wound closure options are available. Prior to closing the wound, it is important to irrigate the wound copiously with sterile saline using a bulb syringe. A pulse lavage may also be used to irrigate the wound for specific cases such as total joint arthroplasty or contaminated open fractures. Typically, deep fascial layers are closed using a large caliber, absorbable, braided suture (e.g., 1 Vicryl). The more superficial subcutaneous tissue layer is closed using a smaller caliber, absorbable, braided suture (e.g., 2-0 Vicryl). The skin is closed with a subcuticular closure using a small-caliber, absorbable, nonbraided monofilament suture (e.g., 4-0 Biosyn) or skin staples. Nylon suture may also be used for reapproximating the skin edges with the use of horizontal or vertical mattress knots.

XVI. Dressing the wound can be accomplished using other options; the preference of the attending is usually followed. In general, the closed wound is cleaned with saline and dried thoroughly prior to applying a dressing. A subcuticular closure is typically dressed with Steri-Strips followed by a nonadherent petroleum jelly (Vaseline)–impregnated gauze (i.e., Adaptic), whereas wounds closed with skin staples are dressed with Adaptic only. At this point, the operative site is covered with a combination of 4 × 4 gauze pads, ABD pads, and tape. Foam or Medipore tape is frequently used to minimize the amount of patient discomfort at the time of tape removal. It is important to place the tape without any skin tension to avoid shearing of the skin when changing the dressing. If an Ace bandage is applied, ask the attending if the entire limb should be wrapped (to reduce the risk of distal swelling) or just the surgical site. It is paramount that the limb is completely dry and the bandage is not wrapped too tightly to avoid blistering or skin necrosis.

CHAPTER 2

Arthroscopic Subacromial Decompression

Karen J. Boselli   and   David L. Glaser

Case Study

A 46-year-old, right hand–dominant female presents with right shoulder pain, which has gradually developed over the past 2 months. She describes pain at the "top" of her shoulder, radiating down her upper arm but not below the elbow. She complains of only mild difficulty with overhead lifting activities. The pain is worse with activities such as combing her hair or reaching for her back pocket. Recently, she has also started to experience night pain. She has tried nonsteroidal anti-inflammatory medications, with minimal relief. She completed an 8-week course of physical therapy, prior to which she received two cortisone injections; the first provided 1 month of relief and the second only 2 weeks. A scapular outlet radiograph and a magnetic resonance imaging scan are presented in Figure 2-1.

BACKGROUND

I. Impingement syndrome is a term used to describe the common condition that involves impingement of the humeral head and rotator cuff beneath the coracoacromial (CA) arch of the shoulder.

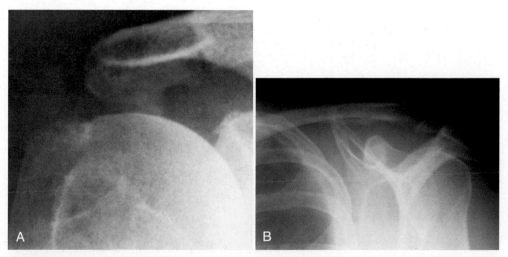

Figure 2-1
A, Anteroposterior view with 30-degree caudal tilt. **B,** Scapular (supraspinatus) outlet view. (*A, From DeLee JC, Drez D, Miller MD [eds]: DeLee & Drez's Orthopaedic Sports Medicine: Principles and Practice, 2nd ed. Philadelphia, Saunders, 2003; B, from Canale ST: Campbell's Operative Orthopaedics, 10th ed. Philadelphia, Mosby, 2003.*)

II. **Anatomy**

A. The rotator cuff consists of four muscles originating from the scapula and inserting on the humeral head: anteriorly, the subscapularis (originating at the subscapular fossa and inserting on the lesser tuberosity); superiorly, the supraspinatus (originating at the supraspinatus fossa and inserting on the greater tuberosity); and posteriorly, the infraspinatus (originating at the infraspinatus fossa and inserting on the greater tuberosity), and the teres minor (originating at the lateral border of the scapula and inserting on the greater tuberosity).

B. The CA arch consists of the coracoid process, acromion, and the CA ligament (Fig. 2-2). This osseoligamentous complex overlies the head of the humerus, preventing upward displacement from the glenoid fossa.

C. The subacromial bursa separates the supraspinatus tendon from the overlying CA arch and the deep surface of the deltoid muscle.

D. With the arm in a neutral position, the greater tuberosity (where the supraspinatus tendon inserts) lies anterior to the CA arch. With forward flexion and internal rotation, the subacromial bursa and supraspinatus tendon become entrapped between the anterior acromion/coracoid and greater tuberosity.

III. Charles Neer, MD, popularized the concept of impingement in 1972, after performing a cadaveric study that demonstrated a characteristic ridge of bone on the undersurface of the anterior process of the acromion. He proposed that these spurs were caused by repeated impingement of the rotator cuff and humeral head. He noticed that the anterior one third of the acromion seemed to be the offending structure in most cases.

IV. The impingement of the humeral head and rotator cuff leads to a series of changes within the shoulder. Neer described a continuum of impingement, starting with chronic bursitis and progressing to complete tears of the rotator cuff. His three stages are outlined in Table 2-1.

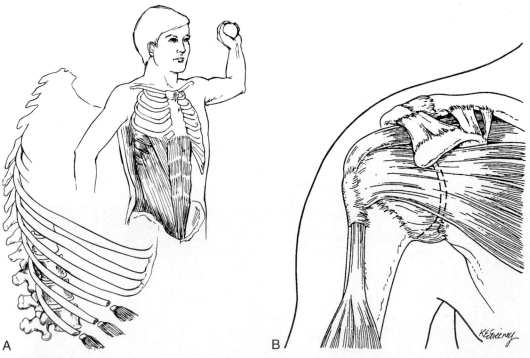

A   B

Figure 2-2
A, The coracoacromial (CA) arch, created by the coracoid, acromion, and CA ligament. **B,** The position of the rotator cuff musculature beneath the arch is demonstrated. (*A, From Krishan SG, Hawkins RJ: Rotator cuff and impingement lesions in adult and adolescent athletes. In DeLee JC, Drez D, Miller MD [eds]: DeLee & Drez's Orthopaedic Sports Medicine: Principles and Practice, 2nd ed. Philadelphia, Saunders, 2003; B, redrawn from Matsen FA III, Arntz CT: Subacromial impingement. In Rockwood CA Jr, Matsen FA III [eds]: The Shoulder. Philadelphia, Saunders, 1990.*)

TABLE 2-1 Stages of Subacromial Impingement Syndrome

Stage	Age (years)	Pathology	Clinical Course	Treatment
I	<25	Edema and hemorrhage	Reversible	Conservative
II	25–40	Fibrosis and tendinitis	Activity-related pain	Therapy/acromioplasty
III	>40	Acromioclavicular spur and rotator cuff tear	Progressive disability	Acromioplasty/repair

Data from Azar FM: Shoulder and elbow injuries. In Canale ST (ed): Campbell's Operative Orthopaedics, 10th ed. Philadelphia, Mosby, 2003.

A. Stage I occurs in younger individuals and involves edema and hemorrhage within the subacromial bursa. The patient may have palpable tenderness at the greater tuberosity and anterior edge of the acromion, with painful abduction between 60 and 120 degrees.

B. Stage II involves chronic inflammation with thickening and fibrosis of the subacromial bursa, biceps tendon, and supraspinatus tendon. Symptoms are generally not reversible with activity modification. Pain interferes with sleep, work, and activities of daily living.

C. Stage III is chronic impingement, resulting in rotator cuff tears, biceps tendon ruptures, and bony changes. Patients typically complain of significant night pain and weakness. Range of motion (ROM) may be limited, muscle atrophy may be present on physical examination, and radiographic changes may be present at the anterior acromion and humeral head.

TREATMENT PROTOCOLS

I. **Treatment Considerations**

A. Patient age

B. Activity level

C. Presence or absence of concomitant rotator cuff tear

D. Presence or absence of other associated shoulder pathology, especially instability

E. Source of pain. For an arthroscopic subacromial decompression to be successful, impingement syndrome must be the primary source of the patient's pain.

F. Differential diagnosis, which includes acromioclavicular (AC) arthritis, glenohumeral arthritis, rotator cuff tear, instability (with secondary impingement), early adhesive capsulitis, and calcific tendinitis. Cervical spondylosis with nerve root irritation and suprascapular nerve injury can also mimic the symptoms of impingement.

II. **Initial Approach**

A. Clinical presentation

1. History. Patients with impingement syndrome provide a history of insidious onset of pain exacerbated by overhead activities. Pain is often referred to the deltoid insertion. Other symptoms may include night pain and pain with internal rotation (such as reaching for the back pocket).

2. Physical examination. A thorough examination of the shoulder *and* neck is necessary to correctly diagnose impingement syndrome.

a. Check ROM bilaterally and test the strength of each of the rotator cuff muscles. Patients with impingement syndrome may have weakness of flexion, abduction, and external rotation due to pain. They may also have weakness secondary to a rotator cuff tear.

b. Check for impingement signs, using the following provocative maneuvers. These signs are highly sensitive but not very specific for diagnosing impingement syndrome.

(1) Neer's sign is pain with maximum passive shoulder elevation and internal rotation, with the scapula held stabilized.

(2) Hawkins' sign is pain with passive forward elevation to 90 degrees and maximum internal rotation with the elbow flexed to 90 degrees.

(3) Neer's impingement test involves injection of the subacromial space with local anesthetic, and observing for a decrease in pain with these provocative tests. Relief of symptoms is a positive impingement test and is suggestive of impingement syndrome.

B. Radiographic features

1. Plain radiographs may show spurring of the acromion or calcification of the CA ligament.

2. A 30-degree anteroposterior caudal tilt view can be used to visualize anterior-inferior acromial spurs.

3. A scapular outlet or supraspinatus outlet view can be used to demonstrate the morphology of the acromion. The patient is positioned for a scapular lateral view (or Y view), with the beam tilted 5 to 10 degrees caudally (Fig. 2-3; see Fig. 2-1A).

   a. Type I = flat
   b. Type II = curved
   c. Type III = hooked

4. Magnetic resonance imaging is frequently used to rule out any concomitant shoulder pathology, such as a rotator cuff or labral tears.

III. **Nonoperative Treatment Options**

A. Nonoperative treatment must *always* be attempted first in the management of impingement syndrome. Two thirds of patients can have significant relief with nonoperative measures, and 91% of patients with a type I acromion have a satisfactory result.

B. Options include:

1. Nonsteroidal anti-inflammatory drugs or acetaminophen
2. Activity modification, avoiding forward flexion beyond 90 degrees
3. Physical therapy including rotator cuff strengthening and scapular stabilization
4. ROM exercises
5. Corticosteroid injections

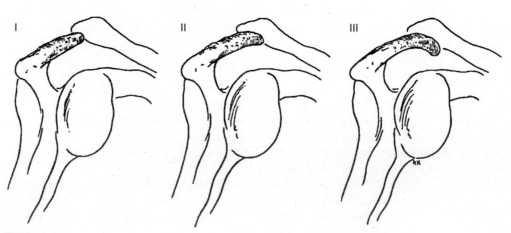

Figure 2-3
Diagram of the three types of acromial morphology, based on the scapular outlet view. *(Redrawn from Jobe CM: Gross anatomy of the shoulder. In Rockwood CA Jr, Matsen FA III [eds]: The Shoulder. Philadelphia, Saunders, 1990.)*

TREATMENT ALGORITHM

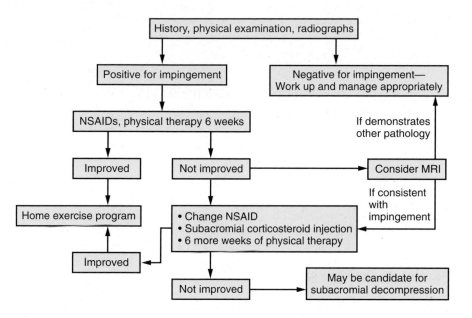

SURGICAL ALTERNATIVES AND INDICATIONS FOR ARTHROSCOPIC SUBACROMIAL DECOMPRESSION

I. Open acromioplasty is the only surgical alternative to arthroscopic subacromial decompression.

II. **Operative Treatment**

A. Arthroscopic acromioplasty provides objective good to excellent results in more than 70% of patients, with subjective satisfactory results in more than 90% of patients.

B. Arthroscopic treatment is often favored due to minimal soft tissue trauma, excellent surgical visualization, and easier rehabilitation.

C. The use of arthroscopy for subacromial decompression also allows the surgeon to identify additional pathology and perform additional procedures such as rotator cuff repair or distal clavicle excision.

D. Operative treatment should be considered for the following patients:

1. Patients with chronic impingement who have failed at least 3 to 4 months of nonoperative treatment. Some believe that surgery should be delayed until the patient has failed at least 9 months of nonoperative treatment.

2. Patients whose pain is relieved with impingement test

3. Younger patients with refractory stage II impingement. Subacromial decompression should be approached with caution in younger athletic individuals, because primary impingement syndrome is less common in patients younger than 25 years of age. Usually, these patients have secondary impingement due to altered shoulder kinematics without any primary pathology in the subacromial space.

4. Patients undergoing other procedures for conditions in which impingement is likely

The impingement test is conducted in the office by injecting 5 mL of lidocaine into the subacromial space of the patient's affected shoulder. The patient is re-examined 5 minutes postinjection to see if there is relief of his or her symptoms. Symptom relief indicates a positive impingement test.

RELATIVE CONTRAINDICATIONS

I. Medically unstable patients

II. Massive, irreparable rotator cuff tear. Disruption of the CA arch in patients with massive, irreparable rotator cuff tears can lead to superior migration of the humeral head and rotator cuff arthropathy.

III. Internal rotation contracture. This should be corrected prior to surgery. Patients with restricted motion, especially those with an internal rotation contracture, may have a suboptimal outcome following subacromial decompression. The patient's inability to externally rotate worsens the impingement due to the tendency of the greater tuberosity to impinge on the acromion even after surgery.

IV. Glenohumeral degenerative joint disease

GENERAL PRINCIPLES OF SUBACROMIAL DECOMPRESSION

I. The main principles of the original procedure, as described by Neer, are as follows:
   A. Resection of the CA ligament
   B. Removal of the anterior lip of the acromion
   C. Removal of the part of the acromion anterior to the anterior border of the clavicle
II. Although initially described by Neer as an open procedure, the basic principles of the arthroscopic procedure are unchanged.

COMPONENTS OF THE PROCEDURE

Positioning, Prepping, and Draping

Documenting the range of motion of both shoulders once the patient is under anesthesia is recommended.

I. After induction of anesthesia, both upper extremities are examined for ROM and stability. Some surgeons request that you record the preoperative ROM.
II. The patient is placed in the beach chair or lateral decubitus position. (See Chapter 4 for details on the lateral decubitus position.)
III. If the patient is placed in the beach chair position, the torso should be approximately 45 degrees relative to the horizontal and the arm and shoulder, completely off the edge of the table to allow full shoulder ROM. The head, neck, and body should be appropriately stabilized (Figs. 2-4 and 2-5).
IV. Patients are typically placed under general anesthesia for the procedure, but this is often coupled with regional anesthesia in the form of an interscalene nerve block of the affected side.

Propionibacter acnes bacteria commonly colonize the skin of the axilla and are a potential source of postoperative infection.

V. The skin should be shaved over the surgical site (anterosuperior approach), as well as the axilla.
VI. The patient is prepped and draped according to the standard surgical principles described in Chapter 1.
VII. Once the draping is completed and the skin incision has been marked, place Ioban over the exposed skin.

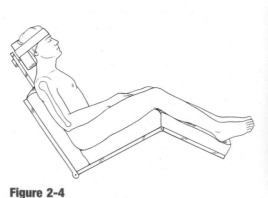

Figure 2-4
Beach chair position. *(From Canale ST [ed]: Campbell's Operative Orthopaedics, 10th ed. Philadelphia, Mosby, 2003.)*

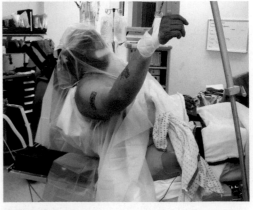

Figure 2-5
Beach chair position with the arm suspended for prepping.

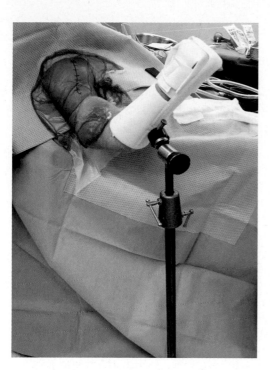

Figure 2-6
Fully draped-out shoulder with extremity held in mechanical arm-holding device.

VIII. Several points during the procedure require the arm to be held or supported. This can be done using an assistant, padded Mayo stand, or a mechanical arm-holding device. The mechanical arm-holding device has become the most popular way to support the arm (Fig. 2-6). It consists of a sterile articulated extension that attaches to the arm at the level of the wrist and forearm via a sterile disposable sleeve. The extension connects to a universal ball joint that is suspended from the operating table. A foot pedal allows the ball joint to be unlocked and the arm to be placed in the optimal position. Releasing the pedal locks the ball joint and arm in the selected position.

Does your attending have a preference regarding patient position?

Establishing the Portals

Mark out the superficial bony anatomy including the spine of the scapula, acromion, distal clavicle, AC joint, and coracoid process (Fig. 2-7).

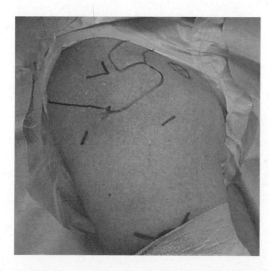

Figure 2-7
Superficial bony anatomy is identified and marked on the patient including the acromion, the acromioclavicular joint, and the coracoid process. The anticipated location of the posterior and lateral portals have also been marked. *(From Miller M, Cooper D, Warner J [eds]: Review of Sports Medicine and Arthroscopy, 2nd ed. Philadelphia, Saunders, 2002.)*

Applied Surgical Anatomy

Does your attending vary the location of the anterior portal based on the type of procedure (e.g., subacromial decompression vs. distal clavicle excision vs. rotator cuff repair)?

Remember that the scapula is oriented 30 degrees anterior to the coronal plane, and therefore this is the direction in which the trochar should be inserted.

I. For routine subacromial decompression, three portals are generally used: anterior, posterior, and lateral (Fig. 2-8).

II. The exact location of the posterior portal varies depending on what needs to be visualized during the case. It is generally considered the "viewing portal" and lies approximately 2 cm medial and 2 to 4 cm inferior to posterolateral tip of the acromion. In this location, feel for the soft spot of the glenohumeral joint while internally and externally rotating the humeral head. This is the interval between the infraspinatus and teres minor and is the location where the arthroscope should enter the joint.

III. The anterior portal is usually the "instrument portal" and should be created under direct visualization from the joint. However, its anticipated location should be marked on the skin to have a rough idea of the location. This is usually about 2 cm medial and 1 cm inferior to the anterolateral border of the acromion (or halfway between the tip of the acromion and the coracoid process). In general, it is in line with the AC joint.

IV. Some surgeons may inject a mixture of lidocaine and epinephrine at the portal sites prior to incision to minimize bleeding. Others inject saline into the joint with a spinal needle prior to introducing the trochar to distend the joint and minimize the risk of trauma to the articular cartilage.

V. The posterior incision is made with an 11-blade. Using the blunt trochar and cannula, gently "pop" through the deltoid fascia. Aim toward the coracoid (slightly medial), keeping the hand parallel to the lateral border of the acromion and parallel to the floor. Gently "pop" through the capsule to enter the glenohumeral joint.

VI. Remove the blunt trochar from the cannula and insert the camera. Focus the camera on the anterior glenohumeral joint, and try to visualize the "triangle" where the anterior portal will be formed—between the glenoid labrum (medial), the tendon of long head of the biceps (superior), and the middle glenohumeral ligament and tendon of the subscapularis (inferior) (Fig. 2-9). Using a spinal needle, enter the skin at the location previously marked, and aim toward the center

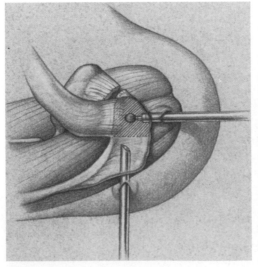

Figure 2-8
The posterior and lateral portals used for arthroscopic subacromial decompression. Note that the lateral portal is in line with the posterior border of the clavicle. (*From Harner CD: Arthroscopic subacromial decompression. Op Tech Orthop 1:229–234, 1991.*)

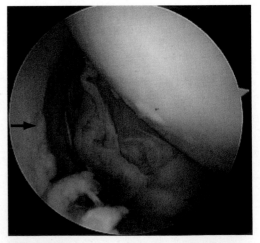

Figure 2-9
Location of the anterior portal, as viewed through an arthroscope with the patient in the lateral decubitus position. The humeral head is in the upper right corner, the long head of the biceps is marked with a *thick arrow*, and the middle glenohumeral ligament is marked with a *thin arrow*. The portal should be placed in the center of this triangle.

of this triangle until the capsule is pierced. Remove the needle, make the anterior incision with an 11-blade, and use a blunt trochar or plastic cannula to enter the joint through the same location.

VII. Mark the lateral portal prior to the start of the procedure, usually with the use of a spinal needle, under direct visualization of the subacromial space. Place it about 3 to 4 cm lateral to the lateral edge of the acromion, in line with the posterior border of the clavicle. To perform successful subacromial decompression, the lateral portal must allow for full triangulation of the undersurface of acromion; this is why it is important to establish the portal under direct visualization.

Diagnostic Arthroscopy and Subacromial Decompression

I. During the diagnostic arthroscopy, the scope should be in the posterior portal. Most surgeons have their own systematic way of inspecting the entire joint for any abnormalities—this inspection should include the biceps tendon, glenohumeral articulation, glenohumeral ligaments, subscapularis tendon, glenoid labrum, rotator cuff, and axillary/subscapular recess.

II. After completion of the diagnostic portion of the procedure, it is necessary to insert the scope into the subacromial space. Remove all instruments from the joint and place the blunt trochar back into the cannula.

III. Insert the instrument through the posterior portal, aiming superiorly toward the posterior acromion—the trochar will gently hit bone. Pull back the instrument slightly, aim the instrument slightly inferior, and gently slide into the subacromial space. Sweep the trochar back and forth across undersurface of the acromion to help remove any adhesions of the subacromial bursa.

IV. Some surgeons drive the trochar all the way across the subacromial space and through the anterior portal until the instrument exits at the skin. A plastic cannula can then be inserted over the instrument and easily drawn back into the subacromial space. Other surgeons prefer to insert the anterior cannula directly into the subacromial space through the previously established anterior incision.

V. A shaver is placed through the plastic cannula into the anterior portal, and an initial limited bursectomy is performed. This initial bursectomy is necessary for patients with an inflamed, thickened bursa to clear the field of vision and establish a lateral portal. Be careful with the shaver, because it can easily cause bleeding from a hyperemic bursa.

VI. After the initial bursectomy, the lateral portal can be established. Starting from the previously marked skin entry point, use a spinal needle to approximate the angle of entry. The skin marking, however, is not "set in stone"; the angle of the spinal needle should be adjusted to allow for full triangulation of the acromion and the skin incision should be modified accordingly.

VII. From the lateral portal, use the shaver or electrocautery device to complete the bursectomy. Methodically sweep the instrument back and forth to clear the tissue. Below the bursa, expose the rotator cuff to check for any bursal-sided tears (Fig. 2-10).

VIII. After completion of the bursectomy, there should be improved visualization of the anterior acromion, AC joint, and CA ligament. The undersurface of the acromion, however, is still covered by periosteum—the entire undersurface of the anterolateral acromion must now be cleared of soft tissue using electrocautery. The anterior acromial surface must carefully be exposed by removal of any deep deltoid attachments. This allows for visualization of any anterior-inferior acromial osteophytes.

IX. The CA ligament should also be sectioned or detached from its acromial attachment using the shaver or electrocautery. This is most easily accomplished with the instrument in the lateral portal. Be aware that the acromial branch of the thoracoacromial artery, which lies near the anteromedial acromion, can be injured during sectioning of the CA ligament. If the anterior cannula has been placed

PLACE THE ARM IN ADDUCTION TO MINIMIZE THE RISK TO THE MUSCULOCUTANEOUS NERVE DURING ESTABLISHMENT OF THE ANTERIOR PORTAL.

REMEMBER THAT THE AXILLARY NERVE ENTERS THE DEEP SURFACE OF THE DELTOID ABOUT 5 CM LATERAL AND DISTAL TO THE ACROMION.

Remember that the lateral portal is the main instrument portal for the acromioplasty—it must be placed so that *full* triangulation of the undersurface of the anterior acromion can be performed.

BLEEDING FROM THE ACROMIAL BRANCH OF THE THORACOACROMIAL ARTERY CAN OCCUR DURING SECTIONING OF THE CORACOACROMIAL LIGAMENT.

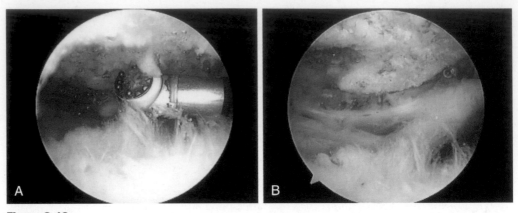

Figure 2-10
A, Completion of bursectomy with electrocautery. **B,** Exposure of bony ridge along the anterior acromion.

properly at the level of the AC joint, it can be used as a landmark (to prevent any shaving medial to this point).

X. The critical portion of this procedure involves bony resection of the undersurface of the anterior acromion. Adequate biplanar visualization is needed to judge the amount of bone that has been removed. This is achieved with visualization from both the posterior and lateral portals.

    A. Starting with the scope in the posterior portal, a burr is placed through the lateral portal. The acromial resection starts at the anterolateral corner, where the burr is used to remove 5 mm of bone. As the bone is removed, an audible sound from the burr is heard.

    B. After the anterolateral portion is completed, work medially and posteriorly toward the mid-acromion. The amount of bone resected should be tapered toward the mid-acromion (Fig. 2-11).

    C. The burr, which is approximately 5 mm in diameter, can be used to judge the amount of bone that has been removed and the amount of space available.

XI. The scope is now switched to the lateral portal, and the burr placed in the posterior portal. If the instrument is flush with the undersurface of both the anterior and posterior acromion, adequate decompression has been achieved.

XII. If the surfaces are not flush, additional bone needs to be resected. The posterior surface is used as a "cutting block" to indicate the amount of additional anterior bone resection that is necessary—the burr is then taken along the anterior acromion until the entire undersurface is uniplanar.

> All anterior-inferior spurs and osteophytes need to be carefully removed.

Figure 2-11
Burr is entering the subacromial space through the lateral portal, and an anterolateral resection of bone is performed.

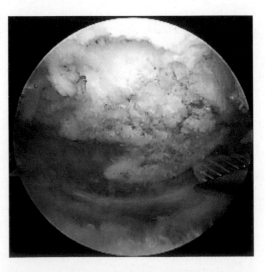

XIII. After completion of the procedure, place the scope back in the lateral portal to examine the subacromial space and confirm adequacy of the decompression. An arthroscopic impingement test can be performed by flexing and internally rotating the shoulder while checking for any remaining sites of impingement. If any such sites remain, they should be addressed with a burr.

XIV. In patients with concomitant symptomatic AC arthritis, the surgeon should perform a distal clavicle excision. The details of this procedure are beyond the scope of this chapter.

Wound Closure

I. The portals are closed using nylon suture or Biosyn. The wound is dressed following the surgical principles outlined in Chapter 1.

II. A sling is provided for comfort.

POSTOPERATIVE CARE AND GENERAL REHABILITATION

I. Patients are generally discharged home on the day of surgery after a period of recovery in the short procedure unit.

II. If the patient has received an interscalene block for pain control, he or she should be warned about the possible increase in pain while the block wears off. Patients should appropriately premedicate with oral narcotics when the block is beginning to diminish. Oral analgesia is usually sufficient for postoperative pain control, and oral antiemetic agents can be provided if necessary.

III. Patients are usually discharged home in a sling and may start pendulum exercises of the shoulder as soon as their surgical pain subsides—usually within 2 days. This helps ensure that some passive ROM is retained in the immediate postoperative period.

IV. Strengthening exercises are delayed until full range of motion has been restored.

COMPLICATIONS

I. **Technical Problems and Pitfalls with Acromioplasty**

A. Adequate bone must be removed to alleviate the impingement. This includes the anterior lip of the acromion and any portion of the acromion that lies anterior to the anterior clavicular border. Inadequate removal occurs more often in arthroscopic than open subacromial decompression.

B. As discussed, when the burr enters the subacromial space from the lateral portal, it must be parallel to the undersurface of the acromion. If the lateral portal is placed too inferiorly, the burr enters the subacromial space at an acute angle to the acromion—this risks bisecting the acromion during bony resection. If the lateral portal is placed too superiorly, the instrument will not be able to reach the anterior surface of the acromion to complete resection of the bony ridge.

C. The CA ligament must be resected and a portion removed to prevent the cut edge from scarring back to acromion.

II. Wound infection

III. Nerve injury

SUGGESTED READINGS

Altchek DW, Warren RF, Wickiewicz TL, et al: Arthroscopic acromioplasty. Techniques and results. J Bone Joint Surg Am 72:1198–1207, 1990.

Bigliani LU, Levine WN: Current concepts review: Subacromial impingement syndrome. J Bone Joint Surg Am 79:1854–1868, 1997.

Bigliani LU, Morrison DS, April EW: The morphology of the acromion and its relationship to rotator cuff tears. Orthop Trans 10:228, 1986.

Gartsman GM, Hasan SS: What's new in shoulder and elbow surgery. J Bone Joint Surg Am 99:230–243, 2006.

Neer CS II: Anterior acromioplasty for the chronic impingement syndrome in the shoulder: A preliminary report. J Bone Joint Surg Am 54:41–50, 1972.

CHAPTER 3

Rotator Cuff Repair

Eric T. Ricchetti   and   Matthew L. Ramsey

Case Study

A 65-year-old, right hand–dominant male presents with a 5-year history of right shoulder pain. He has had gradual progressive difficulty with activities of daily living and is now limited significantly by pain and weakness in his right shoulder. The patient has pain at night, which can interrupt his sleep, and also complains of increased pain with overhead activities. He denies any specific injury that initiated the onset of symptoms and denies any neck pain or associated radiating symptoms (numbness, tingling, pain) down his arms. The patient has tried several nonoperative treatments, including nonsteroidal anti-inflammatory medications; activity modification; physical therapy; and multiple, intermittent corticosteroid injections into his shoulder. These have only provided temporary symptomatic relief, and their effect has lessened as his symptoms have progressed. The man is now retired and lives at home by himself without a caregiver. A coronal magnetic resonance imaging scan is presented in Figure 3-1.

BACKGROUND

I. Rotator cuff disease is a common cause of shoulder pain, with an incidence of rotator cuff tears ranging from 5% to 40%, which increases with age.

II. The rotator cuff consists of four muscles originating from the scapula and inserting on the humeral head: anteriorly, the subscapularis (originating

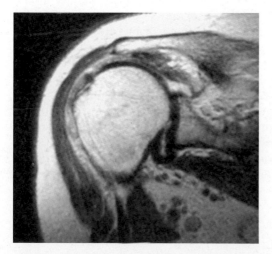

Figure 3-1
Coronal magnetic resonance imaging scan of the right shoulder.

at the subscapular fossa and inserting on the lesser tuberosity); superiorly, the supraspinatus (originating at the supraspinatus fossa and inserting on the greater tuberosity); and posteriorly, the infraspinatus (originating at the infraspinatus fossa and inserting on the greater tuberosity), and the teres minor (originating at the lateral border of the scapula and inserting on the greater tuberosity).

III. Each rotator cuff muscle provides a particular shoulder motion based on its location around the glenohumeral joint.
   A. Subscapularis: internal rotation and adduction
   B. Supraspinatus: abduction
   C. Infraspinatus: external rotation
   D. Teres minor: external rotation

IV. Rotator cuff tears typically occur at the tendinous insertion of the rotator cuff muscles on the humeral head. The supraspinatus is the most commonly torn tendon.

V. Rotator cuff tears can be described based on their depth (partial-thickness or full-thickness), anterior-posterior extent (in centimeters), age (acute, chronic, or acute on chronic), and whether they involve one or more tendons.

VI. Pain, weakness, or both, in the affected shoulder are the most common presenting complaints in patients with rotator cuff tears. Symptoms may begin without an injury or after only minor trauma in patients with chronic degenerative tears. Acute rotator cuff tears may also be associated with a more severe acute event such as a shoulder dislocation in an older patient. Patients typically localize their pain to the anterior or lateral shoulder, and discomfort is usually worsened with use of the arm, particularly overhead activities. Pain is often the worst at night, awakening patients from sleep. Weakness may be from the tear itself or from guarding due to pain. Tear size does not always correlate with function, because patients with large tears can often have good motion and strength.

VII. Physical examination of the affected shoulder may demonstrate muscle atrophy, depending on the chronicity of the injury. Acute tears show no changes, whereas chronic injuries show atrophy in the affected rotator cuff muscles. Active range of motion (ROM) is typically decreased due to either weakness or pain, but passive ROM is usually normal. Strength of the shoulder should also be examined in elevation, abduction, external rotation, and internal rotation to assess for weakness or pain in each of the rotator cuff muscles. Specific changes in ROM and strength can help determine the part of the rotator cuff involved. For example, increased passive external rotation with weak internal rotation (lift-off test and abdominal compression test) suggests a subscapularis tear, whereas weakness in elevation/abduction with passive ROM greater than active ROM suggests a supraspinatus tear. A careful examination of the cervical spine should also be performed to rule out any abnormalities, including radiculopathy and degenerative joint disease, that may cause referred pain or weakness in the shoulder.

VIII. Although rotator cuff tears can be significantly disabling, many patients are asymptomatic and never require treatment. Treatment should therefore be aimed at patients with symptomatic disease. For the majority of patients with symptomatic rotator cuff tears unresponsive to nonoperative treatment, definitive surgical intervention consists of rotator cuff repair.

IX. Approximately 70% to 100% of patients attain adequate pain relief following rotator cuff repair, with functional improvement somewhat less predictable (70% to 80% of patients). Recurrence rates generally increase based on the size of the tear, with single tendon repairs having a 20% recurrence rate and two tendon repairs having a 50% recurrence rate. Results of arthroscopic repair seem to be equivalent to results of open repair.

When a shoulder dislocation occurs in an older patient (>40 years of age), always think about an associated rotator cuff tear (most commonly subscapularis with an anterior dislocation).

If weakness is profound in a patient with a rotator cuff tear following a dislocation or other severe shoulder trauma, always assess for an associated brachial plexus injury (axillary or suprascapular nerve most commonly injured).

Glenohumeral arthritis and adhesive capsulitis (frozen shoulder) are major causes of restriction of both active and passive range of motion in the shoulder.

TREATMENT ALGORITHM

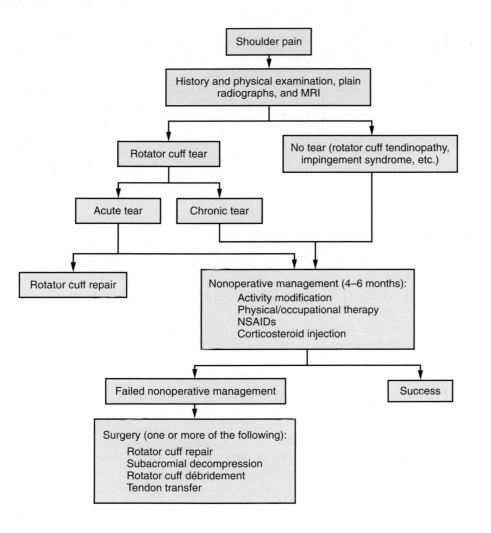

Note: This algorithm is a guideline for management of rotator cuff tears. The decision to ultimately proceed with surgical repair depends on multiple other factors, including patient age and activity level and the status of the rotator cuff (e.g., size and age of tear, amount of tendon retraction, muscle quality), which are evaluated on an individual basis.

What is your attending's treatment algorithm for shoulder pain secondary to a rotator cuff tear?

TREATMENT PROTOCOLS

I. **Treatment Considerations.** All of the considerations below play an important role in the decision-making process of treating patients with rotator cuff tears. For example, older patients with chronic, degenerative tears and a primary complaint of pain tend to be the most responsive to nonoperative treatment. Young, active patients with an acute tear and a primary complaint of weakness are best treated with early (less than 3 months from injury) surgical repair.
   A. Patient age
   B. Activity level
   C. Overall health

D. Status of the rotator cuff: size and age of tear, amount of tendon retraction, and muscle quality
E. Patient expectations

II. **Imaging Modalities**
   A. Plain radiographs should be assessed for the following features:
      1. Cystic changes at greater tuberosity
      2. Humeral head elevation with decreased space between it and the acromion (acromiohumeral distance)
      3. Acromial morphology (e.g., evidence of prominent spurs on the undersurface of the anterior acromion potentially causing impingement)
   B. Arthrography
      1. Once contrast is injected into the glenohumeral joint, plain radiographs are taken.
      2. With a full thickness rotator cuff tear, contrast is seen escaping from the joint through the tear site (geyser sign); however, tear size is difficult to determine, and partial-thickness tears cannot be detected.
      3. This imaging modality was the former gold standard but is less often used due to the availability of magnetic resonance imaging (MRI).
   C. Ultrasound
      1. Advantages: noninvasive, dynamic, inexpensive, and can be performed in an outpatient setting
      2. Disadvantages: operator dependent and unable to assess muscle atrophy or fatty replacement of the muscle
   D. MRI
      1. Imaging study of choice to evaluate the rotator cuff
      2. Highly accurate (93% to 100%) in detecting full-thickness tears; can assess tear size, tendon retraction, muscle atrophy, and related intra-articular pathology
      3. Disadvantages: expensive, patient tolerance (claustrophobia), contraindicated in patients with pacemakers, metal in their eye, or aneurysm clips

III. **Nonoperative Treatment Options**
   A. The literature shows successful nonoperative treatment in 33% to 92% of patients with symptomatic tears, and approximately 50% to 60% of patients report a satisfactory result.
   B. Initial treatment strategy
      1. Nonsteroidal anti-inflammatory drugs or acetaminophen
      2. Activity modification (participating in low-impact activity, avoiding offending motions)
      3. Heat (chronic pain) and cold (acute flare-up) therapy
      4. Physical and occupational therapy
         a. Physical therapy is aimed at eliminating any subtle stiffness and strengthening of the rotator cuff and parascapular muscles.
            (1) Typically a home exercise program can be taught.
            (2) Aqua therapy can be used for exercises and decreasing stress across muscles and joints due to the buoyancy effects of water.
            (3) Ultrasound: heat effect
         b. Occupational therapy is aimed at teaching alternative ways of accomplishing activities of daily living that may be impaired or elicit symptoms.
   C. Subacromial corticosteroid injection
      1. Injections are considered if adequate progress has not been made after 4 to 6 weeks of physical therapy. Usually injected in combination with a local anesthetic (lidocaine and/or bupivacaine).
      2. Steroids can decrease pain that may be limiting a patient's ability to perform exercises.
      3. An injection can be repeated after several months if it gives symptomatic relief, but no more than three injections per year (4-month intervals) should be given.

There are three types of acromion morphologies: type I is flat, type II is curved, and type III is hooked (refer to Chapter 2).

ALWAYS QUESTION PATIENTS REGARDING A HISTORY OF A PACEMAKER, METAL IN THE EYE, ANEURYSM CLIPS, OR OTHER METAL IMPLANTS IN THE BODY PRIOR TO OBTAINING A MAGNETIC RESONANCE IMAGING (MRI) SCAN.

INTRA-ARTICULAR STEROIDS MAY INCREASE ENDOGENOUS GLUCOSE LEVELS POSTINJECTION; THEREFORE, PATIENTS WITH DIABETES SHOULD BE MADE AWARE THAT CLOSE POSTINJECTION GLUCOSE MONITORING MAY BE REQUIRED.

SURGICAL PROCEDURES COMMONLY PERFORMED WITH ROTATOR CUFF REPAIR AND SURGICAL ALTERNATIVES TO ROTATOR CUFF REPAIR

I. **Subacromial Decompression**
   A. Subacromial impingement is frequently seen in association with rotator cuff tears. Irritation or inflammation from this contact may be a contributing cause of pain and tendon injury in patients with rotator cuff tears and, therefore, should also be addressed at the time of surgery. The coracoacromial (CA) ligament should be preserved in patients with an irreparable or large rotator cuff tear, however, if concerned about the healing potential of the repair. Refer to Chapter 2 for details regarding subacromial impingement and decompression.
   B. If performed, subacromial decompression is typically done before the rotator cuff repair.

II. **Acromioclavicular (AC) Joint Resection (Distal Clavicle Excision)**
   A. The AC joint is frequently found to be symptomatic in older patients with rotator cuff tears due to arthritic changes. Symptoms include tenderness to palpation over the AC joint, as well as pain with cross-body adduction of the shoulder. Arthritic changes are noted on plain radiographs and/or MRI. Imaging findings alone, however, are not sufficient to justify surgery because many patients with arthritic changes are asymptomatic.
   B. A symptomatic AC joint can be surgically addressed (open or arthroscopically) at the time of rotator cuff surgery with a distal clavicle excision that acts to remove one end of the irritating joint surface.

III. **Long Head of the Biceps Tenotomy or Tenodesis**
   A. Subacromial impingement from rotator cuff disease can affect the long head of the biceps tendon, leading to potential irritation or inflammation that may be a pain generator in addition to the rotator cuff. The biceps tendon can also become symptomatically painful from instability within the bicipital groove, traumatic injury, or primary age-related degeneration with or without impingement.
   B. Symptoms include tenderness to palpation over the location of the long head of the biceps in the bicipital groove.
   C. A symptomatic long head of the biceps tendon can be surgically addressed (open or arthroscopically) at the time of rotator cuff surgery by performing a tenotomy (detachment of the tendon origin from the superior labrum and glenoid) or a tenodesis (the tendon origin is released and sutured or anchored to the proximal humerus, typically in the bicipital groove).

IV. **Rotator Cuff Débridement**
   A. Débridement is considered an option for partial-thickness rotator cuff tears in which the tear extends only partially through the depth of the tendon. It may be either on the outer, bursal side of the tendon or on the inner, articular side of the tendon.
      1. The degenerated or frayed tendon is débrided away (typically arthroscopically) and can be performed with or without subacromial decompression.
      2. Débridement is typically only considered in tears that are less than 50% of tendon thickness, whereas tears that are more than 50% are more likely to be surgically repaired.
   B. Débridement has also been used as a surgical option in combination with subacromial decompression (without CA ligament resection) in patients with irreparable rotator cuff tears.

V. **Tendon Transfer**
   A. Tendon transfer may be considered in patients with refractory pain and weakness and an irreparable rotator cuff tear with an otherwise normal glenohumeral joint. The goal is to restore overhead function.
   B. When tendon transfer is used for irreparable anterosuperior rotator cuff defects (subscapularis), a pectoralis major transfer can be performed, whereas for irreparable posterosuperior rotator cuff defects (supraspinatus/infraspinatus/teres minor), a latissimus dorsi transfer can be performed.

The coracoacromial ligament may be a primary restraint to superior elevation of the humeral head in patients with significant rotator cuff deficiency, such as those with irreparable rotator cuff tears. Therefore, resection may lead to superior elevation of the humeral head and further worsening of shoulder function.

Distal clavicle osteolysis, commonly seen in weight lifters, is another cause of acromioclavicular joint tenderness.

Acromioclavicular (AC) joint stability is a result of a series of surrounding ligaments. The AC ligaments encircle the joint and primarily provide anterior-posterior stability. The coracoclavicular ligaments (the conoid [medially] and the trapezoid [laterally]) run from the coracoid to the distal clavicle and primarily provide vertical and medial-lateral stability.

BE CAREFUL NOT TO RESECT TOO MUCH OF THE DISTAL CLAVICLE DURING A DISTAL CLAVICLE EXCISION BECAUSE THIS CAN DESTABILIZE THE BONE BY VIOLATING THE STABILIZING LIGAMENTS OF THE CLAVICLE. THE LIMIT OF EXCISION IS TYPICALLY LESS THAN 2 CM.

Does your attending always perform a subacromial decompression when a rotator cuff tear is present? When does he or she consider débridement alone or tendon transfers versus surgical repair for a rotator cuff tear?

Pain is typically the principal indication for surgery in patients failing nonoperative management, because pain relief is more reliably achieved than improvement in function.

C. Tendon transfers typically work only for patients with mild to moderate weakness. If a patient has severe weakness or paralysis with inability to raise his or her arm overhead, a tendon transfer will not likely restore effective overhead function.

SURGICAL INDICATIONS FOR ROTATOR CUFF REPAIR

I. Failed nonoperative treatment (minimum 3 to 4 months)
II. Failed surgical alternative
    A. Subacromial decompression (avoid CA ligament resection in patients with large or irreparable rotator cuff tears; previously mentioned).
    B. Rotator cuff débridement
III. Prominent or progressive rotator cuff weakness
IV. Acute, full-thickness tear in young, active patient
V. Acute subscapularis rupture. This is commonly seen in patients older than 40 years of age who sustain an anterior shoulder dislocation.

RELATIVE CONTRAINDICATIONS TO ROTATOR CUFF REPAIR

I. Current or recent infection
II. Massive, irreparable rotator cuff tear
III. Advanced glenohumeral arthritis requiring arthroplasty
IV. Medically instability. The patient is unable to safely tolerate the stress of surgery.

GENERAL PRINCIPLES OF ROTATOR CUFF REPAIR

I. The rotator cuff plays an important role as a dynamic stabilizer of the shoulder, providing humeral head depression, humeral rotation, shoulder abduction, and glenohumeral joint compression.
    A. Its role in creating a compressive effect at the glenohumeral joint (i.e., pulling the humeral head into the glenoid) helps provide a stable glenohumeral fulcrum during active arm motion. This fulcrum allows the deltoid muscle to act as an effective abductor and elevator of the shoulder, rather than simply pulling the humeral head superiorly.
    B. If the compressive effect is significantly lost due to a rotator cuff tear, the resultant loss of a stable fulcrum and superior subluxation of the humeral head may prevent effective arm elevation.
II. The rotator cuff also has an integral role in maintaining force couples in multiple planes of the shoulder. For example, balanced force couples in the transverse plane exist between the subscapularis anteriorly and the infraspinatus and teres minor posteriorly. Disruption of these couples by a significant rotator cuff tear can potentially result in abnormal shoulder kinematics that, again, lead to an unstable fulcrum at the glenohumeral joint, abnormal humeral head excursion, and impaired shoulder function.
III. The goal of rotator cuff repair is to restore the insertion of the torn tendon(s) on the greater and/or lesser tuberosities of the humeral head, with the aim of decreasing shoulder pain and/or improving function.
IV. Tears that are not repaired may potentially progress in size, leading to irreversible changes in the muscle-tendon unit, including tendon retraction, tissue thinning, muscular atrophy, and fatty replacement. Early repair of acute tears or prompt repair of more chronic tears that fail nonoperative management can help avoid these problems.
V. Regardless of technique, the rate-limiting step for recovery from rotator cuff surgery is the successful healing of the rotator cuff tendon back to bone. Although improvement in both pain and function have been shown even when the tendon does not heal following rotator cuff repair, the most optimal results occur when the rotator cuff successfully heals.

VI. Tendon mobilization, or freeing of the scarred tendon from adhesions to surrounding structures, is as important as the surgical repair of the torn tendon(s) to the tuberosity. This allows the muscle-tendon unit to properly glide and function, preventing postoperative stiffness and excessive tension on the repair that could lead to rerupture.

VII. In open surgery, the anterior deltoid origin is taken down to gain access to the rotator cuff. A secure repair of the deltoid is essential, because one of the most troublesome complications of open rotator cuff repair is damage to or detachment of the deltoid. Arthroscopic rotator cuff repair has the advantage of not violating the deltoid and avoiding these potential complications.

COMPONENTS OF THE OPEN PROCEDURE

The following steps have been focused to describe repair of a full-thickness supraspinatus tear, the most commonly torn rotator cuff tendon. In general, similar steps are also used for repairs of anterior or posterior rotator cuff tears or multitendon tears.

Positioning, Prepping, and Draping

I. The patient is positioned in the beach chair position (refer to Chapter 2 for details on positioning).

II. Prepping and draping is done according to the surgical principles outlined in Chapter 1.

Surgical Approach and Applied Surgical Anatomy

I. The most common approach for open rotator cuff repair is the anterosuperior approach. For patients undergoing revision surgery with a prior anterosuperior incision, the previously made incision should be used.

II. The skin incision is made approximately 6 to 10 cm along Langer's lines, extending from approximately 2 cm lateral to the coracoid anteriorly to the lateral aspect of the anterior one to two thirds of the acromion posteriorly (Fig. 3-2).

III. Following the skin incision, subcutaneous flaps are raised and the deltoid is exposed. A 3- to 5-cm deltoid split is made along the direction of the

> IN A MINI-OPEN APPROACH FOR ROTATOR CUFF REPAIR, THE DELTOID MUSCLE IS SPLIT THROUGH A SMALL OPEN INCISION WITHOUT TAKING DOWN THE ORIGIN AND AVOIDING THE NEED FOR DELTOID REPAIR. HOWEVER, INADVERTENT INJURY TO THE DELTOID DUE TO EXCESSIVE RETRACTION MAY OCCUR.

> MOST OPEN REPAIRS OF SUBSCAPULARIS TEARS ARE PERFORMED USING THE DELTOPECTORAL APPROACH BECAUSE IT PROVIDES MORE ANTERIOR EXPOSURE.

The deltoid is composed of three heads with anterior, lateral, and posterior fibers. It originates from the clavicle anteriorly, acromion laterally, and scapular spine posteriorly and inserts on the deltoid tuberosity of the humerus. The muscle is innervated by the axillary nerve. The deltoid split from the anterolateral corner of the acromion takes advantage of the natural separation between the anterior and lateral fibers.

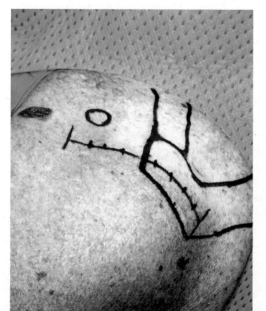

Figure 3-2
Anterosuperior incision marked out.

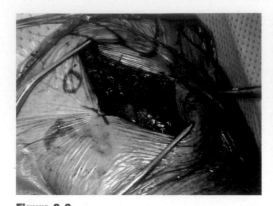

Figure 3-3
Deltoid exposure and split.

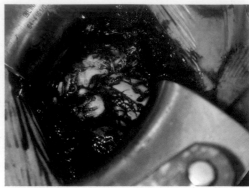

Figure 3-4
Exposed rotator cuff tear.

> THE DELTOID SPLIT CAN BE MOVED MORE POSTERIORLY, STARTING AT THE MIDDLE OF THE ACROMION, FOR LARGER TEARS THAT EXTEND MORE POSTERIORLY. EXTENSION OF THE DELTOID MUSCLE SPLIT MUST NOT BE MADE MORE THAN 5 CM DISTALLY TO AVOID DENERVATION OF THE MUSCLE.

deltoid fibers from the anterolateral corner of the acromion, moving distally. A stay suture is placed at the end of the split to prevent extension. Split extension can potentially lead to axillary nerve damage because the nerve passes approximately 5 to 6 cm distal to the lateral edge of the acromion (Fig. 3-3).

IV. The deltoid origin is then elevated off the anterior acromion. This is elevated as far medially as the start of the AC joint and is dissected around the anterior edge of the acromion laterally. The anteroinferior acromion is exposed to elevate the entire CA ligament with the anterior deltoid origin, so that both structures stay together as one flap for later repair.

V. With the anterior acromion exposed, an acromioplasty can be performed if there are any prominent spurs on the undersurface of the anterior acromion. An osteotome or saw is used to remove excess bone and create a smooth, flat undersurface. The acromioplasty also exposes the AC joint, and a distal clavicle excision can be performed if the AC joint was tender preoperatively.

VI. The subacromial bursa is removed to directly visualize the rotator cuff and the site of the tear (Fig. 3-4).

Tendon Edge Débridement and Tendon Mobilization

I. Débridement and mobilization of the torn rotator cuff tendon is performed to allow the retracted tendon to be repaired back to its insertion site on the greater tuberosity tension-free. Mobilization occurs by freeing all adhesions between the torn tendon and the surrounding tissues.

> AVOID GOING MEDIAL TO THE BASE OF THE CORACOID BECAUSE OF THE RISK OF SUPRASCAPULAR NERVE INJURY.

A. The torn tendon edges are débrided to remove any bursal or fibrous tissue and stimulate healing. This usually removes 1 to 2 mm of tissue and should leave behind a thick tendon edge that can hold sutures.

B. With the edge prepared, temporary sutures are placed at the torn end to provide traction while mobilizing the tendon.

C. The bursal side of the tendon is first released during mobilization, separating the tendon from the acromion and the deltoid. This may include dividing the coracohumeral ligament and releasing the tendon from the base of the coracoid if the tendon is scarred to these structures.

D. If the supraspinatus is torn and medially retracted, it may be scarred to the medial aspect of the adjacent rotator cuff tendons (subscapularis anteriorly and infraspinatus posteriorly). The intervals between these two tendons and the supraspinatus should be released.

> AVOID GOING MORE THAN 1 CM MEDIAL TO THE GLENOID RIM BECAUSE OF THE RISK OF SUPRASCAPULAR NERVE INJURY.

E. The articular side of the tendon is mobilized by releasing capsular attachments that may be tethering the tendon (Figs. 3-5 and 3-6).

II. If the tendon of the long head of the biceps is noted to be significantly damaged, a tenotomy or tenodesis to the proximal humerus is performed at this point.

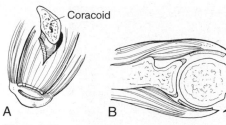

Figure 3-5
Schematic of tendon mobilization. **A,** Mobilization from the base of the coracoid on the bursal side of the tendon. **B,** Mobilization on the articular side of the tendon by releasing capsular attachments. *(From Miller M, Cooper D, Warner J: Review of Sports Medicine and Arthroscopy, 2nd ed. Philadelphia, Saunders, 2002.)*

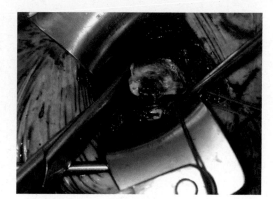

Figure 3-6
Intraoperative view of tendon mobilization.

Rotator Cuff Repair

I. The greater tuberosity is prepared for tendon repair by removing any soft tissue over it and smoothing any irregular bony prominences.

II. The tendon is then repaired to the greater tuberosity with the arm in a neutral position at the side. Heavy, nonabsorbable sutures are used and passed in a transosseous manner through the tendon edge and then through the bone of the greater tuberosity (Fig. 3-7). The sutures should exit the bone at least 2 cm distal to the greater tuberosity to bring the tendon edge down both medially and laterally and restore the normal footprint of the rotator cuff. Simple and/or modified Mason-Allen stitches are used.

III. Once the tendon is repaired back to the greater tuberosity, interval releases that were made between the torn tendon and the intact rotator cuff (subscapularis and infraspinatus) can be sutured closed.

> Suture anchors may also be used to repair the torn tendon back to bone, rather than transosseous sutures. What is your attending's technique for open rotator cuff repair?

Deltoid Repair and Wound Closure

I. Following rotator cuff repair, the shoulder is pulse lavaged with saline with or without antibiotics. The deltoid origin and CA ligament that were taken down together in a flap are then repaired back to bone using heavy, nonabsorbable sutures. A modified Mason-Allen stitch is used to anatomically repair these tissues to the anterior acromion (Fig. 3-8).

II. The deltoid split should be sutured closed.

III. The subcutaneous tissue and skin is closed in standard fashion and the wound is dressed (refer to Chapter 1 for further details).

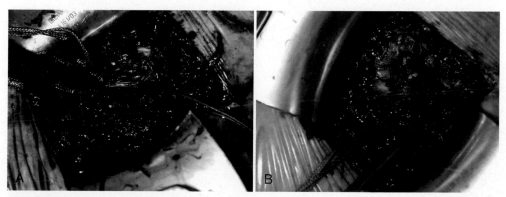

Figure 3-7
Transosseous rotator cuff repair using heavy, nonabsorbable sutures passed through the tendon edge (**A**) and then through the greater tuberosity (**B**).

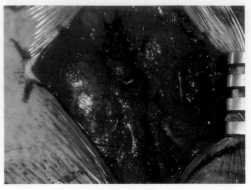

Figure 3-8
Deltoid following repair.

COMPONENTS OF THE ARTHROSCOPIC PROCEDURE

The following steps have been focused to describe repair of a full-thickness supraspinatus tear, the most commonly torn rotator cuff tendon. In general, similar steps are also used for repairs of anterior or posterior rotator cuff tears or multitendon tears.

Positioning, Prepping, and Draping

I. The patient is again placed in the beach chair position. Refer to Chapter 2 for a description of positioning. Chapter 1 outlines the surgical principles used for standard prepping and draping.

II. Shoulder arthroscopy and arthroscopic rotator cuff repair can also be performed in the lateral decubitus position. An inflatable bean bag can be used to place the patient in this position, with the operative extremity facing up. A traction device is then set up on the bed to pull traction on the arm at approximately 30 to 40 degrees of abduction. Usually 10 to 12 pounds of traction are added to open up the glenohumeral joint. (See Chapter 4 for a description of the lateral decubitus position.)

> What is your attending's preferred patient position for arthroscopic rotator cuff repair?

Arthroscopic Portal Placement

I. Multiple portals are used for an arthroscopic rotator cuff repair. Bony landmarks are drawn out on the skin with a marker to establish the location of each portal. These landmarks include the acromion, scapular spine, clavicle, the location of the AC joint, and the coracoid process (Fig. 3-9).

II. Anterior, posterior, and lateral portals are in general always used during arthroscopy, and additional portals are added as necessary for rotator cuff repair. The posterior portal is used for evaluation of the glenohumeral joint and subacromial space with the arthroscope. When used during arthroscopic rotator cuff repair, the anterior portal is primarily used for instrumentation and suture passing in the subacromial space. Refer to Chapter 2 on establishing arthroscopic portals. The lateral portal is placed in the subacromial space and is also used for instrumentation and suture passing during rotator cuff repair. It is a primary portal for knot tying.

III. Anterolateral and posterolateral portals are added if needed and are placed 1 to 2 cm anterior or posterior to the lateral portal, respectively. These portals are used for instrumentation and suture management during rotator cuff repair.

Diagnostic Arthroscopy and Additional Procedures

I. All arthroscopic rotator cuff repairs begin with a thorough inspection of the glenohumeral joint to identify the rotator cuff tear, as well as to identify and treat other pathology.

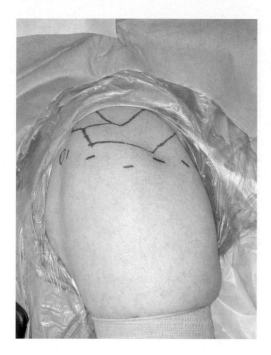

Figure 3-9
Bony landmarks and arthroscopic portals marked out on skin prior to incision. *(From Miller M, Cooper D, Warner J: Review of Sports Medicine and Arthroscopy, 2nd ed. Philadelphia, Saunders, 2002.)*

A. The posterior portal is established and the arthroscope is placed in the glenohumeral joint. All areas of the glenohumeral joint should be inspected in a systematic fashion.

B. The origin of the long head of the biceps at the superior glenoid and labrum is often the first structure identified. Other significant structures to identify include the labrum, glenohumeral ligaments, rotator cuff tendons, and the articular surfaces of the glenoid and humeral head. An articular-sided or full-thickness supraspinatus tear can be seen superolaterally, off the tendon's insertion on the humeral head (Fig. 3-10).

II. After the glenohumeral joint has been fully inspected and other pathology has been addressed, the arthroscope is placed in the subacromial space for evaluation. The subacromial space is also initially entered through the posterior portal.

III. For most chronic and acute full-thickness rotator cuff tears, a subacromial decompression is performed. Viewing from the posterior portal, with an arthroscopic shaver placed in the subacromial space through the lateral portal, a subacromial bursectomy is performed. Removing the bursa allows full visualization of the rotator cuff tear and also exposes the undersurface of the acromion (Fig. 3-11).

AS IN THE OPEN PROCEDURE, IF THE TENDON OF THE LONG HEAD OF THE BICEPS APPEARS TO BE SIGNIFICANTLY DAMAGED DURING INTRA-ARTICULAR INSPECTION, AN ARTHROSCOPIC TENOTOMY OR TENODESIS TO THE PROXIMAL HUMERUS CAN BE PERFORMED.

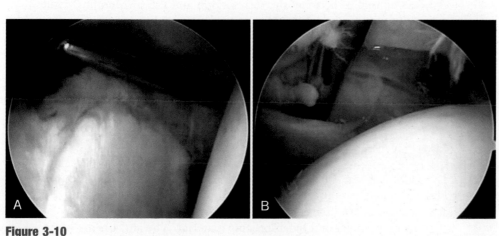

Figure 3-10
Arthroscopic views from the glenohumeral joint of a rotator cuff tear with uncovering of the glenoid (**A**) and humeral head (**B**).

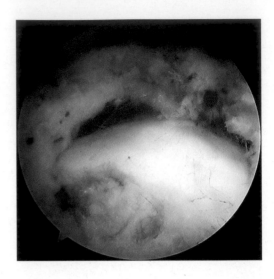

Figure 3-11
Arthroscopic view from the subacromial space of a rotator cuff tear with uncovering of the humeral head.

> **FOR LARGE CHRONIC ROTATOR CUFF TEARS (TWO AND THREE TENDONS) WHERE TENDON HEALING IS NOT GUARANTEED, MAINTAINING THE INTEGRITY OF THE CORACOACROMIAL (CA) ARCH IS CRITICAL. IN THIS CIRCUMSTANCE, AN ACROMIOPLASTY SHOULD NOT BE PERFORMED IF IT REQUIRES RELEASE OF THE CA LIGAMENT.**

IV. The undersurface of the acromion is further cleaned off using the shaver or an arthroscopic radiofrequency device, and the CA ligament can be released off the anterior acromion if not contraindicated.

V. If there are any prominent spurs on the undersurface of the anterior acromion making it curved or hooked in shape, an anterior acromioplasty is performed. This is done using an arthroscopic burr placed in the lateral and/or posterior portals. The burr is used to shave away the excess bone anteriorly, creating a smooth, flat undersurface of the acromion.

VI. As in the open procedure, the acromioplasty also exposes the AC joint, and a distal clavicle excision can be performed arthroscopically if the AC joint is symptomatic preoperatively. (Refer to Chapter 2 for details on subacromial decompression.)

Tendon Edge Débridement and Tendon Mobilization

I. Débridement of the torn tendon edges can be done following the subacromial decompression using the arthroscopic shaver. Any bursal or fibrous tissue should be removed to stimulate healing and leave behind a thick tendon edge that can hold sutures.

II. Depending on the size and mobility of the tear, tendon mobilization is performed to allow the retracted tendon to be repaired back to its insertion site on the greater tuberosity tension-free. Similar to the open procedure, mobilization occurs by freeing all adhesions between the torn tendon and the surrounding tissues.

> **AS IN THE OPEN PROCEDURE, AVOID GOING TOO MEDIAL DURING THE ARTHROSCOPIC RELEASES BECAUSE OF THE RISK OF SUPRASCAPULAR NERVE INJURY.**

   A. Traction sutures can be placed at the tendon edges or an arthroscopic grasping device can be used to provide traction while mobilizing the tendon.
   B. Using a shaver or small periosteal elevator through the lateral portal, subacromial adhesions are released to mobilize the bursal side of the tendon.
   C. Intra-articular or capsulolabral adhesions are released by re-entering the glenohumeral joint with the arthroscope in the posterior portal and using similar instrumentation to mobilize the articular side of the tendon.

Rotator Cuff Repair

I. The rotator cuff tear should be optimally visualized and mobilized at this point, and based on the tear pattern, the appropriate repair technique is determined.

II. Suture anchors are typically used to repair the tendon back to bone and can be made of metal or a bioabsorbable material. The anchors are placed at the greater tuberosity, just off the articular surface of the humeral head, and have suture loaded in them that can be passed through the tendon for repair.

A. The greater tuberosity is prepared for anchor placement with an arthroscopic shaver and/or burr to remove any soft tissue and smooth any irregular bony prominences. Aggressive decortication of the tuberosity is not necessary and can weaken the strength of the anchors in the tuberosity.

B. Suture anchors are placed, typically through the anterolateral portal. A spinal needle can be used to determine the correct orientation of anchor placement prior to making the portal.

C. Depending on the size and pattern of the rotator cuff tear, one or more anchors are used and placed approximately 1 cm apart, starting from the point of least tension and moving toward the point of greatest tension (typically posterior to anterior). The anchors are loaded with a heavy, nonabsorbable suture prior to placement and are either screwed or malleted into the bone.

III. A number of different arthroscopic techniques and instruments are available to facilitate suture passing through the torn rotator cuff tendon prior to tying. The details of these procedures are beyond the scope of this chapter; however, tear pattern often dictates the techniques and instruments used. All of the available portals may be needed to facilitate suture passing, with the arthroscope typically placed in the posterior or lateral portal.

IV. Once all sutures have been passed, they can be sequentially tied to bring the torn tendon back to the greater tuberosity to be held via the anchors. Just as with the open procedure, the goal is to restore the normal footprint of the rotator cuff. The tendon is generally repaired with the arm in a neutral position at the side if possible.

V. Several arthroscopic knot-tying techniques can be used to secure the suture; however, the details of these techniques are beyond the scope of this chapter. In general, sliding knots must be made outside of the shoulder and then passed into the subacromial space through one of the portals with an arthroscopic knot pusher. Once down on the tendon, the knots are then tightened, locked, and the suture cut.

VI. Depending on tear pattern and size, different knot types may be used including simple, horizontal mattress, and modified Mason-Allen stitches. In addition, newer techniques, such as double row repairs and transosseous-equivalent repairs, are continually being developed in order to best restore the normal footprint of the rotator cuff.

VII. Once all sutures have been tied, stability of the repair should be confirmed by visualization through both the subacromial space (tendon outer surface) and glenohumeral joint (tendon undersurface) prior to closure (Fig. 3-12).

> What is your attending's technique for arthroscopic rotator cuff repair? When does he/she convert to an open repair?

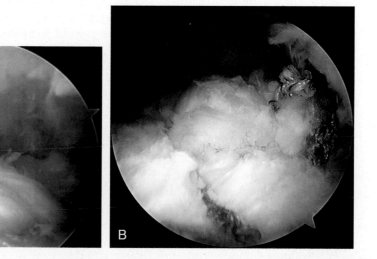

Figure 3-12

Arthroscopic views from the subacromial space of the rotator cuff tears following repair, in Figure 3-10 (**A**) and Figure 3-11 (**B**).

Portal Closure

The arthroscopic portals are closed in standard fashion, and the wounds are dressed (refer to Chapter 1).

POSTOPERATIVE CARE AND GENERAL REHABILITATION

> CAUTION MAY BE NEEDED IN PATIENTS UNDERGOING ARTHROSCOPIC ROTATOR CUFF REPAIR. THEY MAY HAVE LESS DISCOMFORT POSTOPERATIVELY COMPARED WITH THOSE UNDERGOING MORE TRADITIONAL OPEN REPAIR AND MAY WANT TO DO MUCH MORE WITH THE SHOULDER THAN IS INITIALLY DESIRED.

I. Most patients, whether undergoing open or arthroscopic surgery, can go home the day of surgery. Patients should remain overnight for observation if their pain is not adequately controlled.

II. Initial postoperative pain management is best achieved with oral narcotics and/or an interscalene nerve block placed just prior to surgery. Patient-controlled analgesia may be used if the patient remains in the hospital overnight.

III. Shoulder rehabilitation following rotator cuff repair has some variations depending on the size of the tear and the quality of the repair. In addition, the period of shoulder immobilization may vary based on the same factors, as well as surgeon preference. However, some general guidelines are as follows:

A. The first week after surgery, the arm remains in the abduction sling at all times when out in public or in bed. The sling can be removed only for showering, dressing, and for gentle shoulder pendulum exercises. Active ROM exercises can only be done with the hand, wrist, and elbow.

B. Passive shoulder ROM exercises are started as early as 2 to 4 weeks after surgery. These include passive supine forward flexion and passive supine external rotation, with continued pendulums. For smaller tears with good-quality tissue, some surgeons may start these passive exercises immediately after surgery.

C. The shoulder is protected in the sling for up to 4 to 6 weeks after surgery, with large tears protected longer.

D. Active assisted and active ROM exercises are started anywhere from 6 to 10 weeks postoperatively. Exercises begin in the supine position and progress to the seated or standing position. All planes of motion are used at this point, including forward flexion, abduction, external rotation, and gentle internal rotation. The contralateral arm or a cane is used for active assisted activities. Caution is essential as the patient progresses from passive to active assisted to active ROM to avoid compromising the repair. Exercises should not be painful, and progress to active ROM should be stopped or slowed if pain is encountered.

E. By week 10, a strengthening program can generally be started. Comfortable, active ROM must be achieved prior to beginning strengthening. Resistance bands are first used for strengthening, with progression to light free weights and eventually machines as tolerated. Again, overaggressive or premature strengthening should be avoided to prevent compromising the repair, with pain serving as a guide.

> What is your attending's rehabilitation protocol following rotator cuff repair?

IV. Return to sports activities and/or manual labor varies depending on the size of the tear, quality of the repair, and rehabilitation potential of the patient, but may take 6 to 9 months. Complete healing of the repair and return of full strength may take more than 12 months.

COMPLICATIONS

I. Persistent pain (e.g., inadequate subacromial decompression, AC joint arthritis, painful long head of the biceps)

II. Infection

III. Incomplete healing of rotator cuff tear

IV. Recurrent rotator cuff tear

V. Stiffness, adhesive capsulitis (frozen shoulder)

VI. Deltoid detachment or denervation

VII. Nerve injury (axillary, suprascapular)

SUGGESTED READINGS

Craig EV: Master Techniques in Orthopaedic Surgery: The Shoulder, 2nd ed. Philadelphia, Lippincott Williams & Wilkins, 2003.

Iannotti JP, Williams GR: Disorders of the Shoulder: Diagnosis and Management, 2nd ed. Philadelphia, Lippincott Williams & Wilkins, 2007.

Norris TR: Orthopaedic Knowledge Update: Shoulder and Elbow 2. Rosemont, IL, American Academy of Orthopaedic Surgeons, 2002.

CHAPTER 4

Bankart Repair: Open and Arthroscopic

Andrew F. Kuntz   and   Joseph A. Abboud

Case Study

A 29-year-old, right hand–dominant female who works as a teacher presents as an out-patient for evaluation. Two weeks prior to her appointment, she dislocated her right shoulder while changing her clothes. At that time, closed reduction of her shoulder was successfully performed in the local emergency department, and she was placed in a sling for immobilization. History reveals approximately six previous dislocations, with the first occurring 8 years earlier following a fall down stairs. On physical examination, there is no gross deformity about the shoulder. Range of motion is unable to be fully tested due to patient guarding. Anterior apprehension and relocation tests are positive. Otherwise, there is no evidence of rotator cuff or cervical spine pathology, and her neurovascular examination is intact. Radiographs following the most recent glenohumeral reduction reveal no fractures or bony abnormality. A magnetic resonance arthrogram obtained subsequent to her recent dislocation is shown in Figure 4-1.

BACKGROUND

I. **General**
   A. Glenohumeral anatomy and biomechanics may result in significant joint insta-bility. The glenohumeral joint is the most mobile large joint in the body and is the most frequently dislocated. Shoulder dislocations account for approxi-mately 50% of all native joint dislocations.
   B. Most shoulder dislocations are anterior, occurring eight to nine times more frequently than posterior dislocation. Inferior (luxatio erecta) and superior dislocations are very rare.

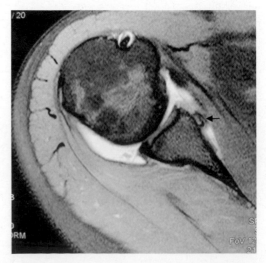

Figure 4-1
Axial cut from a magnetic resonance arthrogram showing a medially displaced Bankart lesion *(arrow)*.

C. Traumatic injury is responsible for approximately 95% of all dislocations. A direct blow to the shoulder, or in the case of an anterior dislocation, trauma to the arm with the shoulder in a position of abduction, extension, and external rotation are the most common mechanisms.

D. The recurrence rate is multifactorial and is related to age at initial injury and the amount of force required for dislocation. Several studies have shown greater than 90% recurrence in patients younger than 20 years of age at initial dislocation. This number decreases to 10% in patients older than 40 years of age.

II. **Shoulder Anatomy**

A. The glenohumeral joint gains little stability from the bony anatomy. Only 25% of the humeral head articulates with the flat glenoid at one time. Therefore, joint stability is a function of both static and dynamic stabilizers. Static stabilizers include the labrum, capsule, and associated ligamentous structures, negative intra-articular joint pressure, and adhesive and cohesive forces of the synovial fluid. Dynamic stability is a function of the rotator cuff, biceps tendons, and periscapular muscles.

B. The glenoid labrum deepens the glenoid 50%. This improves contact between the humeral head and glenoid so that 75% of the humeral head is in contact with the glenoid and labrum at a given time.

C. The shoulder capsule is thin and lax with little inherent stability. However, three capsular thickenings/ligaments play an integral role in providing shoulder stability (Fig. 4-2). The superior glenohumeral ligament serves as a restraint

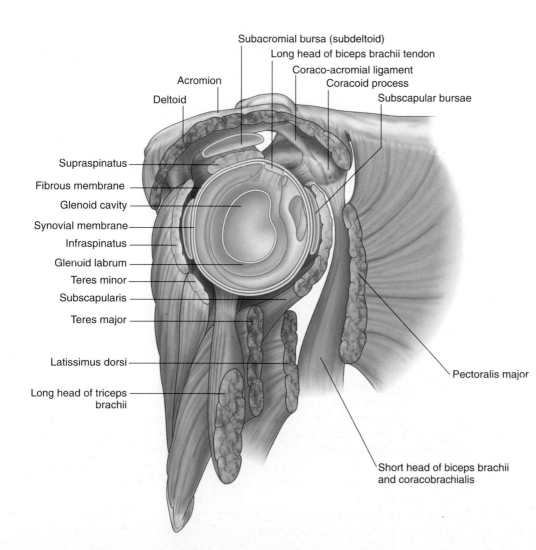

Figure 4-2

Lateral view of right glenohumeral joint and surrounding muscles with proximal end of humerus removed. *(From Drake RL, Vogl W, Mitchell AWM: Gray's Anatomy for Students. Philadelphia, Churchill Livingstone, 2005.)*

to inferior translation and anterior/posterior stress with the arm at 0 degrees of abduction. The middle glenohumeral ligament limits external rotation with arm in midabduction. Once the arm is abducted greater than 45 degrees, the anterior inferior glenohumeral ligament complex acts to limit anterior and posterior humeral head translation.

D. The rotator cuff, a dynamic stabilizer, provides a compressive force to the glenohumeral joint throughout its range of motion.

III. **Bankart Lesion**

A. No single pathologic lesion is responsible for recurrent shoulder instability. In 1906, Perthes described detachment of the anterior glenoid labrum as the "essential" lesion of instability. In 1938, Bankart described two types of acute shoulder dislocations, including forced anterior translation of the humeral head. He found that following this mechanism, tearing the anterior glenoid labrum and detachment of the capsule and periosteum from the scapular neck was common. From this description, traumatic detachment of the glenoid labrum came to be known as the "Bankart lesion."

B. Although not an "essential" lesion for shoulder instability, the Bankart lesion is found in up to 97% of shoulders following traumatic dislocation.

> A Bankart lesion is the traumatic detachment of the anterior-inferior glenoid labrum. With this lesion, there is also disruption of the anterior capsuloligamentous complex.

TREATMENT ALGORITHM

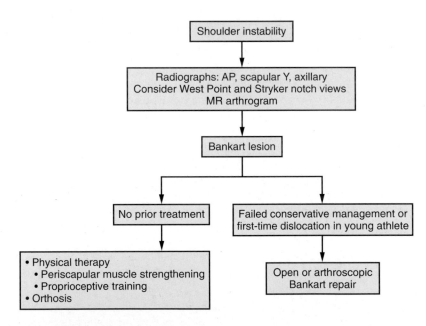

TREATMENT PROTOCOLS

I. **History and Physical Examination**

A. Patient evaluation in the emergency department or outpatient setting is critical in formulating a treatment plan following acute shoulder dislocation or recurrent instability. Examination begins by obtaining a history with a focus on determining the number and frequency of previous dislocations as well as arm position, amount of force, and activity resulting in dislocation.

B. Along with obtaining the proper history, a physical examination is always performed. When examining a patient with an acute shoulder dislocation, the following physical examination components are essential:

1. Observation of shoulder and extremity resting position. Anterior dislocations typically result in humeral external rotation, whereas posterior dislocations result in internal rotation.

2. Inspection and palpation about the shoulder may reveal a depression beneath the lateral deltoid and/or prominence of the humeral head anteriorly.

3. Careful and thorough neurovascular examination must be documented for all patients presenting with a shoulder dislocation. This must include evaluation of the motor function of the axillary nerve through demonstration of deltoid contraction. Evaluation of axillary nerve sensory function alone is unreliable and potentially misleading.

C. In the outpatient setting, physical examination of a patient with recurrent instability should include the following components:
   1. Evaluation of the cervical spine
   2. Comparison to the contralateral shoulder, assuming there is no history of bilateral instability
   3. Inspection for muscle atrophy and/or asymmetry
   4. Palpation for tenderness
   5. Active and passive range of motion assessment in all planes of motion (including observation for possible scapular winging)
   6. Strength testing
   7. Neurovascular assessment
   8. Provocative tests for shoulder instability:
      a. Load and shift test. This demonstrates anterior/posterior translation of the humerus.
      b. Sulcus test. This demonstrates inferior translation of the humerus as a result of longitudinal humeral traction.
      c. Anterior apprehension test. This test is performed with the patient lying supine with the arm in 90 degrees of abduction. Beginning with the arm in neutral rotation, external rotation causes patient apprehension because the tendency of the humeral head is to subluxate/dislocate anteriorly. This maneuver should be performed carefully to avoid in-office dislocation.
      d. Jobe's relocation test. Applying a posterior-directed force over the humeral head during an apprehension test provides comfort and relief for the patient.

II. **Radiographic Evaluation**
   A. An acute shoulder dislocation requires evaluation with three views of the shoulder, including anteroposterior (AP), transscapular, and axillary views. The axillary view is critical in ruling out dislocation and confirming reduction. If an axillary view or equivalent (Velpeau view) cannot be obtained, computed tomography (CT) imaging of the shoulder is required.
   B. Several other specialized radiographic views may be helpful in determining treatment for a patient with recurrent shoulder instability. These include:
      1. Both an AP radiograph with the shoulder in internal rotation and a Stryker notch view can be useful in the evaluation for the presence of a Hill-Sachs lesion.
      2. The West Point view is useful in evaluating the glenohumeral joint for fracture and/or calcification of the anterior inferior glenoid rim.
   C. A CT can be helpful in further evaluating the presence and extent of a Hill-Sachs lesion and/or a glenoid rim fracture.
   D. Magnetic resonance arthrography has become the imaging study of choice in the setting of shoulder instability as it gives the best minimally invasive evaluation of the soft tissues about the shoulder. Injection of contrast medium into the glenohumeral joint serves to delineate the soft tissue structures, increasing the ability to diagnose defects of the labrum and capsule.

III. **Classification**
   A. There is no formal classification system used to categorize Bankart lesions and/or shoulder instability. As a result, glenohumeral instability should be described using the following parameters:
      1. Direction: unidirectional, bidirectional, or multidirectional
      2. Subluxation versus dislocation
      3. Temporal: acute, subacute, or chronic (>6 weeks)

> **ALWAYS ASSESS THE MOTOR FUNCTION OF THE AXILLARY NERVE IN A PATIENT WITH AN ACUTE GLENOHUMERAL DISLOCATION.**

> **NEVER ACCEPT INADEQUATE IMAGING OF THE SHOULDER. AN AXILLARY OR EQUIVALENT VIEW IS MANDATORY WHEN EVALUATING A PATIENT WITH AN ACUTE GLENOHUMERAL DISLOCATION.**

> A Hill-Sachs lesion is a depression fracture of the posterior lateral humeral head, resulting from the humeral head resting on the anterior glenoid rim secondary to an anterior dislocation. This lesion is present following 35% to 40% of first-time dislocations, as well as in 80% of recurrent dislocations.

> A Bankart lesion associated with a glenoid rim fracture is referred to as a bony Bankart lesion.

4. Amount of force required for dislocation
5. Patient age
6. Patient mental status
7. Patient comorbidities

B. Bankart lesions typically involve only detachment of the anterior-inferior glenoid labrum, as well as disruption of the anterior capsuloligamentous structures. Occasionally, there is osseous involvement with an associated anterior-inferior glenoid rim fracture.

IV. **Treatment of Acute Glenohumeral Dislocation**

A. Management of an acute shoulder dislocation should focus on prompt, atraumatic joint reduction. Reduction should be performed following intra-articular local anesthetic injection or conscious sedation. Many reduction techniques have been described; however, use of traction and countertraction is often successful.

B. Following shoulder manipulation, joint reduction must be confirmed radiographically. Subsequently, the patient should have the shoulder immobilized temporarily. Classic immobilization includes a sling and swathe. With this method of immobilization, length of immobilization has no effect on rate of recurrence. Recently, there has been interest in the effectiveness of immobilization in a position of humeral external rotation in reducing recurrence rate. This is based on the finding that immobilization in adduction and internal rotation results in separation and displacement of the anterior labrum.

C. The patient should follow up with an orthopaedic surgeon within 1 week following an acute shoulder dislocation and successful relocation. At that point, further imaging such as CT and/or magnetic resonance imaging (MRI) may be ordered to assess for a Bankart lesion, soft tissue disruption, and bony pathology.

V. **Nonoperative Treatment Alternatives**

A. Rehabilitation and physical therapy, with a focus on periscapular muscle strengthening, are the principal nonoperative treatments for recurrent shoulder instability in patients with Bankart lesions. A successful combination of periscapular muscle strengthening and proprioceptive training can result in the ability to function without surgical intervention.

B. Orthoses that limit shoulder abduction and external rotation are also available and can be used to supplement physical therapy and rehabilitation.

> What is your attending's immobilization protocol following an acute shoulder dislocation?

SURGICAL ALTERNATIVES

I. Alternative surgical options typically address shoulder instability and not labrum or capsule pathology. The following listed procedures are alternatives that were historically popular for treating patients with anterior shoulder instability.

II. **Putti-Platt Procedure**

A. In this procedure, the subscapularis tendon and joint capsule are incised vertically, the lateral capsule is sutured to the glenoid labrum, the medial capsule is imbricated, and then the subscapularis is advanced laterally.

B. Currently, the Putti-Platt procedure is rarely indicated due to enhanced understanding of shoulder biomechanics and the common occurrence of severe postoperative posterior glenoid wear.

III. **Magnuson and Stack Procedure**

A. Anterior shoulder instability is addressed with advancement of the anterior capsule and subscapularis tendon laterally on the humerus.

B. One of the main disadvantages of the Magnuson and Stack procedure is the common external rotation deficit postoperatively.

IV. **Latarjet Procedure**

A. Anterior inferior glenoid rim fractures can increase anterior shoulder instability. When a large portion of the glenoid is involved (>25% of glenoid surface area), surgical intervention to address the bony defect is indicated. Due to the altered glenoid appearance, the "inverted pear" analogy has been used to describe this situation.

B. The Latarjet procedure involves transfer of the entire coracoid process to the anterior glenoid to address local bone loss.

C. Despite this, some surgeons have used this procedure successfully for primary treatment of instability without bone loss.

V. **Bristow Procedure**

A. The Bristow procedure is a modification of the Latarjet procedure and involves transfer of only the tip of the coracoid to the anterior glenoid rim.

B. Indications for this procedure also include shoulder instability in the presence of an anterior inferior glenoid osseous defect.

SURGICAL INDICATIONS FOR BANKART REPAIR

I. Shoulder instability with evidence of a Bankart lesion on MRI

II. Failed nonoperative treatment

A. Physical therapy and/or rehabilitation

B. Orthoses

III. Shoulder instability that prevents return to activity

IV. Single anterior shoulder dislocation in a young (<25-year-old) athlete

A. This is a controversial concept and may be considered a relative indication for operative treatment.

B. Many surgeons believe that Bankart repair is indicated following first-time dislocation in this population due to the high incidence of recurrence. Additionally, although not absent, surgical risks have decreased with the increased use of arthroscopic technique.

> Does your attending operate on patients with a Bankart lesion following a single shoulder dislocation? If not, then what rehabilitation protocol is used?

RELATIVE CONTRAINDICATIONS TO BANKART REPAIR

I. Current or recent infection

II. Multidirectional instability

III. Significant glenohumeral arthritis

IV. Voluntary subluxation and/or psychological issues that contribute to shoulder instability (absolute contraindication)

V. Medical comorbidities that preclude surgical treatment

GENERAL PRINCIPLES OF BANKART REPAIR SURGERY

I. The major goal of Bankart repair surgery is to restore function of the static stabilizers of the shoulder in order to reduce the incidence of recurrent shoulder instability. Bankart repair attempts to restore the anterior-inferior labrum so that it can act as a "bumper" to avoid anterior humeral head translation.

II. Open repair of a Bankart lesion is a time-tested procedure with an overall success rate of 90% to 95%. This procedure involves an anterior approach to the shoulder to repair the capsulolabral structures to the glenoid through use of drill holes or suture anchors.

III. The decision to repair a Bankart lesion arthroscopically is one based on surgeon experience and comfort. In general, there is a steep learning curve associated with arthroscopic surgical fixation of these lesions. Compared with open Bankart repair, arthroscopic surgery has the advantage of being able to achieve anatomic labral repair without surgical takedown of the subscapularis tendon. As a result, patients typically do not experience a decrease in external rotation as they may after open surgery. Additionally, arthroscopic surgery is typically associated with less postoperative pain and a shorter hospital course. The main disadvantage of arthroscopic surgery is historically higher rates of recurrence. However, with improving instrumentation and arthroscopic fixation anchors, recurrence rates are approaching that of open surgery.

> The major goal of Bankart repair surgery is to restore function of the static stabilizers of the shoulder, whereas the goal of rehabilitation is to restore dynamic stability.

IV. Regardless of whether a Bankart repair is performed as an open or arthroscopic procedure, an examination of shoulder stability is performed under anesthesia prior to starting surgery. The examination as described earlier is performed on the operative shoulder and compared to the contralateral side. Under anesthesia, joint stability can be assessed in the absence of patient guarding.

V. Most surgeons begin with diagnostic arthroscopy of the affected shoulder, regardless of whether the Bankart repair is performed open or arthroscopically. Diagnosis of lesions such as a large anterior inferior glenoid defect or an engaging Hill-Sachs lesion (in which a Hill-Sachs lesion engages the glenoid during range of motion, resulting in instability) often require open treatment. Humeral avulsion of the glenohumeral ligaments (HAGL lesion) must also be treated with an open procedure. However, a superior labrum anterior posterior (SLAP) lesion, which may be concomitantly present, must be addressed arthroscopically. (Refer to Chapter 2 for diagnostic arthroscopy.)

COMPONENTS OF OPEN BANKART REPAIR

Refer to Chapter 2 for details regarding patient positioning, prepping, and draping for the beach chair position. Also, refer to Chapter 6 for the anterior surgical approach to the shoulder. The procedure by which the labrum is attached to the glenoid rim is the same technique used for the arthroscopic method described below.

COMPONENTS OF ARTHROSCOPIC BANKART REPAIR

Patient Positioning, Prepping, and Draping

I. Prior to beginning an arthroscopic Bankart repair, the anesthesiologist may provide an interscalene nerve block to decrease postoperative pain. The procedure is typically performed under general anesthesia.

II. Arthroscopic Bankart repair can be performed using the beach chair or lateral decubitus position. This chapter focuses on using the lateral decubitus position.

III. For the lateral decubitus position, the patient is placed on a bean bag on a standard operating room table. In a coordinated effort involving the anesthesiologist, nursing staff, and the surgeon, the patient is rolled into the lateral decubitus position with the operative extremity oriented toward the ceiling. The contralateral arm is placed on an armboard and an axillary roll is placed under the nonoperative arm. The lower extremity that rests against the table should be padded at the level of the proximal fibula and ankle. For female patients, care must be taken to avoid undue pressure on the breasts. Entrapment of the genitalia during positioning must be avoided in male patients. Once the patient is in proper position, the bean bag is connected to suction. The operative extremity is then suspended using a candy cane and prepped in the usual fashion (Fig. 4-3). (Refer to Chapter 1 for surgical principles for prepping and draping.)

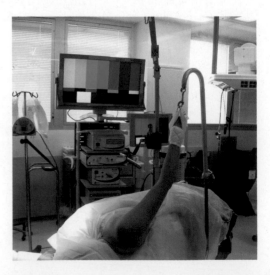

Figure 4-3
Patient positioning in the lateral decubitus position. Once properly positioned, the arm is suspended for prepping.

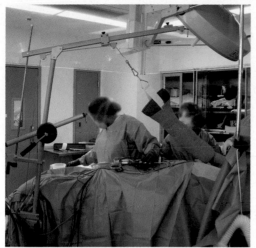

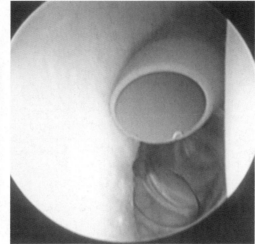

Figure 4-4
Traction is applied to the operative extremity to
provide joint distraction. Here the arm is placed in
a sterile sling and secured in place using Coban.

Figure 4-5
Intra-articular view of dual anterior portals with
the inferior portal placed just proximal to the
subscapularis tendon. (*From Miller M, Cooper D,
Warner J: Review of Sports Medicine and Arthroscopy,
2nd ed. Philadelphia, Saunders, 2002.*)

IV. With the shoulder prepped and draped, the operative extremity is placed in a distraction arm holder (Fig. 4-4). The arm holder is then connected to the traction
setup and approximately 10 to 12 pounds of traction is applied.

Establishment of Arthroscopic Portals and Diagnostic Arthroscopy

I. Refer to Chapter 2 for establishing arthroscopic portals and diagnostic
arthroscopy.
II. In addition to the standard arthroscopic portals, Bankart repair often requires a
second anterior portal inferior and medial to the previous portal. This portal is
placed at the superior aspect of the subscapularis tendon. There should be a
minimum of 3 cm between the anterosuperior and anteroinferior portals to avoid
overcrowding of instruments (Fig. 4-5).

Bankart Lesion Repair

I. Once the diagnostic arthroscopy is complete, the size of the Bankart lesion must
be assessed.
II. The labrum is mobilized from the anterior neck of the scapula (Fig. 4-6). This
can be performed with arthroscopic instruments, a rasp, or with a Cobb elevator.

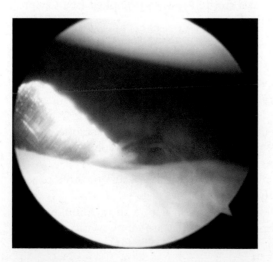

Figure 4-6
Mobilization of the anterior inferior labrum from the
anterior scapular neck is accomplished with a Cobb
elevator.

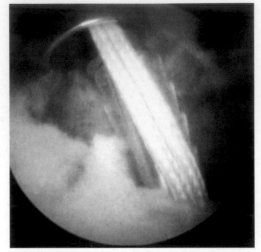

Figure 4-7

Anchor placement. A bioabsorbable suture anchor is inserted through the anterior canula.

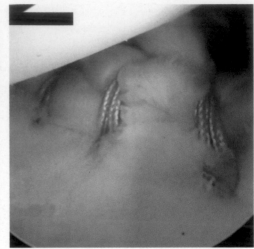

Figure 4-8

Completed Bankart repair with anterior glenoid labrum secured in anatomic position with three suture anchors.

> **SUTURE ANCHORS MUST BE PLACED AT THE PERIPHERY OF THE GLENOID ARTICULAR SURFACE. THE TENDENCY IS TO PLACE ANCHORS TOO FAR MEDIALLY.**

The labrum must be released at least to the 6 o'clock position to perform an anatomic repair with proper tension.

III. The glenoid rim is often sclerotic, and therefore preparation may be necessary. This is accomplished with a shaver or burr until the subchondral bone is exposed and a bleeding bed of bone for labral adherence is established.

IV. The first suture anchor is placed as far inferior on the glenoid rim as possible through the anteroinferior portal (Fig. 4-7). Anchor placement is critical, with optimal placement at the articular surface edge.

V. Depending on the type of anchor used, one or both limbs of the suture are retrieved through the anteroinferior portal. A suture-passing device is then used to capture the capsulolabral tissue with the retrieved suture. The suture is tied to secure the capsulolabral tissue to the glenoid.

VI. The previous steps are repeated as additional anchors are placed along the glenoid face, from inferior to superior. Commonly, three anchors are required. However, the number of anchors required to achieve a stable repair is determined by the size of the lesion (Fig. 4-8).

VII. Once all anchors have been placed and the labrum and associated capsule are secured to the glenoid, laxity of the anterior capsule is assessed and capsular placation is performed as needed.

Portal Closure

The portals are closed in standard fashion, and a sterile dressing is applied (see Chapter 1). A sling is used to immobilize the limb postoperatively.

POSTOPERATIVE CARE

I. Most patients, whether undergoing open or arthroscopic surgery, can go home the day of surgery. Patients should remain overnight for observation if their pain is not adequately controlled.

II. Initial postoperative pain management is best achieved with oral narcotics and/or an interscalene nerve block placed just prior to surgery. Patient-controlled analgesia may be used if the patient remains in the hospital overnight.

III. Shoulder rehabilitation following Bankart repair typically occurs in three phases, with each phase lasting approximately one month.

A. The first phase involves shoulder immobilization with a sling. Shoulder pendulum exercises are started postoperative day 1, as are elbow, wrist, and hand range-of-motion (ROM) exercises. Patients must avoid shoulder abduction and external rotation.

B. The second phase involves full shoulder active ROM exercises with protected abduction and external rotation.

C. The final phase of rehabilitation includes periscapular muscle strengthening.

IV. Rehabilitation following open Bankart repair is typically more aggressive to avoid excessive stiffness. Exercises follow the same progression as outlined above; however, active assisted ROM begins during the first postoperative week.

V. Full return to activity and sports can be expected at approximately 6 months after surgery.

COMPLICATIONS

I. Infection

II. Recurrent shoulder instability. This can be a result of the following:
   A. Failure of labral repair
   B. Nonanatomic labral repair secondary to inadequate immobilization

III. Axillary or musculocutaneous nerve damage

IV. Humeral head articular surface damage. This occurs from prominent metal suture anchors on the glenoid articular surface.

V. Loose suture anchor in the glenohumeral joint

VI. Reactive synovitis or bone cyst formation. This occurs secondary to bioabsorbable suture anchors.

SUGGESTED READINGS

Bottoni CR: Anterior instability. In Johnson DL, Mair SD (eds): Clinical Sports Medicine. Philadelphia, Mosby, 2006, pp 189–199.

Pearle AD, Cordasco FA: Shoulder instability. In Vaccaro AR (ed): Orthopaedic Knowledge Update 8. Rosemont, IL, American Association of Orthopaedic Surgeons, 2005, pp 283–294.

Phillips BB: Recurrent dislocations, Shoulder section. In Canale ST (ed): Campbell's Operative Orthopaedics, 10th ed. Philadelphia, Mosby, 2003, pp 2397–2422.

Su B, Levine WN: Arthroscopic Bankart repair. J Am Acad Orthop Surg 13:487–490, 2005.

CHAPTER 5

Arthroscopic Superior Labrum Anterior Posterior (SLAP) Repair

Brent B. Wiesel   and   G. Russell Huffman

Case Study

A 30-year-old, left hand–dominant male presents with a 6-month history of left shoulder pain, which began after he landed on his left arm while playing ice hockey. The pain is activity related and exacerbated by the use of his left arm for overhead activities or throwing. His symptoms have progressed to the point where he can no longer participate in recreational hockey and softball. A brief course of nonsteroidal anti-inflammatory medications failed to relieve his pain fully, and physical therapy has exacerbated his symptoms. On physical examination, he has full range of motion and no atrophy about the left shoulder. He has positive O'Brien and Mayo sheer tests. He has pain but no apprehension when his arm is placed in abduction and external rotation, and his pain is relieved when a posteriorly directed force is applied to his anterior shoulder. Radiographs of the left shoulder are normal and a coronal oblique T1-weighted magnetic resonance imaging scan with intra-articular contrast is shown in Figure 5-1.

BACKGROUND

I. Injuries to the intra-articular attachment of the long head of the biceps tendon were originally described by Andrews et al in 1985. This entity was further defined and classified by Snyder et al in 1990. The authors described four types of pathologic lesions and named them superior labral anterior and posterior (SLAP) tears.

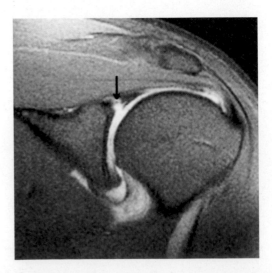

Figure 5-1
Coronal oblique T1-weighted magnetic resonance imaging scan with intra-articular contrast of the left shoulder. *(From Miller MD, Osborne JR, Warner JJP, Fu FH [eds]: Shoulder Arthroscopy in MRI—Arthroscopy Correlative Atlas. Philadelphia, Saunders, 1997.)*

II. Since that time, SLAP tears have been increasingly recognized as a common cause of shoulder pain in throwing athletes, as well as any young individual who suffers a traction or compression injury to the shoulder.

III. In overhead throwing athletes, there are two mechanisms that combine to result in injury to the posterosuperior glenoid labrum:

A. The inciting event is proposed by some to arise from excessive traction on the posterior inferior joint capsule during the follow-through phase of throwing. This repetitive microtrauma may lead to hypertrophy of the posterior band of the inferior glenohumeral ligament.

1. This thickening of the posterior inferior capsule can be demonstrated on physical examination as a loss of glenohumeral internal rotation with the arm in 90 degrees of abduction and the scapula stabilized to prevent scapulothoracic motion.

2. The posterior capsular abnormality initiates a chain of pathologic motion that results in abnormal posterior-superior translation of the humeral head during the late-cocking phase of throwing. This translation places increased stress on the superior labrum and biceps anchor and can lead to type II SLAP tears. This is known as the peel-back mechanism.

B. The second mechanism is that of internal impingement. In positions of glenohumeral abduction and external rotation (e.g., the late cocking phase of throwing), the posterior superior rotator cuff and humeral head articular margin come in contact with the posterosuperior glenoid labrum. With repetition, this contact leads to type II tears of the posterosuperior glenoid labrum and articular-sided rotator cuff tears. This is further exacerbated in the presence of posterior inferior glenohumeral capsular contracture.

TREATMENT PROTOCOLS

I. **History and Physical Examination**

A. The presentation of patients with SLAP lesions can be quite variable, and the diagnosis should be considered in all patients younger than 50 years of age with intra-articular shoulder pain.

B. The most common presenting symptom is shoulder pain with a clear history of an injury or inciting event.

C. Most injuries typically occur from falls on an outstretched hand, weight lifting, eccentric abduction and external rotation, automobile accidents, contact sports, and overhead sports (baseball, softball, volleyball, tennis, swimming).

D. Patients may also describe mechanical symptoms (catching or popping) with overhead activity.

E. Throwing athletes with SLAP tears often present with shoulder pain and a loss of accuracy and velocity.

F. On physical examination, it is important to rule out other common causes of shoulder pain such as impingement, instability, and acromioclavicular joint pathology.

G. We have found the O'Brien, Mayo sheer, and apprehension tests to be the most useful physical examination maneuvers in diagnosing SLAP tears.

1. For the O'Brien test (active biceps compression test), the patient places the arm in 90 degrees of forward flexion, 20 degrees of adduction, and active full internal rotation (thumb pointing toward floor). The examiner then provides a downward force on the patient's forearm as the patient raises his or her arm toward the ceiling. If this reproduces the patient's shoulder pain, the patient is asked to full externally rotate the arm (thumb pointing toward ceiling), and the downward force is reapplied. For a positive test, the pain is experienced with the arm in internal rotation and is relieved with external rotation.

2. In the Mayo sheer test (also known as the dynamic labral sheer test), the patient's elbow is placed at his or her side and flexed 90 degrees. The exam-

iner then puts the arm in maximal passive external rotation and gradually abducts the arm while placing a hand over the posterior aspect of the shoulder to stabilize the scapula. A patient with a positive test experiences increasing pain with abduction between 60 and 120 degrees. A positive test may include pain, pain and a click, or simply a click.

3. Although Jobe's apprehension testing is classically used to diagnose shoulder instability, patients with SLAP tears often have pain without a sensation of instability when the arm is placed in the abducted, externally rotated position. This test is most easily performed with the patient supine on an examination table to stabilize the scapula. This pain is relieved if a posteriorly directed force is applied to the humeral head.

H. Intra-articular local anesthetic is helpful in localizing symptoms to the glenohumeral joint. Three milliliters of anesthetic is injected anteriorly through the rotator interval and provocative testing is repeated. If the examination returns to normal (with the exception of mechanical symptoms) after administration of local anesthetic, then even with negative imaging modalities, the diagnosis of glenoid labrum tears may be made based on patient demographics, history, and physical examination.

I. Overhead athletes with SLAP lesions typically exhibit increased glenohumeral external rotation and diminished internal rotation compared with the contralateral shoulder in 90 degrees of shoulder abduction. A shift in rotational arc is normal; however, a decrease in the total rotational arc compared to the contralateral shoulder is manifested as excessively diminished internal rotation (i.e., to a greater degree than the gain in external rotation). This is known as a glenohumeral internal rotational deficit (GIRD) and can precipitate an injury to the thrower's superior glenoid labrum, rotator cuff, and elbow.

II. **Imaging**

A. Patients with SLAP tears typically do not have any abnormalities on plain radiographs, although a small subset of patients may have concurrent acromioclavicular joint sprains at the time of the glenoid labrum tear.

B. Magnetic resonance imaging (MRI) is the most useful imaging modality for the evaluation of SLAP tears.

1. The diagnosis is made when fluid is visualized between the superior glenoid rim and the labrum on the oblique coronal images.

2. The addition of intra-articular contrast has been reported to increase the sensitivity of MRI in detecting SLAP tears.

3. We have found that a clear history of a traumatic event in a patient younger than 40 years of age and pain on provocative physical examination testing to be more sensitive in making the diagnosis than MRI scans, even when the MRI is interpreted by experienced musculoskeletal radiologists. However, the specificity of the MRI remains high, and this is a useful adjunct to define the tear and associated injuries.

III. **Nonoperative Treatment**

A. Rest, activity modification, preservation of motion, and periscapular and rotator cuff strengthening are initially indicated for SLAP tears.

B. However, the symptoms from glenoid labrum tears often do not improve with nonoperative treatment. In many cases physical therapy exacerbates the patient's pain.

C. In a patient with a possible SLAP tear, but an uncharacteristic history or physical examination, a trial of physical therapy is warranted, because many of the other potential diagnoses improve with therapy. If the patient's pain does not improve, then it is more likely that they have a SLAP tear.

D. For overhead athletes with an internal rotation deficit, sidelying sleeper stretches that isolate the posterior capsule both preoperatively and postoperatively are important.

TREATMENT ALGORITHM

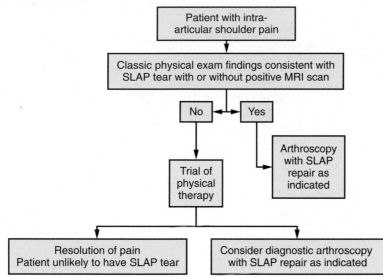

SURGICAL INDICATIONS AND CONTRAINDICATIONS

I. **Indications**

   A. Arthroscopic SLAP repair is indicated in patients younger than 40 years of age with the characteristic history and physical examination findings of a SLAP tear.

   B. For patients with intra-articular shoulder pain without the characteristic physical examination findings, who have failed conservative treatment, including a trial of physical therapy, arthroscopy of the involved shoulder is indicated. A SLAP tear can then be appropriately addressed if identified at the time of surgery.

II. **Contraindications**

   A. Patients with asymptomatic lesions found incidentally on MRI scans should not undergo SLAP repair.

   B. SLAP lesions found at the time of shoulder arthroscopy to treat other pathology should generally either be left alone or addressed with débridement. This is especially true in patients older than 40 years of age and those without the characteristic finds of a SLAP tear on physical examination.

GENERAL PRINCIPLES OF SLAP REPAIR

I. Classification of SLAP tears is performed intraoperatively using the classification described by Snyder et al (Fig. 5-2).

II. SLAP tears are treated with arthroscopic fixation only. Open repair is not an option for treatment of tears requiring surgical intervention.

III. The operative management of tears is based on their classification.

   A. Type I tears involve fraying or degeneration of the superior labrum without detachment of the labrum or the biceps anchor. Treatment consists of débridement of the frayed tissue.

   B. Type II tears consist of detachment of the superior labrum and biceps anchor from the glenoid rim. Treatment consists of anatomic repair of the labral-biceps anchor complex back to the glenoid rim using suture anchors as described below.

   C. In Type III tears there is detachment of the superior labrum from the glenoid rim without involvement of the biceps anchor. These tears can be débrided unless the tear involves greater than one third the width of the labrum, in which case the labrum is repaired in a manner similar to type II tears.

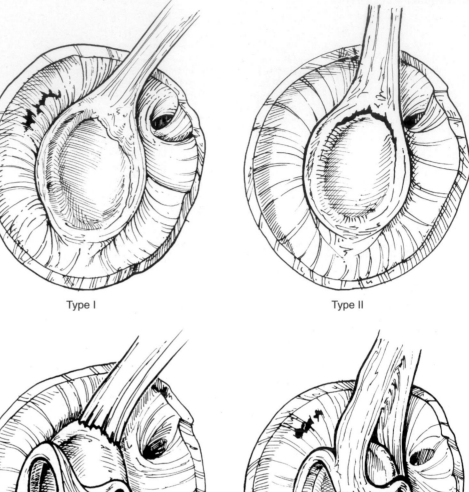

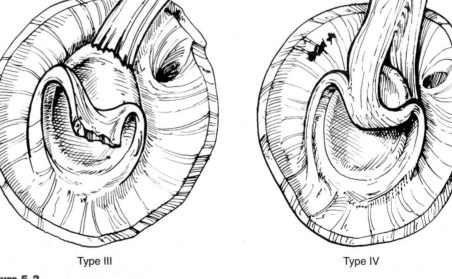

Figure 5-2
The classification of arthroscopic superior labrum anterior posterior (SLAP) tears as described by Snyder et al. *(Adapted from Miller MD, Osborne JR, Warner JJP, Fu FH [eds]: Shoulder Arthroscopy in MRI—Arthroscopy Correlative Atlas. Philadelphia, Saunders, 1997.)*

    D. Type IV tears involve a bucket-handle tear of the superior labrum extending into the biceps tendon.
       1. If the tear of the biceps tendon involves less than one third of the tendon, it can be debrided and the labral component can be managed like a type III tear.
       2. If more than one third of the biceps is involved but the tendon appears healthy, the biceps split is repaired with side-to-side sutures and the labrum is repaired to the glenoid rim. If the biceps tendon is degenerative, than a biceps tenodesis or tenotomy should be performed.
  IV. In patients older than 40 years of age, SLAP tears are often encountered at the time of arthroscopy for the treatment of other shoulder pathology (especially

rotator cuff disease). In these patients, the tear should not be addressed if the biceps anchor is stable and the biceps tendon is in good condition. If there is instability of the biceps anchor or degeneration of the tendon, a biceps tenotomy or tenodesis should be considered.

COMPONENTS OF THE PROCEDURE

Note that all arthroscopic photos demonstrating the operative technique are of the left shoulder viewed from the posterior portal in the lateral decubitus position. SLAP repair, like other arthroscopic shoulder procedures, may be performed in either the beach chair or lateral decubitus position. We use the lateral decubitus position because the traction applied to the arm creates a larger working area within the joint and allows superior access to the posterior labrum when needed.

Positioning, Prepping, and Draping

  I. Refer to Chapter 4 for complete details on lateral decubitus positioning.
 II. The patient is prepped and draped in standard fashion using the surgical principles described in Chapter 1.

Portal Placement and Diagnostic Arthroscopy

  I. Prior to incision, we use a skin marker to define the posterior lateral and anterior lateral borders of the acromion. The V is defined by the posterior border of the clavicle and the anterior border of the scapular spine (in the region of the arthroscopic portal described by Neviaser), and the coracoid process.
 II. A standard posterior portal is established. In cases in which a posterior glenoid labrum tear is suspected, the posterior incision is placed more laterally in line with the lateral border of the acromion process.
III. A spinal needle is then used to localize the anterior rotator interval portal, which is established via an outside-in technique. On the skin surface the portal is located slightly lateral and superior to the coracoid process and is roughly in line with and inferior to the acromioclavicular joint. The portal should enter the joint in the triangle defined by the biceps tendon and the superior border of the subscapularis muscle. We prefer to make a skin incision using an 11-blade scalpel and then penetrate the joint capsule with a metal switching stick that can be used as a probe during the diagnostic arthroscopy (Fig. 5-3).
 IV. A standard diagnostic arthroscopy is performed (see Chapter 2).
  V. If a SLAP lesion is suspected, the attachment of the biceps tendon to the superior glenoid rim is carefully examined by placing the probe at the attachment site and using it to pull the biceps tendon superiorly (Fig. 5-4).

> **CARE MUST BE TAKEN WHEN ARTHROSCOPICALLY DIAGNOSING ABNORMALITIES OF THE BICEPS ANCHOR BECAUSE SOME PATIENTS HAVE NONPATHOLOGIC REDUNDANCY IN THIS AREA. GENERALLY, IF THE GLENOID RIM THAT IS EXPOSED WHEN SUPERIOR TRACTION IS APPLIED TO THE BICEPS TENDON IS COVERED WITH CARTILAGE, THEN IT IS THE PATIENT'S NATURAL ANATOMY. IF TRACTION ON THE PROXIMAL BICEPS EXPOSES BONE, THEN THIS IS A PATHOLOGIC FINDING INDICATIVE OF A SLAP LESION.**

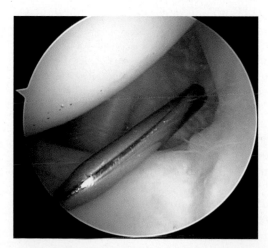

Figure 5-3
A switching stick is used to establish the anterior interval portal via an outside-in technique.

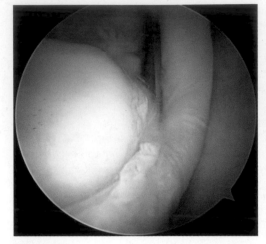

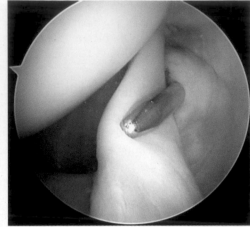

Figure 5-4

Probing of the biceps attachment demonstrates a type II arthroscopic superior labrum anterior posterior (SLAP) tear.

Figure 5-5

The probe is placed on the superior aspect of the biceps tendon and used to pull the tendon into the joint to check for degeneration or subluxation.

What are your attending's indications for a biceps tenotomy versus a tenodesis for proximal biceps pathology?

VI. For all patients with biceps anchor pathology, it is important to examine the proximal biceps tendon closely. To do this, the probe is placed on the superior surface of the tendon and an inferior and medially directed force is applied to pull the proximal portion of the tendon into the joint for inspection. Significant fraying of the portion of the tendon that resides in the bicipital groove or medial subluxation of the tendon over the superior border of the subscapularis might direct the surgeon to perform a biceps tenodesis or tenotomy instead of a SLAP repair (Fig. 5-5).

VII. If a SLAP lesion is identified, it is classified and the decision is made as to whether it is reparable. If a repair is to be performed, the number and location of the anchors are determined.

SLAP Repair

I. If the SLAP lesion is to be repaired, a 6-mm arthroscopic cannula is introduced over the switching stick in the anterior portal.

II. An anterior superior portal is then established via an outside-in technique.

A. This portal is located just off the anterior lateral edge of the acromion and enters the joint just anterior to the leading edge of the supraspinatus tendon behind the biceps tendon in the rotator interval. A 5-mm cannula is introduced via this portal (Figs. 5-6 and 5-7). With this technique, the supraspinatus tendon is not violated.

TO PROTECT THE LABRUM DURING THIS STEP, IT IS IMPORTANT THAT THE SHAVER'S TEETH ARE ORIENTED ONLY TOWARD THE GLENOID.

B. However, for more posterior glenoid labrum lesions, a direct lateral portal in the myotendinous junction of the supraspinatus may be necessary (portal of Wilmington). When used, this portal must be small and medially placed (just against the acromial edge) to prevent injury to the supraspinatus tendon.

III. A 4.2-mm arthroscopic meniscal shaver is then inserted via the anterior superior portal and used to debride any frayed tissue. The shaver is then placed between the superior labrum and the glenoid rim and run at high speed on forward to create a bed of fresh bone where the labrum will attach (Fig. 5-8). Preparation of the superior glenoid articular margin may also be performed with an arthroscopic burr.

The dense bone of the glenoid rim allows the anchors used in this location to be smaller in size (3 to 4 mm) than those inserted into the humeral head for rotator cuff repairs (5 to 8 mm).

IV. An arthroscopic anchor is then inserted via the anterior superior cannula and placed on the glenoid rim at the posterior aspect of the tear (Fig. 5-9). We prefer to use the Mini-Revo anchor (Linvatec, Largo, Florida).

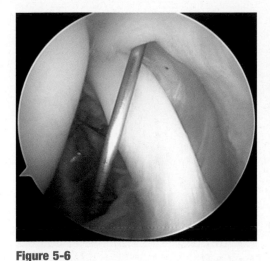

Figure 5-6
A spinal needle is used to localize the anterior superior portal just anterior to the leading edge of the supraspinatus tendon but posterior to the biceps tendon.

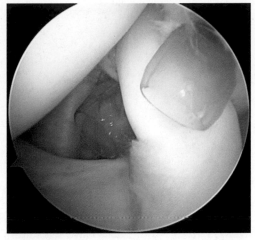

Figure 5-7
A 6-mm cannula is placed through the anterior portal and a 5-mm cannula is placed via the anterior superior portal.

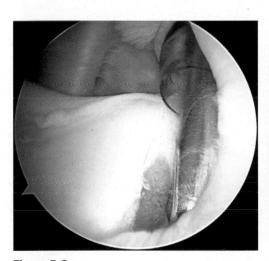

Figure 5-8
An arthroscopic shaver is used to create a bed of exposed bone where the labrum will be reattached.

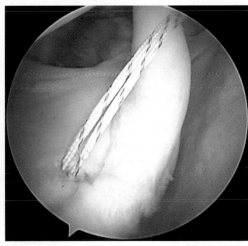

Figure 5-9
A suture anchor is placed on the glenoid rim at the posterior aspect of the tear.

V. The suture strand that is closest to the labrum is retrieved through the anterior cannula using a crochet hook (Fig. 5-10).

VI. An 18-gauge spinal needle is inserted via Neviaser's portal (located at the apex of the V formed by the distal clavicle and the spine of the scapula) and passed through the joint capsule and the superior labrum above the anchor. It is important that the surgeon be able to identify the needle between the capsule and the superior labrum. This is accomplished by passing the needle through the capsule and then backing it up slightly and passing it through the labrum instead of passing it through both structures in a continuous manner (Figs. 5-11 and 5-12).

VII. An 0-Prolene suture is then threaded through the spinal needle and retrieved out the anterior portal using the crochet hook (Fig. 5-13).

VIII. The strand of suture from the anchor is then attached to the Prolene suture via a simple knot, and the Prolene and anchor suture strands are pulled back into the joint, through the labrum and out Neviaser's portal along with the spinal needle.

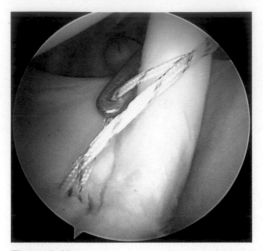

Figure 5-10
The suture strand closest to the labral tissue is retrieved out the anterior portal using a crochet hook. This will be the post-strand for the arthroscopic knot.

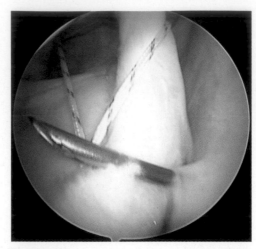

Figure 5-11
A spinal needle is inserted through the superior capsule via Neviaser's portal.

What type of knot does your attending prefer to fix the superior labrum?

IX. The suture is pulled out the anterior superior cannula. Because this strand passes through the labrum, it serves as the post for an arthroscopic sliding knot (Fig. 5-14).

X. An arthroscopic knot of the surgeon's preference is tied via the anterior lateral cannula and used to compress the labrum to the glenoid rim (Fig. 5-15).

XI. The steps are repeated to place as many anchors as needed moving from posterior to anterior along the glenoid rim. In general, two to three anchors are used for isolated SLAP repairs.

XII. If the tear extends anterior to the biceps tendon, the anchors can generally be inserted via the anterior portal and a penetrating grasper can be inserted via the same cannula to pass the post-strand through the labrum in place of the spinal needle.

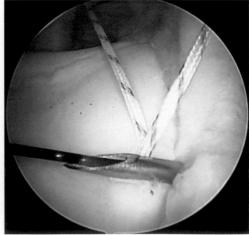

Figure 5-12
The needle is then directed through the superior labrum.

Figure 5-13
An 0-Prolene suture is threaded down the needle and retrieved out the anterior portal.

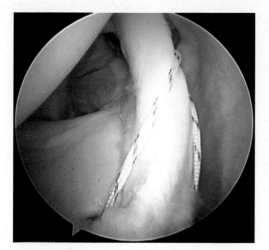

Figure 5-14
The suture is used to shuttle the post-strand of the suture anchor through the labral tissue. The post-strand is then retrieved out the anterior superior portal.

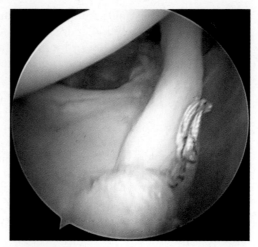

Figure 5-15
An arthroscopic knot is used to secure the labrum to the glenoid rim.

Wound Closure

The arthroscopic portals are closed in standard fashion, and a sterile dressing is applied (see Chapter 1). The arm is placed in a sling for postoperative immobilization (Fig. 5-16).

POSTOPERATIVE MANAGEMENT

I. All SLAP repairs are performed on an outpatient basis.
II. The patient is instructed to keep the operative arm in a sling for 3 weeks except when performing active finger, wrist, and elbow range of motion exercises and gentle Codman exercises of the shoulder.
III. At 3 weeks, the sling is discontinued and the patient begins a passive range-of-motion program with the therapist.
IV. Once full range of motion has been regained, generally at 6 weeks, the patient begins a progressive strengthening program.
V. The patient is allowed to return to sports at 3 months unless they are involved in overhead throwing.

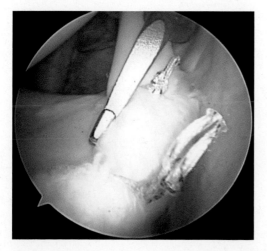

Figure 5-16
Following completion of the repair, the biceps attachment is probed to make sure that it is secure. This repair required two anchors that were both placed via the anterior superior cannula.

What postoperative protocol does your attending follow after an arthroscopic superior labrum anterior posterior repair?

VI. Gentle throwing is initiated at 4 months and the patient progresses to competitive throwing between 6 and 9 months after surgery.

VII. For overhead athletes with preoperative internal rotation deficits, it is important to emphasize posterior capsular stretching throughout the postoperative course.

COMPLICATIONS

I. Shoulder stiffness. For this reason, it is important to begin early pendulum exercises followed by passive range of motion with a therapist at 3 weeks.

II. Continued pain. In this situation, it is important to consider alternative diagnoses.

III. Infection

SUGGESTED READINGS

Andrews JR, Carson WG Jr, McLeod WD: Glenoid labrum tears related to the long head of the biceps. Am J Sports Med 13:337–341, 1985.

Burkhart SS: Superior labrum anterior and posterior lesions. In Norris TR (ed): Orthopaedic Knowledge Update Shoulder and Elbow 2. Rosemont, IL, American Academy of Orthopaedic Surgeons, 2002, pp 543–549.

Burkhart SS, Morgan CD, Kibler WB: The disabled throwing shoulder: spectrum of pathology. Part II: Evaluation and treatment of SLAP lesions in throwers. Arthroscopy 19:531–539, 2003.

Mileski RA, Snyder SJ: Superior labral lesions in the shoulder: Pathoanatomy and surgical management. J Am Acad Orthop Surg 6:121–131, 1998.

Neviaser TJ: Arthroscopy of the shoulder. Orthop Clin North Am 18:361–372, 1987.

Snyder SJ, Karzel RP, Del Pizzo W, et al: SLAP lesions of the shoulder. Arthroscopy 6:274–279, 1990.

Tennet TD, Beach WR, Meyers JF: A review of special tests associated with shoulder examination. Part II: Laxity, instability and superior labral anterior and posterior (SLAP) lesions. Am J Sports Med 31:301–307, 2003.

CHAPTER 6

Total Shoulder Arthroplasty

Eric T. Ricchetti   and   Matthew L. Ramsey

Case Study

A 70-year-old, right hand–dominant female presents with a 5-year history of right shoulder pain. She has had gradual progressive difficulty with activities of daily living and is now limited significantly by pain and stiffness in her right shoulder. The patient has pain at night, which keeps her awake on a regular basis. She denies any specific injury that initiated the onset of her symptoms and denies any neck pain or associated radiating symptoms (numbness, tingling, pain) down her arms. She has tried several nonoperative treatments, including nonsteroidal anti-inflammatory medications; activity modification; physical therapy; and multiple, intermittent corticosteroid injections into her shoulder. These have provided her only with temporary symptomatic relief, and their effect has lessened as her symptoms have progressed. She is now retired and lives at home by herself without a caretaker. True anteroposterior and axillary lateral views of her right shoulder are presented in Figure 6-1.

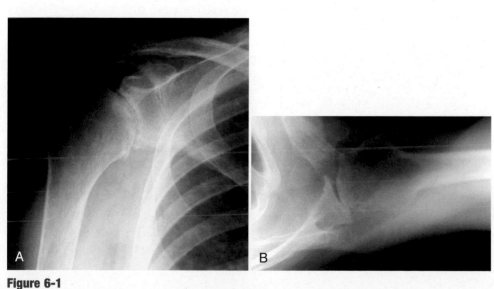

Figure 6-1
True views of the shoulder. **A,** Anteroposterior. **B,** Axillary lateral.

BACKGROUND

I. Arthritis, by definition, means intra-articular inflammation, although inflammation may not always be present in the disease. The term is more accurately described as articular cartilage degeneration, which may be a result of several different causes. The most common etiology of glenohumeral arthritis is osteoarthritis, but other diseases, such as rheumatoid or inflammatory arthritis, osteonecrosis, rotator cuff arthropathy, and post-traumatic or postsurgical arthritis, can also be a cause. The different etiologies of glenohumeral arthritis may dictate different treatment options, but total shoulder arthroplasty (TSA) may be a final surgical option in all forms of the disease.

II. Glenohumeral arthritis occurs in as many as 20% of adults and is much less common than arthritis of the hip or knee. Osteoarthritis, the most common form, occurs more often in women than men, and is more likely in patients older than 60 years of age.

III. Pain in the affected shoulder is the most common presenting complaint in patients with glenohumeral arthritis. Shoulder stiffness is also a frequent problem, and patients may note a sensation of crepitus with shoulder movement. Symptoms usually begin gradually and are chronic and progressive. Discomfort is typically worsened with activity, and patients may awaken at night from pain, particularly if they sleep on the affected shoulder. Functional limitations may be evident, including an inability to perform overhead activities or reach behind the back or under the opposite axilla with the affected arm. In the case of inflammatory arthritis, the associated synovitis may cause considerable swelling and inflammation.

> Adhesive capsulitis (frozen shoulder) is another major cause of restriction of both active and passive range of motion in the shoulder and must be ruled out.

> A patient's inability to externally rotate includes the following differential diagnosis: (1) posterior dislocation of the shoulder, (2) adhesive capsulitis, or (3) glenohumeral arthritis.

IV. Physical examination of the affected shoulder may demonstrate mild shoulder atrophy from disuse. Although often nonspecific, posterior joint line tenderness is typical in osteoarthritis, while anterior and lateral tenderness is seen more frequently in inflammatory arthritis. Range of motion (ROM), both active and passive, is typically restricted in glenohumeral arthritis, usually in multiple planes. Decreased external rotation is commonly seen in osteoarthritis from anterior capsular contracture and articular derangement. Specific patterns of restricted motion may also be related to prior trauma or surgery, such as a loss of external rotation in patients with previous surgical stabilization for anterior shoulder instability. Pain and crepitus in the glenohumeral joint may be elicited with active or passive motion. Muscle strength testing should assess the rotator cuff, deltoid, and other shoulder girdle muscles. A careful examination of the cervical spine should also be performed to rule out any abnormalities, including radiculopathy and degenerative joint disease that may cause referred pain, stiffness, or weakness in the shoulder.

V. For the majority of patients with painful arthritis unresponsive to nonoperative treatment, definitive surgical intervention consists of TSA. Although TSA can provide both pain relief and improvement of function, pain relief is more reliably achieved. Therefore, pain relief, not restoration of function, should be the primary goal of surgery. Shoulder replacement can be performed to replace both the humeral head and glenoid (TSA) or the humeral head alone (hemiarthroplasty), depending on the degree of glenoid degeneration, integrity of the rotator cuff, and age of the patient.

VI. Approximately 90% or more of patients can be expected to attain good or excellent pain relief following TSA, and prosthesis survivorship is greater than 90% at 10 years.

VII. Newer prostheses include the humeral head resurfacing implant without a stem and the reverse shoulder prosthesis used in patients with irreparable rotator cuff deficiency. However, long-term results are still needed to determine the ultimate utility of these implants.

TREATMENT ALGORITHM

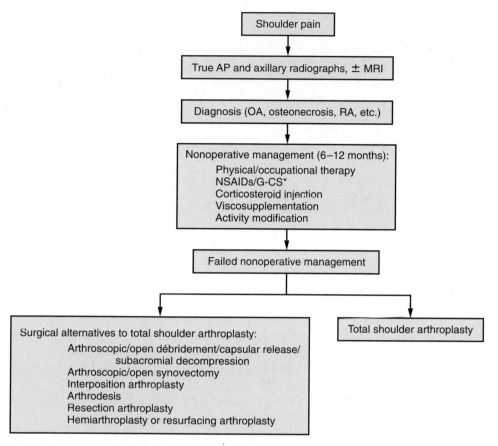

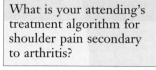

What is your attending's treatment algorithm for shoulder pain secondary to arthritis?

*Glucosamine–chondroitin sulfate

TREATMENT PROTOCOLS

I. **Treatment Considerations.** All of the following considerations play an important role in the decision making process of treating patients with glenohumeral arthritis:
   A. Patient age
   B. Activity level
   C. Overall health
   D. Degree of joint involvement
   E. Integrity of the rotator cuff
   F. Patient expectations

II. **Nonoperative Treatment Options**
   A. Initial treatment strategy
      1. Nonsteroidal anti-inflammatory drugs or acetaminophen
      2. Glucosamine–chondroitin sulfate oral supplementation
      3. Activity modification (e.g., low-impact activity, discontinuation of manual labor)
      4. Weight loss
      5. Heat (chronic arthritic pain) and cold (acute flare-up) therapy
      6. Physical, occupational, and aqua therapy
         a. Physical therapy and aqua therapy are aimed at regaining motion and strength. These techniques typically include gentle passive motion/ stretching and isometric strengthening (deltoid, rotator cuff, scapular muscles). Aqua therapy decreases stress across muscles and joints because of the buoyancy effects of water.
         b. Ultrasound: heat effect

THERAPY CAN BE CHALLENGING IF THE ARTICULAR SURFACE IS SEVERELY DEGENERATED, BECAUSE STRETCHING AND STRENGTHENING ACROSS A COMPROMISED ARTICULAR SURFACE CAN INCREASE SYMPTOMS.

INTRA-ARTICULAR STEROIDS MAY INCREASE ENDOGENOUS GLUCOSE LEVELS POSTINJECTION. THEREFORE, PATIENTS WITH DIABETES SHOULD BE MADE AWARE THAT CLOSE POSTINJECTION GLUCOSE MONITORING MAY BE REQUIRED.

VISCOSUPPLEMENTATION IS CURRENTLY NOT FDA APPROVED FOR USE IN OSTEOARTHRITIS OF THE SHOULDER. THE PATIENT MUST BE INFORMED OF THIS OFF-LABEL USE OF THE PRODUCT IF ITS USE IS BEING CONSIDERED.

The following make up the borders of the rotator interval: supraspinatus superiorly, subscapularis inferiorly, coracoid process medially, and long head of the biceps and humeral head laterally.

The coracoacromial ligament may be a primary restraint to superior elevation of the humeral head in patients with significant rotator cuff deficiency, such as those with irreparable rotator cuff tears. Therefore, resection may lead to superior elevation of the humeral head and further worsening of shoulder function.

c. Occupational therapy is aimed at teaching alternative ways of accomplishing activities of daily living (ADLs) that may be impaired and providing assistive devices.

B. Intra-articular corticosteroid injections
   1. Corticosteroids are considered if initial treatments have been ineffective, but are of variable benefit.
   2. Typically, these are more useful for symptomatic relief in inflammatory arthritis than in osteoarthritis.
   3. Injections can be performed at 4-month intervals (no more than 3 per year) if they are helpful.

C. Intra-articular hyaluronic acid injections (viscosupplementation)
   1. This is an alternative for patients who have been unresponsive to other nonoperative therapies, but results are variable, with fewer data on its use in the shoulder than in the hip and knee.
   2. It involves a series of three to five injections administered 1 week apart.

SURGICAL ALTERNATIVES TO TOTAL SHOULDER ARTHROPLASTY

I. **Arthroscopic Procedures**
   A. Débridement
      1. Indicated for mild to moderate glenohumeral arthritis without structural alteration of the joint. Patients with mechanical symptoms due to loose bodies, degenerative labral tears, or small humeral head lesions from osteonecrosis are most likely to benefit from this treatment.
      2. Débridement has a limited role in the absence of true mechanical symptoms and its benefit is not as clear as in the knee.
      3. Arthroscopy may have an additional diagnostic benefit by revealing previously unrecognized degenerative changes.
   B. Capsular releases
      1. Indicated for mild to moderate glenohumeral arthritis associated with limited motion, particularly external rotation.
      2. Anterior capsulolabral structures are released for decreased external rotation, including the rotator interval, while posterior capsulolabral structures are released for decreased internal rotation.
      3. Passive manipulation under anesthesia is also performed after soft tissue releases to further increase motion and disrupt tight tissues. This technique, however, is not effective as an isolated procedure for chronic loss of motion from osteoarthritis.
   C. Subacromial decompression
      1. Some pain complaints in patients with arthritic shoulders may be due to inflammation or bursitis in the subacromial space, or acromial impingement.
      2. Subacromial decompression can include a subacromial bursectomy, coracoacromial (CA) ligament resection, and anterior acromioplasty.
   D. Synovectomy
      1. Can be used in patients with early stage inflammatory arthropathies or osteoarthritis with synovitis
      2. Can provide pain relief and improved function, but the synovitis can recur, requiring a repeat procedure
      3. May protect the rotator cuff from attritional tearing that can occur with chronic inflammatory arthritis

II. **Open Procedures**
   A. Resection arthroplasty
      1. Resection arthroplasty is indicated for more severe infections, fractures, or failed TSA. The humeral head is resected and a pseudoarthrosis forms that allows some shoulder function.
      2. Function is generally better if the rotator cuff attachments to the proximal humerus can be preserved.

B. Interposition arthroplasty and biologic glenoid resurfacing
   1. Use of a biologic tissue placed between the humeral head and glenoid; the more modern technique of glenoid resurfacing involves suturing the biologic tissue directly to the glenoid, with or without humeral head replacement (hemiarthroplasty) or resurfacing.
      a. Biologic tissue choices: anterior capsule, autogenous fascia lata, Achilles tendon allograft, human dermal collagen allograft, or meniscal allograft
      b. A surface replacement implant may be used for the humeral head that removes minimal bone (lacks the intramedullary stem of a traditional humeral head replacement).
   2. Indications
      a. Young, active patients who may wear out or loosen a standard shoulder replacement
      b. Rheumatoid arthritis patients
      c. Patients with rotator cuff tear arthropathy or irreparable cuffs and eccentric glenoid wear
      d. Revision arthroplasties with glenoid removal and poor glenoid bone stock
C. Arthrodesis (surgical fusion)
   1. Indicated as a salvage procedure in patients with recurrent or indolent infection, significant loss of deltoid and/or rotator cuff function, other severe soft tissue deficiencies (e.g., CA arch deficiency), brachial plexus palsy, persistent symptomatic instability, or multiple failed surgeries.
   2. The recommended position of shoulder fusion is 30 degrees of abduction, 30 degrees of forward flexion, and 30 degrees of internal rotation.

> What surgical alternatives would your attending consider for a given pattern of arthritis?

SURGICAL INDICATIONS FOR TOTAL SHOULDER ARTHROPLASTY

I. **End-Stage Degenerative Joint Disease**
  A. Most common etiologies
    1. Osteoarthritis
    2. Osteonecrosis (Fig. 6-2)
    3. Rheumatoid arthritis
    4. Post-traumatic arthritis
    5. Arthritis of dislocation
    6. Postsurgical arthritis (e.g., postinstability stabilization)
    7. Rotator cuff arthropathy

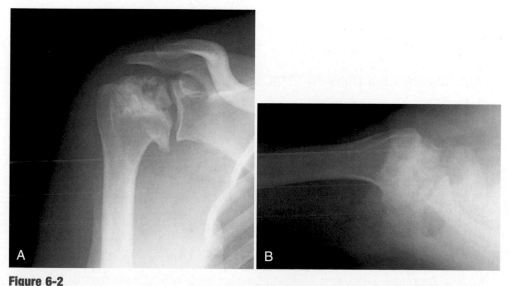

Figure 6-2
True views of a shoulder with end-stage osteonecrosis. **A,** Anteroposterior. **B,** Axillary lateral.

B. Other etiologies that may result in end-stage joint deterioration
 1. Crystalline arthritis
  a. Calcium pyrophosphate dehydrate deposition disease
  b. Gout
  c. Apatite deposition disease ("Milwaukee shoulder")
 2. Inflammatory arthritis
  a. Juvenile idiopathic arthritis
  b. Spondyloarthropathies
   (1) Ankylosing spondylitis
   (2) Reiter's syndrome
   (3) Psoriatic arthritis
   (4) Enteropathic arthritis
 3. Dialysis arthropathy
 4. Neuropathic arthropathy (Charcot arthropathy)
 5. Hemophilia arthropathy
 6. Postinfectious arthritis
C. Clinical presentation
 1. Worsening pain over time
 2. Pain that awakens from sleep
 3. Decreased active and passive shoulder ROM (external rotation commonly affected)
 4. Decreased ability to perform ADLs
D. Radiographic features and diagnostic criteria

OSTEOARTHRITIS	RHEUMATOID ARTHRITIS
1. Asymmetric joint space narrowing (typically posterior glenoid wear)	1. Symmetric joint space narrowing (typically central glenoid wear)
2. Sclerosis	2. Periarticular osteopenia/osteoporosis
3. Subchondral cysts	3. Joint erosions
4. Osteophyte formation (inferior humeral head common)	4. Ankylosis

II. **Failed Treatment**
 A. Activity modification (e.g., low-impact activity, discontinuation of manual labor)
 B. Weight loss
 C. Nonsteroidal anti-inflammatory drugs, acetaminophen, and/or glucosamine–chondroitin sulfate
 D. Physical, occupational, or aqua therapy
 E. Heat (chronic arthritic pain) and cold (acute flare-up) therapy
 F. Intra-articular injections (corticosteroids or viscosupplementation)
 G. Previous surgical alternative treatment

RELATIVE CONTRAINDICATIONS TO TOTAL SHOULDER ARTHROPLASTY

 I. Current infection (absolute)
 II. Recent infection
 III. Concomitant rotator cuff and deltoid dysfunction
 IV. Neuropathic arthropathy (Charcot arthropathy)
 V. Severe brachial plexopathy
 VI. Intractable shoulder instability
 VII. Young and active patient. It wears out faster.
 VIII. Medically unstable. The patient is unable to safely tolerate the stress of surgery.

GENERAL PRINCIPLES OF TOTAL SHOULDER ARTHROPLASTY

 I. The glenohumeral joint is a ball-and-socket joint with the greatest ROM of any joint in the body.

II. Although the glenohumeral joint is a congruent articulation with less than 2 mm of mismatch between the radius of curvature of the glenoid and humeral head, only one third of the humeral head is covered by the glenoid.

III. Normal anatomic relationships of the glenoid and humeral head include the following:

A. Glenoid version ranging from 7 degrees of retroversion to 10 degrees of anteversion, with an average of 5 degrees of upward tilt. The glenoid surface is pear-shaped, with the superior half approximately 20% narrower than the inferior half.

B. Humeral head retroversion, relative to the transepicondylar axis of the distal humerus, ranging from 25 to 40 degrees (average, 30 degrees). The articular surface of the humeral head is inclined an average of 130 degrees superiorly relative to the humeral shaft. The center of the humeral head is also offset medially and posteriorly relative to the center of the humeral shaft.

C. The greater tuberosity (GT) and the lesser tuberosity (LT) of the humeral head are located laterally and medially, respectively, to the bicipital groove and are the attachment sites of the rotator cuff tendons (GT: supraspinatus, infraspinatus, teres minor; LT: subscapularis).

D. The GT is 5 to 10 mm below the top of the humeral head.

IV. The goal of TSA is to establish normal relationships about the glenohumeral joint and to restore a smooth articulation between the humeral head and glenoid. This has the primary objective of providing pain relief, with a secondary benefit of increased function. Establishing normal glenohumeral relationships places the rotator cuff and other soft tissues at their most efficient tension and provides optimal results.

V. A TSA consists of a humeral component and a glenoid component. The humeral component is made of metal, typically a cobalt chrome head with a titanium stem, and the glenoid component is made of ultra-high-molecular-weight polyethylene.

VI. The success of TSA is far more dependent on proper soft tissue functioning and balance than hip and knee replacements because the glenohumeral joint has far less bony constraint.

A. The status of the rotator cuff is a key component of proper soft tissue functioning around the prosthesis. If the rotator cuff is deficient and the humeral head shows superior migration on radiographs, the glenoid will not be concentrically loaded following TSA. This leads to eccentric superior wear on the glenoid component and possible mechanical loosening and failure of the glenoid.

B. The glenoid is subjected to significant shear forces due to the lack of bony constraint and a replacement component may loosen prematurely as a result. The glenoid component appears to be the weak link in implant survival, typically wearing out or loosening prior to the humeral component.

> Glenoid component loosening is the most common complication in total shoulder arthroplasty.

VII. The amount of glenoid bone stock available for resurfacing is another important factor in TSA. Significant glenoid erosion may prevent placement of a glenoid component due to a lack of bone stock or may alter glenoid version. Abnormal version must be corrected to neutral during surgery so that the glenohumeral articulation becomes concentric. For example, posterior glenoid wear seen in osteoarthritis is typically corrected to neutral version with anterior reaming, or less commonly with posterior bone grafting.

COMPONENTS OF THE PROCEDURE

Positioning, Prepping, and Draping

I. Once the patient is positioned and under full anesthesia, passive shoulder ROM, particularly external rotation at the side, should be noted.

II. The patient is placed in the beach chair position (see Chapter 2 for details).

III. The operative upper extremity is prepped and draped in standard fashion according to the principles outlined in Chapter 1. Draping should allow access to the

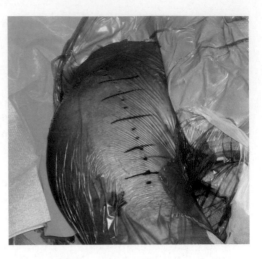

Figure 6-3
Deltopectoral incision marked out.

medial clavicle proximally and to the wrist distally. A Foley catheter should be placed prior to the start of the case.

IV. Mark the skin incision (deltopectoral) using a sterile marker (Fig. 6-3).

Surgical Approach and Applied Surgical Anatomy

The deltoid muscle is innervated by the axillary nerve. The pectoralis major muscle is innervated by the medial and lateral pectoral nerves.

I. The most common approach for TSA is the deltopectoral approach. For patients undergoing revision surgery with a prior deltopectoral incision, the previously made incision should be used.

II. The skin incision is made approximately 10 to 15 cm long, marked from the tip of the coracoid proximally to the deltoid tuberosity distally, and it is centered over the interval between the deltoid laterally and the pectoralis major medially.

III. Once the skin and the subcutaneous tissues have been exposed, the first structures to identify are the cephalic vein, deltoid, and pectoralis major. The cephalic vein rests in a groove between the deltoid (lateral) and pectoralis major (medial), marking the deltopectoral interval (Fig. 6-4).

IV. As a major draining vein of the arm, the cephalic vein should be preserved and can be retracted either medially or laterally. Lateral retraction is generally preferred because of the many branches to the cephalic vein that come in on the lateral side. Medial retraction places less tension on the vein but sacrifices the numerous lateral feeding vessels.

The conjoined tendon originates from the coracoid process. It is composed of the short head of the biceps and the coracobrachialis (both supplied by the musculocutaneous nerve).

V. The cephalic vein and deltoid are retracted laterally and the pectoralis major is retracted medially to expose the underlying clavipectoral fascia and the conjoined tendon (Fig. 6-5).

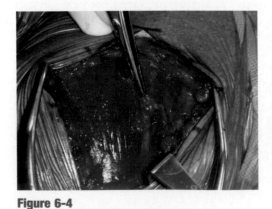

Figure 6-4
Deltopectoral interval exposed with the deltoid laterally (left), pectoralis major medially (right), and the cephalic vein pointed out between the two.

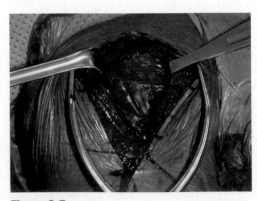

Figure 6-5
Deltoid retracted laterally (left retractor) and the pectoralis major retracted medially (right retractor) to expose the conjoined tendon with the clavipectoral fascia overlying it.

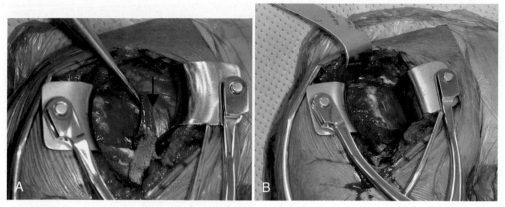

Figure 6-6
Exposure of the subscapularis tendon with the conjoined tendon first mobilized (**A**, *arrow*), then retracted (**B**) medially to expose the subscapularis.

VI. The clavipectoral fascia is then incised just lateral to the conjoined tendon and retracted to expose the subscapularis tendon. The incision should be taken up to, but not through, the CA ligament because of its role in superior restraint of the humeral head (see earlier; Fig. 6-6).

VII. The subscapularis and other rotator cuff muscles can be inspected in this position for evidence of a tear. Rotator cuff tears are rare in association with osteoarthritis (5% to 10%).

VIII. Several important neurovascular structures can be identified in this position as well. The musculocutaneous nerve enters the undersurface of the conjoint tendon approximately 5 to 8 cm distal to the coracoid process and can be digitally palpated, whereas the axillary nerve should be palpated just below the inferior border of the subscapularis tendon as it heads posteriorly through the quadrilateral space. The anterior humeral circumflex vessels also run along the inferior edge of the subscapularis and are clamped, cut, and tied off or coagulated once exposed (Fig. 6-7).

IX. To expose the glenohumeral joint, the subscapularis tendon must be released (Fig. 6-8). Depending on the amount of external rotation loss that is present, the tendon

The quadrilateral space is bordered by the following structures: superior, teres minor; inferior, teres major; medial, long head of the triceps; and lateral, surgical neck of the humerus or lateral head of the triceps. The posterior humeral circumflex artery accompanies the axillary nerve through this space.

The primary blood supply to the humeral head is the arcuate artery, a branch of the anterior humeral circumflex artery.

CARE MUST BE TAKEN TO AVOID INJURY TO THE AXILLARY AND MUSCULOCUTANEOUS NERVES EITHER BY EXCESSIVE RETRACTION OR DIRECT INJURY.

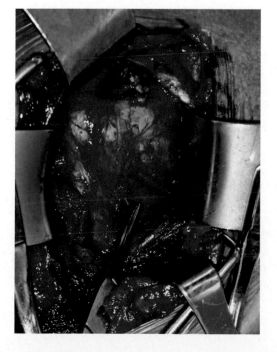

Figure 6-7
Subscapularis tendon exposed with the anterior humeral circumflex vessels pointed out.

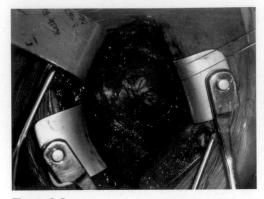

Figure 6-8
Release of the subscapularis tendon.

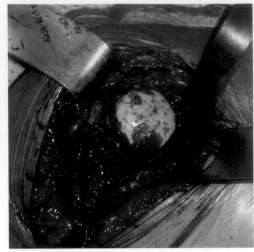

Figure 6-9
Exposure of the humeral head following dislocation.
Note the worn articular surface and presence of
osteophytes.

is released differently. If the deficit is mild (external rotation > 30 degrees at the side), the tendon can be incised intratendinously (approximately 2 cm medial to the LT) and repaired anatomically or an LT osteotomy can be performed with subsequent bone-to-bone repair. For a moderate deficit (−30 degrees < external rotation < 30 degrees), the tendon is released at the LT and advanced and repaired medially at closure. Rarely, a severe deficit is present (external rotation < −30 degrees), and a Z-plasty lengthening of the tendon is performed. However, this procedure weakens the muscle.

X. Release of the anterior and inferior joint capsule also improves external rotation and helps with surgical exposure.

XI. The humeral head can now be dislocated by simultaneous adduction, external rotation, and extension. This exposes the humeral head for preparation and implant insertion (Fig. 6-9).

Humeral Head Preparation

I. Osteophytes are removed from the humeral head to improve exposure and to allow identification of the anatomic neck. This allows the natural version of the humerus to be determined prior to humeral head resection.

II. A humeral head cutting guide is next positioned to make the humeral head osteotomy. Cutting guides can be intramedullary or extramedullary, or a freehand technique can even be used.

III. The humeral head cut is made to recreate the natural version of the humeral head (average, 30 degrees of retroversion) and should exit through the anatomic neck. The cut should be close to the rotator cuff insertions superiorly and posteriorly without violating the insertions (Fig. 6-10).

IV. The humeral canal is prepared and trialed to find the appropriately fitting stem. Canal preparation typically consists of the use of reamers and progressively larger broaches to open up the canal.

V. Trial humeral head sizing allows appropriate sizing of the glenoid component. The trial humeral head should be removed for glenoid exposure and preparation, but the trial stem should be left in place to prevent humeral shaft fracture (Fig. 6-11).

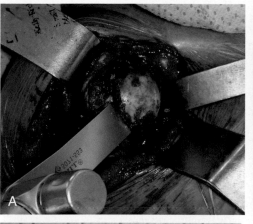

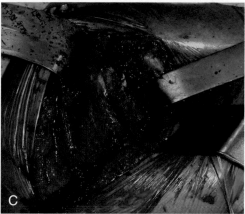

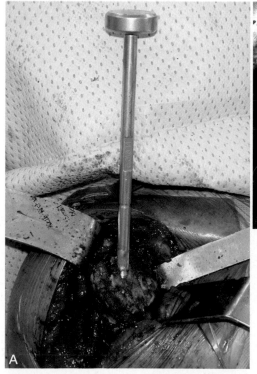

Figure 6-10

A, The humeral head being cut with an oscillating saw. **B,** The cut head removed, and the remaining proximal humerus shown. **C,** The humeral head component should be similar in size to the resected native head when implanted.

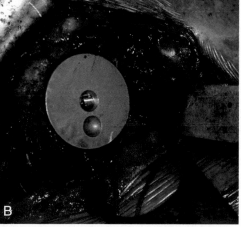

Figure 6-11

A, Humeral canal preparation begins with the use of an entry reamer to find the intramedullary canal. **B,** Once the canal has been prepared, the trial humeral stem can be placed.

Glenoid Exposure and Preparation

I. The arm is abducted, externally rotated, and extended to relax the posterior joint capsule and retract the humerus posteriorly. Any remaining anterior joint capsule should be released off the glenoid to further improve exposure (Fig. 6-12).

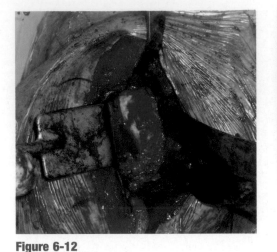

Figure 6-12
Exposure of the glenoid.

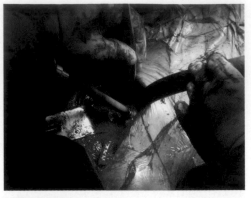

Figure 6-13
Reaming of the glenoid.

The long head of the biceps originates on the superior labrum and supraglenoid tubercle.

II. The labrum is circumferentially removed and the long head of the biceps is released if it is partially torn or tethered in the bicipital groove.

III. The glenoid can now be prepared by reaming to subchondral bone (Fig. 6-13). Neutral version should be recreated. Therefore, an eccentrically worn glenoid should be reamed more opposite the side of wear.

IV. The prepared glenoid should be checked for penetration through the deep cortical bone. If the cortex is violated, bone grafting is needed.

V. Two common glenoid components are currently used, a pegged design and a keeled design, and both are cemented into place. Drilling guides are used to drill holes in the glenoid following reaming to appropriately accept one of the two designs (Fig. 6-14).

MAKE SURE THE CEMENT IS NOT TOO HARD BEFORE CEMENTING IN THE GLENOID COMPONENT.

VI. The cement is ready to use when its consistency is between being too runny and too hard. The cement is placed on the glenoid surface, followed by the glenoid component. The component must be held in position on the glenoid with forceful pressure until the cement has completely hardened to prevent component movement as the cement hardens and expands (Fig. 6-15).

Humeral Head Trialing and Component Placement

I. Once the glenoid is complete, the humerus is redislocated for humeral head trialing.

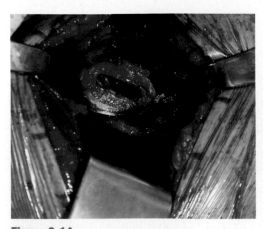

Figure 6-14
Glenoid prepared to accept keeled design following drilling.

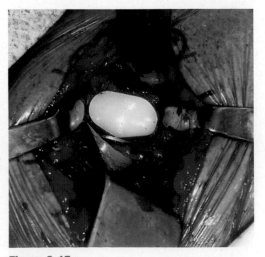

Figure 6-15
Glenoid component in place following cementing.

II. The humeral head component should be similar in size to the resected native head and should be well centered on the cut surface of the proximal humerus, with coverage of the cut surface maximized and overhang of the component minimized.

III. A trial implant is placed and assessed for adequate fit by reducing the humerus and checking for joint laxity and soft tissue tensioning. An ideal prosthesis provides a stable joint with appropriate soft tissue tension. This can be assessed checking posterior translation. The prosthesis should allow for approximately 50% to 100% posterior translation of the head when a posterior force is applied, with spontaneous reduction of the head when the force is removed.

IV. Once the proper sized humeral head is selected, the humeral component is assembled (consisting of both the stem and humeral head) and implanted. The prosthesis can be cemented into place or impacted without cement using a press-fit technique (Fig. 6-16).

V. Patients with poor bone quality and a large diaphysis-to-metaphysis diameter ratio are at increased risk of fracture with press-fit implantation, and should have the humeral prosthesis cemented into place.

> **IT IS CRITICAL THAT ALL OSTEOPHYTES BE REMOVED FROM THE PROXIMAL HUMERUS TO APPROPRIATELY SIZE THE HUMERAL HEAD.**

Wound Closure

I. Once the components have been secured in place, the shoulder is pulse lavaged with saline. A drain may be used to drain the shoulder and minimize the likelihood of a postoperative hemarthrosis.

II. The subscapularis is repaired according to how it was released (see above); tendon-to-tendon (intratendinous) or bone-to-bone (LT osteotomy) anatomic repair, medial repair to bone (LT release with medialization), or Z-plasty and lengthening (Fig. 6-17). The external rotation that can be obtained before tension is placed on the subscapularis repair is noted and used to direct postoperative rehabilitation.

III. Typically, the rotator interval is then closed with a heavy suture, followed by loose closure of the deltopectoral interval with a couple of interrupted sutures.

> Does your attending use a drain postoperatively? Why or why not?

> **IF THE ROTATOR INTERVAL IS CLOSED, THE ARM SHOULD BE HELD IN EXTERNAL ROTATION TO AVOID LIMITING EXTERNAL ROTATION POSTOPERATIVELY.**

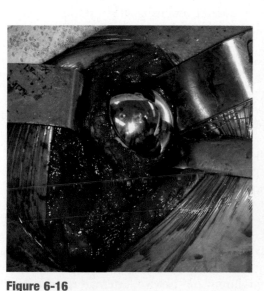

Figure 6-16
Humeral head implant in place.

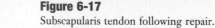

Figure 6-17
Subscapularis tendon following repair.

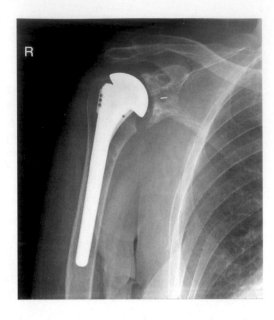

Figure 6-18
Anteroposterior radiograph of a shoulder following total shoulder arthroplasty.

IV. The subcutaneous tissue and skin is closed in standard fashion.

V. A sterile dressing is placed over the incision, and the arm is placed in a sling.

VI. Typically, patients have an anteroposterior radiograph of the shoulder taken postoperatively in the recovery room (Fig. 6-18).

POSTOPERATIVE CARE AND GENERAL REHABILITATION

I. Postoperative management includes pain control and prophylaxis against infection as well deep venous thrombosis.

II. Initial postoperative pain management is best achieved with patient-controlled analgesia and/or an interscalene nerve block placed just prior to surgery.

III. At least 24 hours of postoperative prophylactic antibiotics are administered.

IV. Unless contraindicated, some form of pharmacologic anticoagulation is typically given for deep venous thrombosis prophylaxis. Prophylaxis can be augmented with compression stockings, mechanical compression devices for the lower extremities, and early mobilization.

V. In the typical patient with osteoarthritis, physical therapy is started on postoperative day 1 and is dictated in part by the amount of tension-free external rotation that was obtained following subscapularis repair in the operating room (see previous discussion).

A. The first 6 weeks of therapy consist of daily exercises for hand, wrist, and elbow ROM.

B. Shoulder exercises during this time include pendulums, passive supine forward flexion without limitation, and passive supine external rotation limited to the tension-free amount observed in the operating room (typically about 30 degrees).

VI. The arm is maintained in a sling at all times during the first 2 weeks after surgery, except during physical therapy exercises and personal hygiene. After 2 weeks, the sling can be removed at home, and unweighted ADLs can be performed with the arm at the side.

VII. Three weeks postoperatively, cross-body adduction stretches are added to stretch the posterior capsule, as well as light isometric external rotation strengthening. A 1-pound weight limit is given for ADLs.

VIII. Six weeks postoperatively, internal rotation strengthening is started, external rotation strengthening is advanced, and limits on passive external rotation are eliminated.

> How long does your attending use antibiotics in the postoperative period?

> What does your attending use for deep venous thrombosis prophylaxis in the postoperative period?

IX. Deltoid strengthening begins approximately 3 months after surgery, when the rotator cuff shows adequate strength.

X. Return to sports activities such as golf is permitted at 4 months, but heavy weight lifting activities and vigorous sports should be avoided.

XI. Maximal recovery takes approximately 1 year.

XII. Plain radiographs are taken at yearly intervals to assess for component position and loosening.

COMPLICATIONS

I. Stiffness
II. Instability or dislocation
III. Subscapularis detachment or rupture
IV. Nerve injury (axillary, musculocutaneous, brachial plexus)
V. Glenoid loosening
VI. Periprosthetic fracture (humeral shaft most commonly)
VII. Infection
VIII. Rotator cuff tear

POSTOPERATIVE PHYSICAL THERAPY AND REHABILITATION PROTOCOLS CAN VARY DEPENDING ON THE BONE AND SOFT TISSUE QUALITY AT THE TIME OF SURGERY. RHEUMATOID PATIENTS TYPICALLY HAVE POORER QUALITY BONE AND SOFT TISSUES AND REQUIRE A SLOWER PROGRESSION IN THERAPY AND MORE MOTION RESTRICTION EARLY ON TO ALLOW FOR ADEQUATE HEALING.

SUGGESTED READINGS

Abboud JA, Getz CL, Williams GR: Shoulder arthroplasty. In Garino JP, Beredjiklian PK (eds): Core Knowledge in Orthopaedics: Adult Reconstruction and Arthroplasty. Philadelphia, Elsevier, 2007.

Craig EV: Master Techniques in Orthopaedic Surgery: The Shoulder, 2nd ed. Philadelphia, Lippincott Williams & Wilkins, 2003.

Iannotti JP, Williams GR: Disorders of the Shoulder: Diagnosis and Management, 2nd ed. Philadelphia, Lippincott Williams & Wilkins, 2007.

Norris TR: Orthopaedic Knowledge Update: Shoulder and Elbow 2. Rosemont, IL, American Academy of Orthopaedic Surgeons, 2002.

CHAPTER 7

Cubital Tunnel Release and Ulnar Nerve Transposition

Julia A. Kenniston and David R. Steinberg

Case Study

A 48-year-old, right hand–dominant male, a concert violinist, presents to the clinic complaining of intermittent paresthesias in his right hand affecting his ring and small fingers along with pain at his medial elbow and medial forearm of 6 months' duration. These symptoms affect him mostly after playing his violin and occasionally when he wakes up in the morning. He also reports "clumsiness" in his fingers, which he has never experienced before. He denies trauma to his right arm and any medical problems, including diabetes, hypothyroidism, or history of cancer. He claims to be healthy and exercises regularly and denies smoking or use of alcohol. He is concerned that this problem will affect his career.

BACKGROUND

Carpal tunnel syndrome is seen in 40% of patients with cubital tunnel syndrome.

I. Cubital tunnel syndrome is a phrase used to describe symptoms related to the compression or traction of the ulnar nerve around the elbow. It is the second most common compressive neuropathy in the upper extremity, after carpal tunnel syndrome.

II. Although the cubital tunnel is limited to the elbow, any ulnar neuropathy in the mid-arm to mid-forearm (10 cm proximal and 5 cm distal to elbow joint) is included in the phrase "cubital tunnel syndrome."

III. The cubital tunnel is an anatomic passageway through which the ulnar nerve travels around the elbow with the following anatomic borders:
   A. Anterior: medial epicondyle
   B. Posterior: olecranon
   C. Floor: medial collateral ligament
   D. Roof: arcuate ligament (also known as *cubital tunnel retinaculum* or *triangular ligament*)

IV. **Ulnar Nerve Anatomy** (Fig. 7-1)
   A. The ulnar nerve is derived from the medial cord of the brachial plexus and receives contributions from C8, T1, and occasionally C7.

As it courses down the forearm, the ulnar nerve lies between the flexor carpi ulnaris and the flexor digitorum profundus.

   B. The nerve travels along the anterior arm, traverses the medial intermuscular septum at the arcade of Struthers adjacent to the medial head of the triceps muscle and continues in the posterior compartment. At the elbow, the nerve enters the cubital tunnel and passes between the two heads of the flexor carpi ulnaris (FCU) and exits under the deep flexor pronator aponeurosis to lie deep to the flexor digitorum superficialis (FDS), FCU, and superficial to the flexor digitorum profundus (FDP).
   C. At the medial epicondyle, the sensory fibers to the hand and the motor fibers to the intrinsics are superficial, whereas the motor fibers to the FCU and FDP are deep. This may explain why the FCU and FDP are relatively protected in cubital tunnel syndrome.

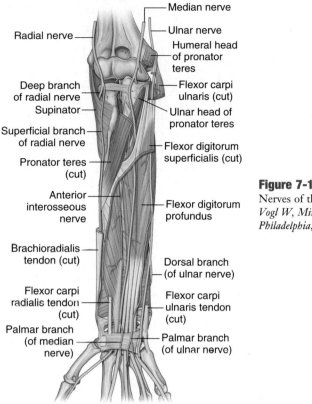

Radial nerve

Deep branch
of radial nerve

Supinator

Superficial branch
of radial nerve

Pronator teres
(cut)

Anterior
interosseous
nerve

Brachioradialis
tendon (cut)

Flexor carpi
radialis tendon
(cut)

Palmar branch
(of median
nerve)

Median nerve

Ulnar nerve

Humeral head
of pronator
teres

Flexor carpi
ulnaris (cut)

Ulnar head of
pronator teres

Flexor digitorum
superficialis (cut)

Flexor digitorum
profundus

Dorsal branch
(of ulnar nerve)

Flexor carpi
ulnaris tendon
(cut)

Palmar branch
(of ulnar nerve)

Figure 7-1

Nerves of the anterior forearm. *(From Drake RL, Vogl W, Mitchell AWM: Gray's Anatomy for Students. Philadelphia, Churchill Livingstone, 2005.)*

D. Anatomic variations exist with regard to ulnar nerve innervation, including sensory branches and the number of muscle motor branches.
   1. Sensory
      a. The dorsal sensory branch emerges approximately 5 cm proximal to the pisiform and supplies the dorsal-ulnar hand and dorsal aspect of the ulnar one and one half digits. This differentiates cubital tunnel syndrome from ulnar tunnel/Guyon's canal nerve compression.
      b. The palmar cutaneous branch of the ulnar nerve is located proximal to Guyon's canal and supplies sensation to the ulnar palm and palmar aspect of the ulnar one and one half digits. This nerve is at risk for injury in a carpal tunnel release.
      c. The palmar branches from the superficial ulnar nerve may also supply sensation to the ulnar palm and palmar aspect of the ulnar one and one half digits.
   2. Motor (the following muscles require motor innervation from the ulnar nerve)
      a. FCU
      b. FDP; digits four and five
      c. Palmaris brevis
      d. Adductor pollicis
      e. Deep head of flexor pollicis brevis
      f. Abductor digit minimi
      g. Flexor digiti minimi brevis
      h. Opponens digit minimi
      i. Third and fourth lumbricals
      j. Dorsal interossei (four muscles)
      k. Palmar interossei (three muscles)
   E. The blood supply is derived from branches of the brachial artery (superior and inferior ulnar collateral artery) and the posterior recurrent ulnar artery, a branch of the ulnar artery.

The ulnar nerve does not innervate any structure in the upper arm.

Figure 7-2
Potential sites of compression of the ulnar nerve at the elbow. *(From Gelberman RH: Operative Nerve Repair and Reconstruction. Philadelphia, JB Lippincott, 1991. Illustration by Elizabeth Roselius, copyright 1991. Reprinted with permission.)*

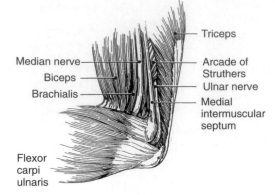

V. **Possible Sites of Compression** (Fig. 7-2)
   A. Area of the intermuscular septum
      1. Arcade of Struthers: musculofascial band 8 to 10 cm proximal to medial epicondyle extending from the medial head of the triceps to the medial intermuscular septum
      2. Medial intermuscular septum: area of the intermuscular septum that becomes thick and flares distally as it inserts onto the medial epicondyle
      3. Medial head of the triceps: may compress the nerve if it becomes hypertrophied (e.g., bodybuilders) or if it snaps over the medial epicondyle, causing friction neuritis
   B. Medial epicondyle. This may cause compression or excessive traction forces on the ulnar nerve by valgus or varus deformity from a previous supracondylar humerus fracture or by osteophytes in an arthritis elbow.
   C. Epicondylar groove
      1. Space-occupying lesion may cause compression with mass effect.
      2. Shallow groove increases risk of nerve subluxation.
      3. External compression may result from leaning on a flexed elbow for a prolonged period of time.
   D. Arcuate ligament: roof of cubital tunnel
   E. Osborne's fascia
      1. Proximal fibrous edge of the FCU
      2. Most common cause of nerve compression
   F. Anconeus epitrochlearis. This accessory muscle arises from the medial olecranon and triceps and inserts into the medial epicondyle. It is found in 10% of patients undergoing cubital tunnel release.
   G. Deep flexor pronator aponeurosis

DIAGNOSIS

I. **Physical Examination**
   A. Check elbow range of motion (ROM) (functional ROM is 30 to 130 degrees) and carrying angle (normal range is 7 to 15 degrees).
   B. Palpate the elbow and cubital tunnel to exclude mass lesions.
   C. Examine the hand for muscle wasting and resting position of digits.
   D. Test muscle function and strength (cross fingers, hand grip, pinch, and Froment sign).
   E. Examine sensation in the hand to differentiate cubital tunnel syndrome from ulnar tunnel syndrome.
   F. Perform threshold testing (Semmes-Weinstein monofilament or vibration testing).
   G. Check innervation density (static and moving two-point discrimination).
   H. Check cervical ROM and associated pain/radiculopathy.

Sidebar notes:

Delayed ulnar neuropathy occurring years after a supracondylar humerus fracture, typically with a progressive valgus deformity, is referred to as *tardy ulnar nerve palsy*.

Osborne's fascia is the most common cause of ulnar nerve compression about the elbow.

Discuss the concept behind threshold and innervation density nerve testing with your physician.

II. **Clinical Findings**
   A. Paresthesia and numbness in the ring and small finger, which may worsen with elbow flexion
   B. Altered threshold testing, which occurs early in disease with changes in monofilament and vibration testing
   C. Decreased two-point sensation, which occurs late in disease and reflects axonal degeneration after chronic nerve compression/traction injury
   D. Tenderness to palpation at the medial elbow
   E. Tinel's sign. Paresthesias in the ulnar nerve distribution with percussion of the nerve at level of the medial epicondyle
   F. Elbow flexion test. Symptoms are reproduced within 3 minutes with elbow in full flexion and wrist in full supination and extension.
   G. Intrinsic muscle weakness and wasting with "clumsy fingers"
      1. Motor symptoms occur after sensory changes and reflect disease progression
      2. Weak grip strength
      3. Wartenberg's sign: inability to adduct the small finger
      4. Froment sign: flexion of thumb interphalangeal joint during attempt to hold paper with thumb and index finger
      5. Inability to cross fingers
      6. Clawing of ring and small finger

III. **Diagnostic Testing**
   A. Electromyography/nerve conduction velocity
      1. Distal latencies
         a. Sensory latencies greater than 3.2 msec
         b. Motor latencies greater than 4.2 msec
         c. Often normal at wrist with cubital tunnel syndrome
      2. Nerve conduction velocity less than 50 m/sec
      3. Abnormal electromyography results: associated with poor surgical outcomes
   B. Imaging studies
      1. Plain radiographs: may reveal osteophytes or other osseous causes of compression
      2. Magnetic resonance imaging: may reveal space-occupying lesions or edema within the nerve or enlargement of the nerve
      3. High-resolution ultrasound: may be useful to evaluate morphologic changes within the ulnar nerve secondary to compression or traction

IV. **Differential Diagnosis**
   A. Cervical disk disease/radiculopathy
   B. Thoracic outlet syndrome
   C. Spinal tumor
   D. Syringomyelia
   E. Amyotrophic lateral sclerosis
   F. Guillain-Barré syndrome
   G. Ulnar tunnel syndrome (Guyon's canal): dorsal hand sensation remaining intact
   H. Systemic causes: diabetes, hypothyroidism, alcoholism, malnutrition, cancer

V. **Treatment Considerations**
   A. Other causes of symptoms: rule out
   B. Concomitant carpal tunnel syndrome: necessary to consider simultaneous release
   C. Patient compliance
   D. Worker's compensation
   E. Occupation
   F. Prognosis
      1. Age
      2. Comorbidities
      3. Duration of nerve compression
      4. Severity of symptoms

With elbow flexion, the volume of the cubital tunnel decreases by 55%, the pressure increases sevenfold, the nerve is placed on traction, and it elongates approximately 5 to 8 mm. These factors exacerbate cubital tunnel symptoms with elbow flexion.

Poor prognosis correlates most closely with intrinsic atrophy.

A Martin-Gruber anastomosis may mask muscular symptoms as motor fibers from the median nerve communicate with the ulnar nerve.

Does your attending require an electromyogram prior to surgery?

5. Worse prognosis with impaired two-point discrimination, severe weakness, and muscle atrophy

TREATMENT ALGORITHM

When does your attending decide to operate?

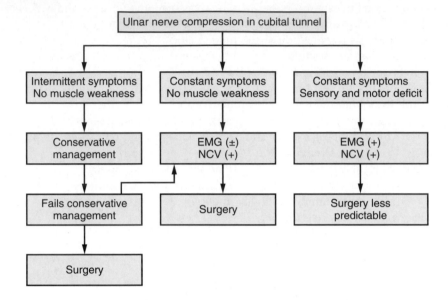

TREATMENT PROTOCOLS

I. **Nonoperative**
   A. Splint elbow in 70 degrees of flexion
   B. Soft elbow padding
   C. Activity modification: avoid repetitive elbow flexion/pronation, direct compression
   D. Nonsteroidal anti-inflammatory drugs

II. **Operative**
   A. In situ decompression: unroof cubital tunnel and release compression sites
      1. Indications
         a. Mild ulnar nerve compression with mild symptoms
         b. Mild slowing on nerve conduction velocity study
         c. No tenderness directly over the bony medial epicondyle
         d. No subluxation of nerve
         e. Normal bony anatomy
      2. Advantages
         a. Minimal damage to vascular supply of the ulnar nerve
         b. No damage to ulnar nerve and branches
         c. No postoperative immobilization required
      3. Disadvantages
         a. Potentially higher recurrence rate
         b. Risk of nerve subluxation
      4. Contraindications
         a. Severe cases of compressive neuropathy (e.g., post-traumatic compression secondary to perineural scarring)
         b. Space-occupying lesion
         c. Chronic subluxation of nerve
   B. Anterior transposition of ulnar nerve
      1. Indications
         a. Unsuitable bed for ulnar nerve
         b. Space occupying mass
         c. Anconeus epitrochlearis

       d. Heterotopic ossification

       e. Significant tension on ulnar nerve with elbow flexion

       f. Exacerbation of symptoms or subluxation of the nerve with elbow flexion

       g. Elbow deformity secondary to valgus elbow or post-traumatic etiology

       h. Valgus instability at elbow

   2. Advantages. This procedure transfers the ulnar nerve to a region of less scar and eliminates tension on the ulnar nerve when the elbow is in flexion by moving the nerve anteriorly.

   3. Disadvantages. This procedure is more technically demanding and has the potential to devascularize the nerve and damage small nerve branches (e.g., FCU proximal motor branch).

   4. Types of anterior transposition

       a. Subcutaneous: places nerve anterior between subcutaneous tissue and muscle

          (1) Less dissection and technically uncomplicated

          (2) Ulnar nerve may be vulnerable in patients with minimal subcutaneous fat

       b. Intramuscular: nerve buried within the flexor-pronator muscle

          (1) Moderate muscle dissection

          (2) Potential for increased scarring as nerve placed within muscle at right angles to fibers and is subject to traction forces

       c. Submuscular: nerve buried deep to flexor-pronator muscle

          (1) More extensive dissection leads to an increased risk of postoperative scar tissue formation.

          (2) Initially the nerve lies in an unscarred anatomic plane not subject to traction forces compared with the intramuscular transposition.

          (3) Postoperative immobilization may increase the risk of forming flexion contractures at the elbow.

 C. Medial epicondylectomy

   1. Indications

       a. Nonunion of epicondyle fracture with cubital tunnel symptoms

       b. Shallow groove for ulnar nerve

       c. Ulnar nerve subluxation

       d. Concomitant medial epicondylitis

   2. Advantages. This procedure results in a more thorough decompression and causes minimal damage to the vascular supply and small nerve branches off the ulnar nerve.

   3. Disadvantages

       a. Allows greater anterior migration of the ulnar nerve with elbow flexion

       b. Potential for elbow instability if collateral ligaments are damaged

       c. Potential for nerve vulnerability at epicondylectomy site

       d. Increased risk of elbow stiffness/flexion contracture

       e. Fails to release potential sites of compression distally

       f. Technically challenging with regards to an accurate amount of bone to excise

   4. Contraindications

       a. Throwing athletes due to increased stresses on the medial elbow

       b. Patients involved in activities requiring intensive movements of elbow flexion-extension

> How does your attending decide which procedure to perform?

GENERAL PRINCIPLES OF ULNAR NERVE DECOMPRESSION AND SUBCUTANEOUS NERVE TRANSPOSITION

   I. The cubital tunnel is the main restraint for the ulnar nerve as it courses around the elbow joint and has multiple potential sites of nerve compression. Maximum strain occurs when the elbow is held in flexion because the volume of the cubital tunnel decreases by 50%.

II. The initial symptoms consist of sensory change and progress to weakness. If muscle atrophy is present, the result from surgical intervention is less predictable.

III. Cubital tunnel syndrome must be differentiated from C8 radiculopathy or ulnar tunnel syndrome to ensure appropriate treatment.

IV. The goal of surgery is to decrease pain and symptoms associated with ulnar neuropathy and to prevent muscular weakness and progression of the disease.

V. It is important to assess all potential compression sites and to completely release the nerve while preventing the creation of new sites.

VI. In situ decompression preserves vascular supply but may not provide a sufficient release, whereas an anterior transposition more thoroughly decompresses the nerve but increases the risk of compression at a new site and subsequent vascular compromise.

COMPONENTS OF THE PROCEDURE

Positioning, Prepping, and Draping

I. The patient is placed in a supine position on the operating table with a hand table attachment.

II. The arm is prepped and draped in standard fashion with the use of a tourniquet. A sterile tourniquet may be used if an adequately sized sterile field cannot be secured (Fig. 7-3). (Refer to Chapter 1 for surgical principles of prepping and draping.)

III. Using a sterile marker, the surgical incision is marked out after identifying the medial epicondyle and the ulnar nerve (Fig. 7-4).

IV. The operative extremity is exsanguinated with an Esmarch and the tourniquet is inflated to the preset value (Fig. 7-5).

Ulnar Nerve Decompression and Subcutaneous Nerve Transposition

I. Make a skin incision midway between the medial epicondyle and the olecranon starting 8 to 10 cm proximal to and 5 to 7 cm distal to the medial epicondyle. The incision is slightly posterior to the ulnar nerve.

II. If possible, identify and protect the posterior branch(es) of the medial antebrachial cutaneous nerve.

> The surgical dissection is carried out 8 to 10 cm proximal to the medial epicondyle to identify the arcade of Struthers. If it is not located within 10 cm, it is unlikely to be the cause of compression and does not need to be released.

> THE MEDIAL ANTEBRACHIAL CUTANEOUS NERVE MAY CROSS THE ELBOW ANYWHERE FROM 6 CM PROXIMAL TO 6 CM DISTAL TO MEDIAL EPICONDYLE. THIS NERVE INNERVATES THE SKIN OVER THE MEDIAL EPICONDYLE AND OLECRANON. DAMAGE TO THIS NERVE MAY CAUSE SCAR TENDERNESS AND NUMBNESS AS WELL AS A PAINFUL NEUROMA.

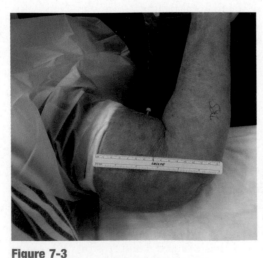

Figure 7-3
Right arm with tourniquet and 1010 drape over a hand table.

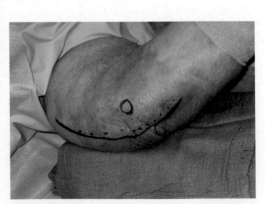

Figure 7-4
Incision marked out with a straight line, the ulnar nerve indicated by a dotted line, and the medial epicondyle indicated by a circle.

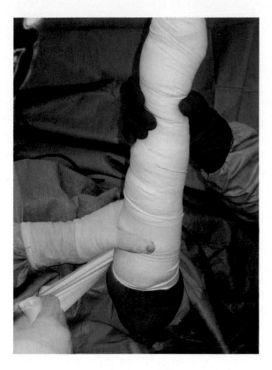

Figure 7-5
Esmarch bandage exsanguination of the limb.

III. Mobilize thick skin flaps to expose the medial intermuscular septum and fascia over the flexor-pronator muscle origin using tenotomy scissors. Next, identify the ulnar nerve.

IV. Incise the fascia immediately posterior to the medial intermuscular septum along the course of the ulnar nerve.

V. Identify Osborne's fascia and divide the fibroaponeurotic covering of the epicondylar groove (Fig. 7-6).

VI. Mobilize the ulnar nerve and protect the branches to the elbow joint, FCU, and FDP. The motor branch of the FCU should be identified and protected while articular branches to the elbow capsule may be sacrificed.

VII. Protect the ulnar nerve while dividing the aponeurosis between the two heads of the FCU. Bluntly dissect the muscle fibers of the two heads of the FCU to ensure that the nerve is completely unroofed and there are no fibrous bands distally causing compression (Figs. 7-7 and 7-8).

> **IT IS IMPERATIVE TO IDENTIFY AND PROTECT THE MOTOR BRANCH TO THE FLEXOR CARPI ULNARIS, BECAUSE IT MAY BE THE ONLY BRANCH INNERVATING THE FLEXOR CARPI ULNARIS.**

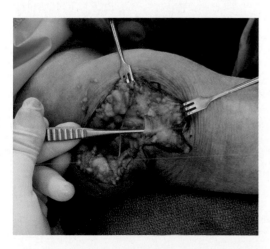

Figure 7-6
Osborne's fascia indicated by forceps.

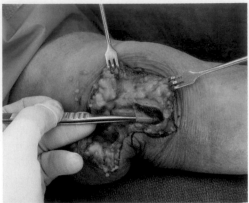

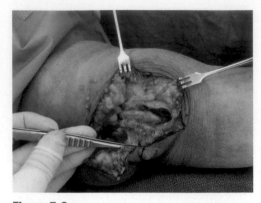

Figure 7-8
Complete in situ release of ulnar nerve.

Figure 7-7
Flexor carpi ulnaris aponeurosis at forceps tips.

VIII. Evaluate the decompression by assessing the nerve in extension and in flexion. If the nerve subluxates in flexion or appears to be stretched tightly over the medial epicondyle, additional surgical procedures should be considered.

IX. Identify the intermuscular septum and mobilize the ulnar nerve proximally; protect the ulnar nerve with a vessel loop.

X. Be sure to identify the leash of vessels at the distal end of the intermuscular septum and cauterize them to prevent excessive bleeding prior to excising a portion of the intermuscular septum and creating a new compression point (Figs. 7-9 and 7-10).

XI. Create a fasciodermal sling from fascia overlying the flexor-pronator muscle. Make sure that the sling is sufficiently large and broad so as to not create a new compression site. Transpose the ulnar nerve anterior to the sling and suture the deep subcutaneous tissue to the fasciodermal sling using absorbable sutures, such as 2-0 Vicryl (Figs. 7-11 and 7-12).

Wound Closure

I. Release the tourniquet and achieve hemostasis with bipolar electrocautery prior to closing the wound.

II. Close the subcutaneous layer in standard fashion (see Chapter 1); close the skin with a subcuticular closure.

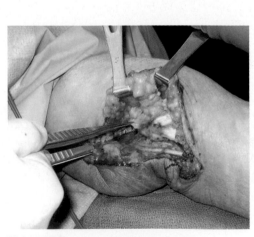

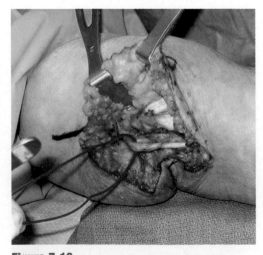

Figure 7-9
Intermuscular septum.

Figure 7-10
Proximal release of ulnar nerve protected with vessel loop.

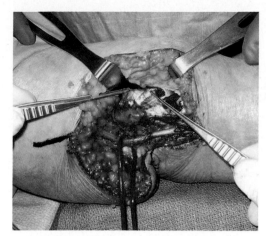

Figure 7-11
Fasciodermal sling.

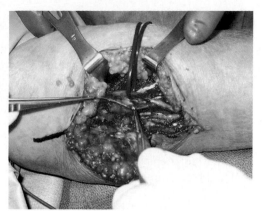

Figure 7-12
Transposition of ulnar nerve anterior to sling.

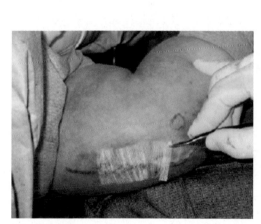

Figure 7-13
Wound closed and Steri-Strips applied.

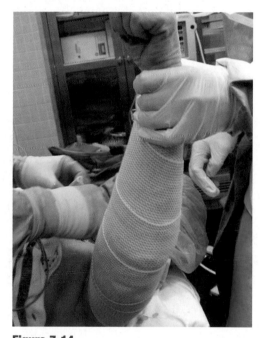

Figure 7-14
Postoperative soft dressing.

   III. Dress the wound in standard fashion, and apply a soft dressing (Figs. 7-13 and 7-14).

   IV. A sling may be used for comfort postoperatively.

POSTOPERATIVE REHABILITATION

     I. **In Situ Decompression/Subcutaneous Transposition/Medial Epicondylectomy**
       A. No immobilization
       B. Early ROM
    II. **Intramuscular Transposition**
       A. Immobilize elbow at 90 degrees flexion with full pronation.
       B. Begin ROM exercises after 1 to 3 weeks of immobilization.
   III. **Submuscular Transposition**
       A. Immobilize elbow at 45 degrees flexion in neutral to slight pronation.
       B. Begin ROM exercises after 1 to 3 weeks of immobilization.

> When does your attending begin to mobilize the elbow? Does he or she like to use a continuous passive motion machine for the elbow?

COMPLICATIONS

    I. Infection
   II. Incomplete release of the ulnar nerve
  III. Creation of a new compression site
  IV. Injury to the posterior branches of medial antebrachial cutaneous nerve
   V. Recurrent ulnar nerve subluxation
  VI. Elbow instability
 VII. Elbow stiffness/flexion contracture
VIII. Medial epicondylitis
  IX. Heterotopic ossification

SUGGESTED READINGS

Bainbridge C: Cubital tunnel syndrome. In Berger RA, Weiss APC (eds): Hand Surgery. Philadelphia, Lippincott Williams & Wilkins, 2004, pp 887–896.

Bozentka DJ: Cubital tunnel syndrome pathophysiology. Clin Orthop 351:90–94, 1998.

Eversmann Jr WW: Medial epicondylectomy for cubital tunnel compression of the ulnar nerve. In Strickland JW (ed): Master Techniques in Orthopaedic Surgery, The Hand. Philadelphia, Lippincott Williams & Wilkins, 1998, pp 293–302.

Posner MA: Compressive ulnar neuropathies at the elbow: I. Etiology and diagnosis. J Am Acad Orthop Surg 6:282–288, 1998.

Posner MA: Compressive ulnar neuropathies at the elbow: II. Treatment. J Am Acad Orthop Surg 6:289–297, 1998.

Szabo RM: Entrapment and compression neuropathies. In Green DP, Hotchkiss R, Pederson W, Wolfe S (eds): Green's Operative Hand Surgery, 4th ed. Philadelphia, Elsevier, 2005, pp 1422–1429.

Terry GC, Zeigler TE: Cubital tunnel syndrome. In Baker CL, Plancher KD (eds): Operative Treatment of Elbow Injuries. New York, Springer, 2002, pp 131–139.

CHAPTER 8

Open Reduction and Internal Fixation of Adult Distal Humerus Fractures

Sameer Nagda and Neil P. Sheth

Case Study

A 53-year-old, right hand–dominant male presents after a fall on a flexed left elbow. He had immediate pain and swelling after the fall, and he complains of numbness in his hand and has difficulty moving his elbow. On physical examination, there are no open wounds but there is significant swelling with a gross deformity of the elbow. Any palpation or motion of his elbow causes severe pain. The forearm and wrist are nontender, and there is no pain with passive stretch of the fingers. The motor examination is intact in the median, ulnar, and radial nerve distribution. Objectively, the sensory examination is intact, and there is a 2+ radial pulse distally. This is an isolated injury with no evidence of tenderness about the proximal humerus and shoulder. Anteroposterior and lateral radiographs of the left elbow are presented in Figure 8-1.

BACKGROUND

 I. Fractures about the elbow include distal humerus, olecranon, coronoid, and radial head fractures. These fractures can be difficult to identify and plain radiographs may often present only subtle findings with significant underlying injuries. This chapter focuses on the diagnosis and treatment of adult distal humerus fractures.
 II. Distal humerus fractures comprise approximately 0.5% of all fractures in adults. Although these fractures are not extremely common, they often present as severe injuries. Patients may be a victim of polytrauma. Thus, evaluation using the Advanced Trauma Life Support (ATLS) protocol is necessary to stabilize the patient and diagnose associated injuries.
 III. There is no universally accepted classification that is widely used for describing distal humerus fractures. The AO and the OTA classifications are the most widely used by trauma surgeons. A type A fracture is extra-articular, a type B fracture partially includes the articular surface, and a type C fracture includes the articular surface with complete dissociation of the articular fragments from the humeral shaft. However, these fractures are better defined with use of a computed tomography (CT) scan.

TREATMENT PROTOCOLS

 I. **Treatment Considerations.** All of these considerations play an important role in the decision-making process of treating patients with a distal humerus fracture.
 A. Patient age (concomitant osteoporosis)
 B. Activity level

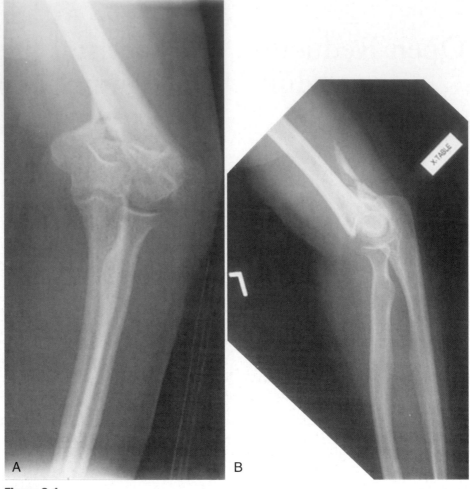

Figure 8-1
Anteroposterior (**A**) and lateral (**B**) views of a closed distal humerus fracture.

C. Arm dominance
D. Intra-articular extension
E. Overall health (able to tolerate surgery)
F. Integrity of the elbow soft tissue envelope
G. Neurovascular status
H. Patient expectations

II. **Initial Evaluation**

A. A thorough history and physical examination are critical to the assessment of elbow fractures. The mechanism of injury can be a fall on an outstretched hand or a fall directly onto the elbow. Typically, an axial load with the arm flexed more than 90 degrees results in a distal humerus fracture.

B. Fractures of the distal humerus that are a result of high-energy trauma require close attention with a high suspicion for possible open injuries. In addition, high-energy fractures result in fracture comminution and intra-articular extension.

C. Patients who sustain this injury due to high-energy trauma require a thorough ATLS evaluation for associated injuries. Assessment of the elbow should document if the fracture is open and the status of the initial neurovascular examina-

The radial nerve courses around the humerus in the radial groove. The nerve pierces the lateral intermuscular septum approximately 13 cm proximal to the level of the joint. Radial nerve injuries are highly associated with Holstein-Lewis type spiral fractures.

tion. With proximal extension of the fracture line, injury to the radial nerve should be suspected.

D. Distal humerus fractures with a spiral component are termed Holstein-Lewis fractures and have a higher rate of associated radial nerve injury.

E. Although compartment syndrome is not commonly associated with these fractures, concomitant neurovascular injury may be present. Early identification of neurovascular injuries results in more emergent operative treatment.

F. Every patient should at minimum have an anteroposterior and lateral radiograph of the involved elbow. Additional oblique radiographs can also help with understanding the fracture pattern. Any fracture that extends into the elbow joint requires a CT scan to help delineate the fracture fragments and develop a more comprehensive preoperative plan.

III. **Nonoperative Treatment Options**

A. Conservative treatment is considered an option when surgical intervention is not possible due to comorbidities.

B. It may be used as a treatment for nondisplaced extra-articular fractures. Nonoperative treatment is contraindicated in cases of neurovascular compromise.

C. Distal humerus fractures can be treated with a long-arm cast with the elbow in no more than 90 degrees of flexion. Flexion of more than 90 degrees can compromise blood vessels and impair distal blood flow and venous return.

D. Radiographs should be obtained after 1 week to demonstrate lack of displacement and confirm adequate position of the distal humerus.

E. The duration of immobilization should be 6 to 8 weeks or until there is radiographic evidence of fracture healing.

F. Patients typically require extensive therapy to regain elbow range of motion (ROM) with loss of terminal extension being the most common residual deficit.

G. Intra-articular fractures are usually not considered for nonoperative treatment due to the increased risk for fracture displacement.

> Does your attending consider any additional patient scenarios as candidates for nonoperative treatment?

SURGICAL ALTERNATIVES TO OPEN REDUCTION AND INTERNAL FIXATION OF DISTAL HUMERUS FRACTURES

I. **Spanning Elbow External Fixator**

A. Used to provide fracture stability for acute high-energy distal humerus fractures

B. Typically used when there is significant soft tissue envelope compromise

C. Treatment of choice for open fractures (grade II and higher)

D. Time to conversion for definitive fracture fixation: should be dictated by the soft tissues

E. Can be left in place for approximately 2 weeks before converting to definitive fixation

II. **Hinged Elbow External Fixator**

A. A treatment modality that provides fracture stability while allowing for elbow ROM

B. Typically used for high-energy distal humerus fractures with soft tissue swelling

C. Can be used as definitive fracture fixation

III. **Total Elbow Arthroplasty**

A. This is considered an option for severely comminuted intra-articular fractures in elderly patients with osteoporotic bone.

B. Elbow replacement has demonstrated good to excellent results with regard to pain relief, elbow ROM, and return of function.

> What surgical alternatives would your attending consider for a given fracture pattern?

TREATMENT ALGORITHM

What is your attending's
treatment algorithm for
distal humerus fractures?

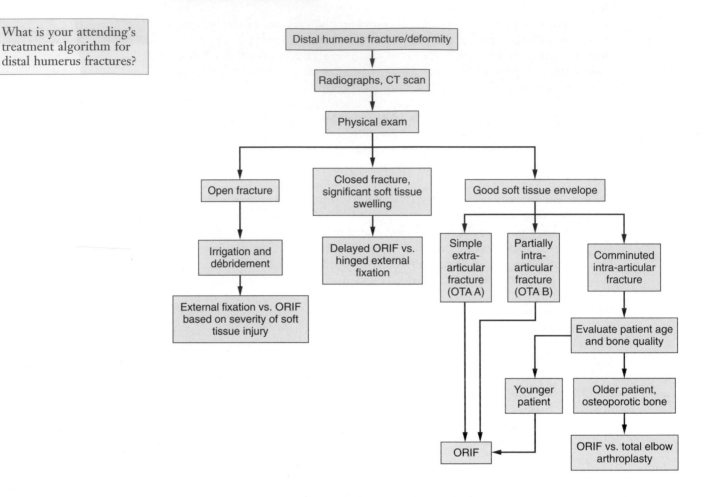

SURGICAL INDICATIONS FOR OPEN REDUCTION AND INTERNAL FIXATION OF DISTAL HUMERUS FRACTURES

    I. Displaced extra-articular distal humerus fractures
   II. Intra-articular humerus fractures
  III. Fractures that have failed nonoperative treatment
  IV. Concomitant neurovascular injury
   V. Distal humerus fractures associated with an elbow dislocation

RELATIVE CONTRAINDICATIONS TO OPEN REDUCTION AND INTERNAL FIXATION OF DISTAL HUMERUS FRACTURES

    I. Current infection (absolute)
   II. Recent infection
  III. Severe soft tissue envelope compromise
  IV. Medically unstable. (Patient is unable to safely tolerate the stress of surgery.)

GENERAL PRINCIPLES OF OPEN REDUCTION AND INTERNAL FIXATION OF DISTAL HUMERUS FRACTURES

    I. The goal of open reduction and internal fixation (ORIF) is to achieve fracture reduction, congruency of the articular surface, and reconstitution of both the medial and lateral humeral columns (Fig. 8-2).

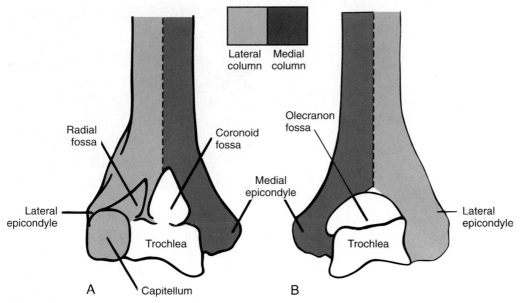

Figure 8-2
Anterior (**A**) and posterior (**B**) views of the medial and lateral columns of the distal third of the humerus. *(From Browner BD, Jupiter JB, Levine AM, Trafton PG [eds]: Skeletal Trauma: Basic Science, Management, and Reconstruction. Philadelphia, Saunders, 2003.)*

II. A construct stable enough to allow early elbow ROM is critical to obtaining a favorable clinical outcome.

III. ORIF achieves rigid internal fixation to avoid shear stress and postoperative fracture displacement.

IV. Distal humerus fractures typically require a preoperative CT scan of the elbow to understand the intra-articular component of the fracture and help with preoperative planning.

V. Preservation of the soft tissue envelope surrounding the elbow is crucial in preventing infection.

VI. The level of swelling and soft tissue injury should be used to determine timing of intervention and conversion to definitive fixation if external fixation is initially chosen for treatment.

VII. Reduction of the medial and lateral condyles should be done first prior to securing them as a single unit to the humeral shaft.

VIII. Distal humerus fracture fixation is typically done using dual plating. The first option utilizes medial and lateral column precontoured plates. The second option includes 90/90 plating where one plate is placed on the medial column and the second plate is placed posteriorly on the lateral column.

COMPONENTS OF THE PROCEDURE

Positioning, Prepping, and Draping

I. Distal humerus fractures can be treated operatively in the prone, supine, or lateral position. In this chapter, we focus on the lateral position with the use of a paint roller.

II. The patient is placed in the lateral position with the unaffected side down. A paint roller is placed at the middle portion of the table on the opposite side of the affected elbow. Place a tourniquet on the arm in standard fashion.

III. The operative elbow is then draped across the body so that the olecranon points toward the ceiling. Standard prepping and draping procedures are followed until a sterile operative field has been attained (See Chapter 1 for surgical principles of

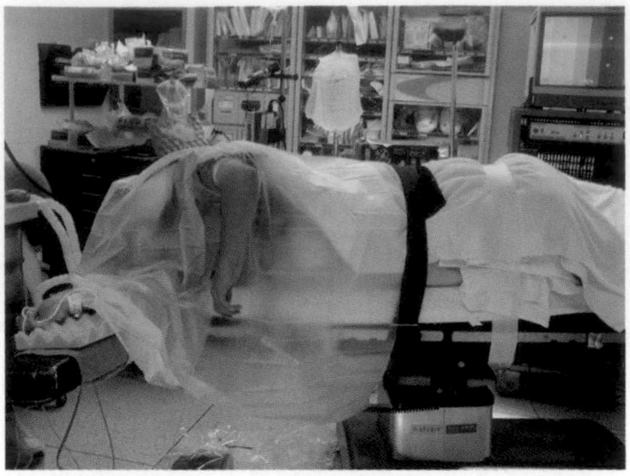

Figure 8-3
Lateral positioning of the elbow using a paint roller. *(From Miller M, Cole B: Textbook of Arthroscopy. Philadelphia, Saunders, 2004.)*

> **THE LATERAL ASPECT OF THE ELBOW IS ALWAYS TOWARD THE HEAD, WHEREAS THE MEDIAL ASPECT OF THE ELBOW IS TOWARD THE FEET WHEN USING THE LATERAL DECUBITUS POSITION.**

prepping and draping.) The incision is marked out using a sterile marker and the tourniquet is inflated prior to starting the procedure (Fig. 8-3).

IV. Prior to making an incision, make sure to be oriented as to what is lateral and medial. Also, make sure that the image intensifier is in the proper location and that adequate radiograph imaging can be obtained.

Surgical Approach

I. A midline incision is made across the dorsal surface extending both proximal and distal to the elbow joint. The incision is slightly curved medial or lateral at the level of the olecranon.

II. Exposure is obtained through the subcutaneous tissues, making sure that thick soft tissue flaps are created.

III. Next, the fascia overlying the triceps tendon is visualized. A longitudinal incision is made in the triceps fascia and it is dissected free from the medial and lateral edges of the tendon.

IV. Next, the ulnar nerve is located on the medial side of the elbow and traced proximally (to the medial intermuscular septum) and distally (to the first motor branch to the flexor carpi ulnaris muscle).

V. Once the nerve is adequately mobilized, a Penrose drain or a rubber vessel loop is placed around the nerve for safe repositioning during the case.

> Does your attending prefer using a different technique to access the elbow joint?

VI. Access to the elbow joint can be gained through several different approaches. In this chapter we discuss the use of a chevron (V-shaped) olecranon osteotomy. The tip of the olecranon is typically predrilled so that the tip can be resecured to the shaft of the ulna prior to wound closure.

VII. After the osteotomy has been completed, the distal humerus as well as the articular surface of the elbow joint can be visualized.

Fracture Reduction

I. Most distal humerus fractures are reduced with provisional fixation using K-wires. The main condylar fragments are secured together so that the entire distal humerus can be re-attached as a unit to the humeral shaft.

II. Once K-wires have allowed for provisional fixation, the fixation construct must be determined. In this chapter, we use the medial and lateral 90/90 plating technique.

III. Regardless of the technique used for fixation, the condylar fragments are secured to the shaft of the humerus using several screws. Interdigitating screws from both medial to lateral and vice versa allow for a more stable fixation construct.

IV. After fracture fixation is adequate via visual inspection, the fracture can be assessed using fluoroscopy. Once sufficient reduction is attained, the elbow can be taken through a ROM to assess fixation stability. This evaluation of intraopera-

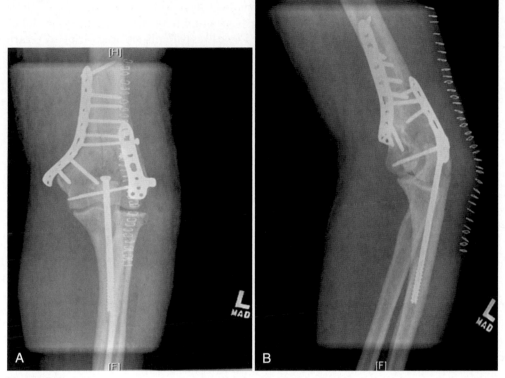

Figure 8-4
Postoperative radiographs demonstrating medial and lateral column fixation with 90/90 plating technique. **A**, Anteroposterior. **B**, Lateral.

    tive stability helps determine the appropriate postoperative rehabilitation protocol.

V. The wound is now irrigated and the olecranon osteotomy is reduced to the ulnar shaft. A 6.3-mm cannulated screw is placed through the predrilled cortex and is used to secure the osteotomy.

VI. In standard fashion, a large-caliber, braided, absorbable suture is used to reapproximate the edges of the triceps fascia over the triceps tendon and the medial and lateral distal humeral plates.

VII. Prior to wound closure, the ulnar nerve is routinely transposed anteriorly at the time of distal humerus fracture fixation. (Refer to Chapter 7 for ulnar nerve transposition technique.)

Wound Closure

I. The wound is closed in layers in standard fashion and the wound is dressed accordingly (see Chapter 1 for wound closure principles).

II. A posterior splint is typically placed for comfort and temporary immobilization of the elbow postoperatively (Fig. 8-4).

POSTOPERATIVE REHABILITATION

I. Most attending physicians place patients in a splint for a short period of time after surgery, typically 10 to 14 days. Caution should be exercised with the length of postoperative immobilization. Elbow stiffness can result fairly quickly with prolonged immobilization. In general, immobilization should not exceed 3 weeks.

II. The staples are removed 14 days postoperatively. The wound should be assessed for any persistent drainage.

III. Once the patient exhibits pain-free ROM, therapy should be focused on regaining full ROM. At a minimum, the functional ROM should be the goal.

IV. In general, patients are made weight bearing as tolerated once there is radiographic evidence of fracture healing. Typically, patients are asked not to return to sporting activities until 6 months postoperatively.

COMPLICATIONS

   I. Wound infection
  II. Septic elbow
 III. Failure of fixation (early or late)
 IV. Ulnar nerve injury (neurapraxia or more severe injury)
  V. Osteotomy nonunion
 VI. Forearm compartment syndrome (rare)

SUGGESTED READINGS

Anglen J: Distal humerus fractures. J Am Acad Orthop Surg 13(5):291–297, 2005.

Cobb TK, Morrey BF: Total elbow arthroplasty as primary treatment for distal humerus fractures in elderly patients. J Bone Joint Surg Am 79:826–832, 1997.

O'Driscoll SW, Jupiter JB, Cohen MS, et al: Difficult elbow fractures: Pearls and pitfalls. Instr Course Lect 52:113–134, 2003.

SECTION II

HAND

CHAPTER 9

Trigger Finger and Trigger Thumb Release

Jonas L. Matzon   and   David R. Steinberg

Case Study

A 55-year-old female with a history of diabetes mellitus presents with left long finger pain. The pain is located in the palm and has been present for several months. She cannot recall any trauma or inciting event. Occasionally, as she flexes or extends the finger, it catches or pops. Her symptoms are worse in the morning when she awakens, and occasionally the long finger is stuck in a flexed position. She finally decided to come to the hand surgeon's office today because the finger has started to lock in flexion (Fig. 9-1). With gentle manipulation, she can massage the finger back into an extended position.

BACKGROUND

I. Trigger finger, or stenosing flexor tenosynovitis, is a very common problem that is characterized by the inability to flex or extend the digit. It can occur in any digit but is most commonly seen in the thumb, followed by the ring, long, small, and index fingers.

II. Primary stenosing flexor tenosynovitis is idiopathic, affects women approximately four times more than men, and is seen in infants. The peak incidence is between 55 and 60 years of age, and involvement of several fingers is not unusual. The lifetime incidence of primary flexor tenosynovitis in adults older than 30 years of age is about 2.2%.

III. Secondary stenosing flexor tenosynovitis occurs in patients with rheumatoid arthritis, diabetes mellitus, hypothyroidism, renal disease, gout, and other connective tissue diseases.

IV. Normally, the flexor tendons (flexor digitorum profundus, flexor digitorum superficialis, flexor pollicis longus) glide through the fibro-osseous flexor pulley system without difficulty in both finger flexion and extension (Fig. 9-2).

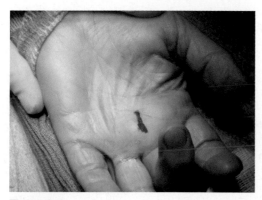

Figure 9-1
Left long finger in trigger position.

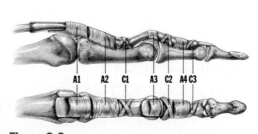

Figure 9-2
Lateral and volar views of the fibro-osseous pulley system. *(From Wolfe SW: Tenosynovitis. In Green DP, Hotchkiss RN, Pederson WC, Wolfe SW [eds]: Green's Operative Hand Surgery, 5th ed. Philadelphia, Churchill Livingstone, 2005.)*

> The A2 and A4 pulleys are vital in preventing tendon bowstringing.

> The A1 pulley is involved in stenosing flexor tenosynovitis.

    A. The pulleys are fascial condensations that overlie the flexor tendon and sheath.

    B. Each digit has five annular and three cruciate pulleys. The thumb has two annular pulleys and one oblique pulley, which is in continuity with the adductor pollicis insertion.

V. However, in trigger finger digits, there is a discrepancy in size between the flexor tendon and the tendon sheath, which leads to mechanical impingement. This is exaggerated during power grip or any finger flexion, when high angular loads occur at the distal edge of the A1 pulley.

VI. There are two types of trigger finger—nodular and diffuse.

    A. Nodular tenosynovitis is caused by thickening of the tendon on the distal edge of the A1 pulley and has a distinct nodule. It responds better to injections and nonsteroidal anti-inflammatory drugs (NSAIDs).

    B. Diffuse tenosynovitis is caused by diffuse thickening of the flexor tenosynovium, and the pathology is not contained to one specific location.

VII. Trigger digits can usually be diagnosed by history and physical examination alone. Patients may complain of stiffness of the fingers, often in the morning on awakening. When triggering or pain is present, patients may localize it to the proximal interphalangeal joint, even though the actual pathology occurs more proximally. On examination, tenderness is usually localized to the palmar base of the involved digit. Depending on the severity of the condition, crepitus, catching, or locking can be felt.

    A. It is important to differentiate between nodular and diffuse stenosing tenosynovitis.

    B. The differential diagnosis includes locking due to impingement of the collateral ligaments on a prominent metacarpal head condyle, flexor digitorum profundus avulsion/rupture, metacarpophalangeal dislocation, and extensor tendon rupture.

VIII. Although triggering has been classified into various systems, no one uniform classification system dictates treatment. The following classification is preferred by Green.

    A. Grade I (pretriggering): pain, history of catching that is not demonstrable, and tenderness over A1 pulley

    B. Grade II (active): demonstrable catching but active extension

    C. Grade III (passive): demonstrable catching requiring passive extension (IIIA) or inability to actively flex (IIIB)

    D. Grade IV (contracture): demonstrable catching with fixed flexion contracture at the proximal interphalangeal joint

IX. **Congenital Trigger Thumb**

    A. Pathology usually involves a thickened tendon as opposed to the annular sheath in adults. Notta's node is the pathologic nodular tendon thickening found at surgery.

    B. Bilateral incidence is 25% to 33%.

    C. If it does not respond to nonsurgical modalities, surgical release is required.

TREATMENT PROTOCOLS

I. **Nonoperative Treatment**

    A. Most primary trigger digits in adults can be treated successfully by nonoperative methods, but this is contraindicated in infants and children.

    B. In mild cases, activity modification and splinting in extension during sleep may be successful.

    C. NSAIDs should be included in the initial treatment of all trigger digits unless contraindicated secondary to patient comorbidities.

D. Splinting
  1. Various splinting techniques have been used. Some hand surgeons advocate immobilizing the metacarpophalangeal joint in 0 to 15 degrees of flexion while allowing free motion at both the proximal and distal interphalangeal joints. Others prefer simple distal interphalangeal immobilization.
  2. Splinting is effective in approximately 55% to 66% of patients but is contraindicated for locked digits.

E. Corticosteroid injection
  1. An injection is indicated in early (usually <4 to 6 months) primary flexor tenosynovitis of a single digit.
  2. Injections are less successful in secondary, diffuse, and chronic flexor tenosynovitis.
  3. A single corticosteroid injection is effective in relieving symptoms in 47% to 87% of patients. If symptoms persist after a single injection, then surgical release is indicated. Some attending hand surgeons perform two or three injections prior to surgical intervention.
  4. Recurrence of triggering following injection is approximately 27% in just 1 year. If symptoms were relieved after injection but then recurred, another injection can be attempted. However, no more than three injections should be given per year.
  5. The injection technique varies per attending surgeon. In general, a 1:1 combination of lidocaine and corticosteroid is injected into the tendon sheath with a 27-gauge needle under sterile conditions (Fig. 9-3).
  6. Many types of corticosteroids exist, but betamethasone is usually preferred because it is water soluble and therefore does not precipitate. It also results in less fat necrosis. Risks of any corticosteroid include transient rises in blood and urine glucose, skin depigmentation, and flare reaction.

II. **Operative Treatment**
  A. Surgical release has a success rate of greater than 90%.
  B. Indications include failed nonoperative treatment, a locked digit, and congenital trigger digits.
  C. Options: open and percutaneous release
    1. Open surgical release of the A1 pulley is the gold standard.
    2. Recently, percutaneous release has gained some popularity, but its use still remains controversial.
      a. This method can be performed in the office, decreasing costs and recovery time.
      b. There is an increased incidence of complications and inadequate release of the A1 pulley.

> How does your attending like to splint trigger digits?

> How many injections does your attending perform prior to progressing to surgical management?

> What type of corticosteroid does your attending prefer for injecting the tendon sheath?

> What are your attending's thoughts regarding the role of percutaneous release?

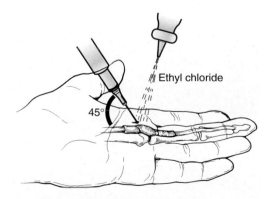
Ethyl chloride

45°

Figure 9-3
Technique for trigger finger injection. *(From Wolfe SW: Tenosynovitis. In Green DP, Hotchkiss RN, Pederson WC, Wolfe SW [eds]: Green's Operative Hand Surgery, 5th ed. Philadelphia, Churchill Livingstone, 2005.)*

TREATMENT ALGORITHM

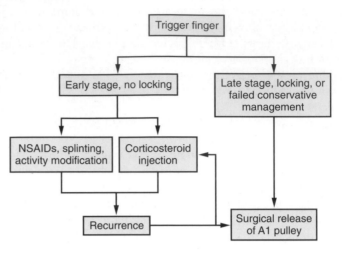

GENERAL PRINCIPLES OF TRIGGER FINGER RELEASE

I. The goal of trigger release is to release the A1 pulley to allow the flexor tendons to glide smoothly.
II. Adequate decompression should prevent recurrence of the trigger finger.

COMPONENTS OF THE PROCEDURE

Positioning, Prepping, and Draping

I. The patient is placed in a supine position with the operative arm placed on a hand table.
II. The hand is prepped and draped in standard fashion (see Chapter 1). Once adequately prepped and draped, a marking pen is used to mark the incision.
    A. Either transverse or longitudinal incisions can be used depending on the surgeon's preference. Typically, however, longitudinal incisions are used for the fingers, while a transverse incision is used for the thumb.
    B. The proximal edge of the A1 pulley almost always coincides with the distal palmar crease in the small and ring rays. The proximal palmar crease indicates the proximal edge of the index ray, while a point half way between the two creases is indicative for the middle ray. For the thumb, the proximal edge of the A1 pulley is directly deep to the metacarpophalangeal joint flexion crease (Figs. 9-4 and 9-5).
III. The arm is exsanguinated (Fig. 9-6), and the tourniquet inflated in standard fashion (see Chapter 1) prior to starting the case.

Figure 9-4
Incisions marked out for left trigger thumb and ring trigger finger release.

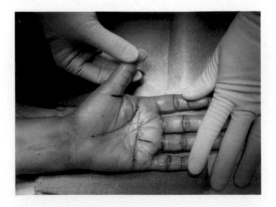

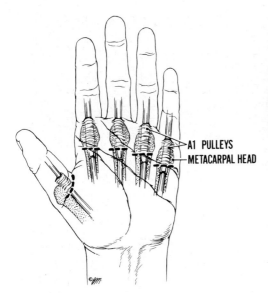

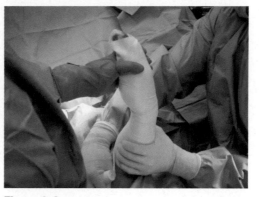

Figure 9-6
Esmarch exsanguination.

Figure 9-5
Incisions with respect to palmar creases. *(From Wolfe SW: Tenosynovitis. In Green DP, Hotchkiss RN, Pederson WC, Wolfe SW [eds]: Green's Operative Hand Surgery, 5th ed. Philadelphia, Churchill Livingstone, 2005.)*

Surgical Release of the A1 Pulley

I. Anesthetize the skin overlying the incision using lidocaine (local injection).

II. Make the skin incision using a 15-blade scalpel.

   A. Care must be taken to avoid crossing any flexor crease with the incision because this can cause contractures on wound healing.

   B. The incision must remain superficial. A deep incision risks injury to the digital neurovascular bundle.

III. After the skin has been incised, use blunt tenotomy scissors to spread longitudinally directly onto the flexor tendon to expose the flexor sheath. Carefully retract the digital neurovascular bundles using small right angle retractors. The proximal and distal edge of the A1 pulley should be directly visualized. If the edges cannot be seen, further blunt dissection is required.

IV. Next, incise the A1 pulley directly over the flexor tendon using a 15-blade. Frequently, there is apparent anatomic continuity between the A1 and A2 pulley, so care must be taken to avoid incising the A2 pulley, which is vital in preventing bowstringing. Often, the palmar aponeurosis pulley (a few millimeters proximal to the A1 pulley) must also be released.

V. Passively flex the digit or have the patient do it actively to confirm that the sheath has been adequately released and that there is no further triggering (Fig. 9-7).

VI. Deflate the tourniquet and achieve meticulous hemostasis by electrocautery.

VII. Close the incision with 5-0 nylon suture using simple or horizontal mattress knots.

WOUND DRESSING AND POSTOPERATIVE CARE

I. The wound is dressed in standard fashion with a soft dressing.

II. The digits are left free, and early finger motion should be encouraged.

III. Sutures are usually removed 7 to 10 days postoperatively.

> **FOR A TRIGGER THUMB RELEASE, THE SUPERFICIAL COURSE OF THE RADIAL DIGITAL NERVE ACROSS THE SURGICAL FIELD MAKES IT EXTREMELY VULNERABLE TO INJURY.**

> Ask your attending to discuss the concept of tendon bowstringing and the role of the A2 and A4 pulleys in preventing this phenomenon.

> Studies have show that as much as 25% of the A2 pulley can be divided without detrimental effect.

Hand

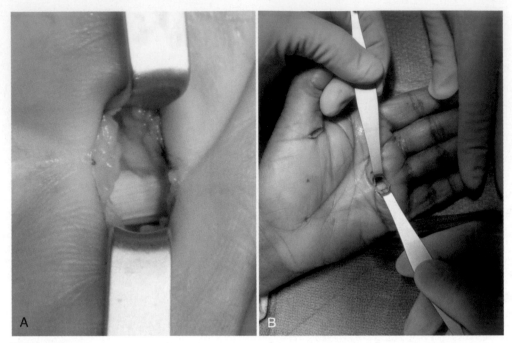

Figure 9-7
Close-up (**A**) and full hand (**B**) views of flexor tendon after A1 pulley release.

COMPLICATIONS

I. The overall incidence of complications is low.

II. The most common complications are digital nerve transection, A2 pulley injury with potential bowstringing, recurrence, painful scars, and reflex sympathetic dystrophy.

SUGGESTED READINGS

Patel MR, Bassini L: Trigger fingers and thumb: When to splint, inject, or operate. J Hand Surg [Am] 17:110–113, 1992.

Saldana MJ: Trigger digits: Diagnosis and treatment. J Am Acad Orthop Surg 9:246–252, 2001.

Tan V, Daluiski A: Tendon. In Beredjiklian PK, Bozentka DJ (eds): Review of Hand Surgery. Philadelphia, Saunders, 2004.

Wolfe SW: Tenosynovitis. In Green DP, Hotchkiss RN, Pederson WC, Wolfe SW (eds): Green's Operative Hand Surgery, 5th ed. Philadelphia, Churchill Livingstone, 2005.

Carpal Tunnel Release

Jonas L. Matzon and David J. Bozentka

C ase Study

A 49-year-old female secretary presents to a hand surgeon complaining of numbness in her right thumb, index, and long fingers, which she has had for several months. She had similar symptoms when she was pregnant approximately 15 years ago, but they resolved following the delivery of her child. The symptoms are worse at night and when she is performing repetitive activities, such as typing. Recently, she has become more concerned regarding her condition because the symptoms have become constant. She also feels more clumsy than usual and has been dropping objects with her right hand (Fig. 10-1).

BACKGROUND

 I. Carpal tunnel syndrome (CTS), or median nerve compression at the wrist, is the most common compression neuropathy.

 II. The carpal canal is defined by the hamate and triquetrum ulnarly, the scaphoid and trapezium radially, and the transverse carpal ligament volarly. The canal contains the median nerve along with nine tendons (four tendons of the flexor digitorum superficialis, four tendons of the flexor digitorum profundus, and one tendon of the flexor pollicis longus). The flexor carpi radialis tendon does not lie within the carpal canal (Fig. 10-2).

 III. The median nerve lies just deep to the transverse carpal ligament. Most commonly, the median nerve gives off the motor recurrent branch radially and beyond the distal edge of the flexor retinaculum, but many variations exist (Fig. 10-3).

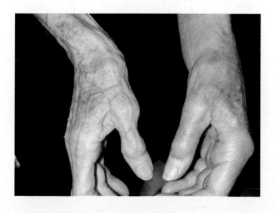

Figure 10-1
Right hand thenar atrophy.

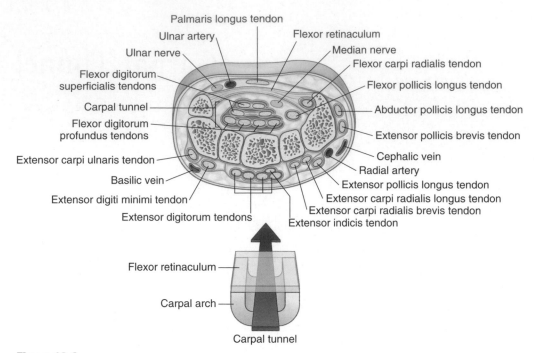

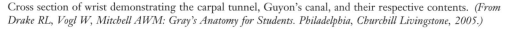

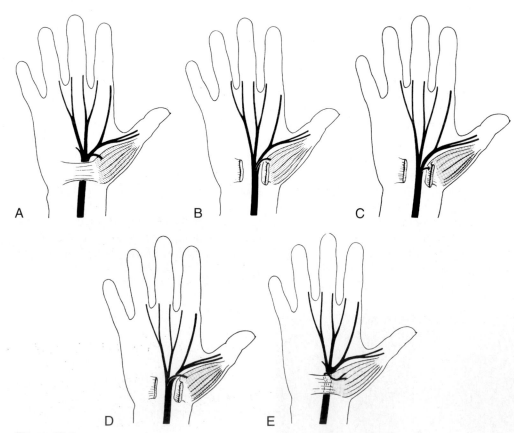

Figure 10-2

Cross section of wrist demonstrating the carpal tunnel, Guyon's canal, and their respective contents. *(From Drake RL, Vogl W, Mitchell AWM: Gray's Anatomy for Students. Philadelphia, Churchill Livingstone, 2005.)*

Figure 10-3

Median nerve variations in the carpal tunnel. **A,** Extraligamentous; **B,** subligamentous; **C,** transligamentous; **D,** ulnar take-off of motor branch; **E,** motor branch lying on top of transverse carpal ligament. *(From Mackinnon SE, Novak CB: Compression neuropathies. In Green DP, Hotchkiss RN, Pederson WC, Wolfe SW [eds]: Green's Operative Hand Surgery, 5th ed. Philadelphia, Churchill Livingstone, 2005.)*

IV. Multiple causes of CTS exist.
   A. Anatomic abnormalities (aberrant muscles, masses)
   B. Inflammatory disorders (gout, rheumatoid arthritis, infection)
   C. Metabolic disease (diabetes mellitus, hypothyroidism)
   D. Fluid imbalances (hemodialysis, pregnancy)
   E. Trauma (hematomas, distal radius fractures, lunate dislocations)
   F. Positional factors (extreme flexion and extension decrease the carpal canal size)
 V. The diagnosis is typically made based on the patient history and physical examination.
VI. Classically, carpal tunnel syndrome presents gradually with pain and paresthesias of the palmar aspect of the radial $3\frac{1}{2}$ digits of the hand.
   A. Symptoms are commonly exacerbated by prolonged or repetitive activities involving the wrist and hand, such as driving or typing.
   B. Pain and numbness are often worse at night.
   C. Chronic or severe compression can result in decreased thumb abduction strength from thenar muscle atrophy and weakness.
   D. Patients may complain of clumsiness and/or weakness, which is usually secondary to decreased sensation but can be related to decreased strength.
VII. **Physical Examination**
   A. Sensory function
      1. Abnormal two-point discrimination is greater than 7 mm.
      2. Semmes-Weinstein monofilament and vibration tests are the most sensitive.
   B. Motor function
      1. Assess for thenar atrophy.
      2. Test abductor pollicis brevis strength.
   C. Provocative maneuvers, which rely on reproduction of symptoms in the median distribution
      1. Tinel's sign: percussion over the median nerve at the wrist
         a. Sensitivity: 60%
         b. Specificity: 67%
      2. Phalen's maneuver: wrist flexion held for 60 seconds
         a. Sensitivity: 75%
         b. Specificity: 47%
      3. Carpal canal compression test: direct compression over the volar aspect of the forearm at the level of the wrist crease for 60 seconds
         a. Sensitivity: 87%
         b. Specificity: 90%
VIII. The diagnosis as well as severity of CTS can be confirmed by electromyogram/ nerve conduction velocity (EMG/NCV).
   A. Distal motor latency greater than 4.0 msec or asymmetry of greater than 1.0 msec between hands
   B. Distal sensory latency greater than 3.5 msec or asymmetry of 0.5 msec between hands
   C. In severe CTS, fibrillation potentials and positive sharp waves in the thenar muscles
IX. **Differential Diagnosis**
   A. Cervical spine radiculopathy
   B. Diffuse peripheral neuropathy
   C. Proximal median nerve neuropathy
   D. Ulnar neuropathy
   E. Thoracic outlet syndrome
   F. Overuse syndromes

ACUTE CARPAL TUNNEL SYNDROME (USUALLY SECONDARY TO FRACTURES AND FRACTURE DISLOCATIONS ABOUT THE WRIST) IS CONSIDERED A SURGICAL EMERGENCY AND REQUIRES IMMEDIATE DECOMPRESSION.

Sensation about the thenar eminence of the palm should be normal because the palmar cutaneous branch of the median nerve originates 5 cm proximal to the carpal tunnel and does not travel within the canal. As a result, the palmar cutaneous branch is not involved.

Ask your attending to discuss the use of two-point discrimination and Semmes-Weinstein filament testing for diagnosing carpal tunnel syndrome.

The carpal compression test is the most sensitive and specific test for diagnosing carpal tunnel syndrome.

When does your attending order electromyograms?

Hand

TREATMENT ALGORITHM

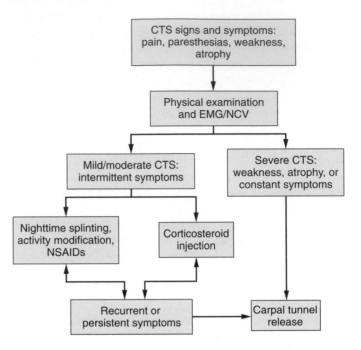

NONOPERATIVE TREATMENT

I. Nonoperative management is the initial mode of treatment in mild to moderate CTS. It is most successful in patients with intermittent symptoms for less than 10 months and with no motor weakness or thenar atrophy.

II. Oral nonsteroidal anti-inflammatory drugs should be considered to help reduce synovitis.

III. Medical management of underlying systemic diseases is an important first step.

IV. Activity modification, ergonometric tips, and nerve gliding exercises can also help treat symptoms of CTS.

V. Splinting

A. The wrist should be immobilized in the neutral position because this maximizes canal size and minimizes canal pressure.

B. The splint is typically worn at night and occasionally during the day during activities that aggravate the symptoms.

C. Because the functional position of the wrist is in 30 degrees of extension, some attending physicians advocate only nighttime splinting.

VI. Corticosteroid injections may be administered into the carpal tunnel.

A. Injections typically result in transient relief in 80% of patients but only 22% remain symptom-free at 18 months.

B. The injection technique varies per the attending surgeon. In general, a 1:1 combination of lidocaine and corticosteroid is injected into the ulnar bursa within the carpal tunnel using a 25-gauge needle. The injection site is 1 cm proximal to the distal wrist flexion crease, ulnar to the palmaris longus tendon, in line with the ring finger, and at a 45-degree angle directed distally (Fig. 10-4).

C. Dexamethasone has been recommended because it has been found to have less deleterious effects if injected directly into the nerve.

> What is your attending's splinting protocol?

> **IF PARESTHESIAS ARE ELICITED, WITHDRAW THE NEEDLE TO PREVENT INJECTING DIRECTLY INTO THE MEDIAN NERVE.**

OPERATIVE INDICATIONS AND TREATMENT OPTIONS

I. Surgical release is indicated in patients with persistent or progressive symptoms despite nonoperative management and in patients with a severe neuropathy. A

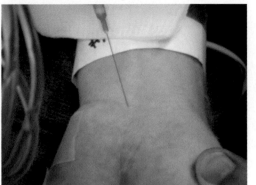

Figure 10-4
Carpal tunnel injection.

severe neuropathy manifests as constant symptoms, motor weakness, or thenar atrophy.

II. Success usually correlates with improved pain and numbness.

III. Postoperative improvement is dependent on severity of the neuropathy. Despite surgical release, EMG values usually do not return to normal postoperatively and may take several months.

IV. Operative options include open and endoscopic release.
   A. Open surgical release of the carpal tunnel remains the gold standard.
   B. Endoscopic release
      1. This was introduced to decrease incision size and surgical dissection, resulting in less postoperative discomfort, with earlier return of grip strength and earlier return to work.
      2. Decreased visualization makes nerve injury and/or incomplete release more common.
      3. Details regarding endoscopic technique are beyond the scope of this book.

CONTRAINDICATIONS TO CARPAL TUNNEL RELEASE

I. Carpal tunnel release is a relatively safe procedure.

II. Contraindications include active infection or medical comorbidities that prevent clearance for surgery.

GENERAL PRINCIPLES OF CARPAL TUNNEL RELEASE

I. The goal of carpal tunnel release is to decompress the median nerve as it travels under the transverse carpal ligament.

II. Be cautious of anatomic variants (e.g., transligamentary recurrent motor branch) to avoid inadvertent nerve injury.

III. The most common cause for failure of carpal tunnel release is inadequate release. The release must extend proximally to the level of the antebrachial fascia to ensure complete decompression of the median nerve.

IV. Hemostasis prior to wound closure is crucial in avoiding hematoma formation and continued nerve compression.

COMPONENTS OF THE PROCEDURE

Positioning, Prepping, and Draping

I. The patient is placed supine on the operating room table with a hand table and is prepped and draped in standard fashion (see Chapter 1).

II. Once the draping is complete, a sterile marker is used to mark the incision (Fig. 10-5).
   A. Incisions may vary per attending surgeon. In general, a straight or slightly curvilinear incision is drawn ulnar to the thenar crease and palmaris longus

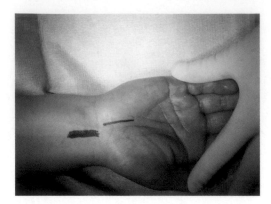

Figure 10-5
Carpal tunnel incision with the proximal mark indicating the location of palmaris longus.

tendon, in line with the long axis of the ring finger, approximately 2 to 3 cm in length, and ending distal to the transverse wrist crease.

B. Do not draw your incision beyond Kaplan's cardinal line to prevent injury to the palmar arch.

III. Exsanguinate the arm and inflate the tourniquet as per the principles outlined in Chapter 1.

Carpal Tunnel Release

I. Anesthetize the skin overlying the incision using a 1:1 mixture of 1% lidocaine and 0.25% bupivacaine (Marcaine), both without epinephrine.

II. Make the skin incision using a 15-blade scalpel just through the dermis until the subcutaneous fat is visualized.

III. Minimize any superficial bleeding using bipolar electrocautery.

IV. Sometimes, muscle fibers are encountered superficially. These are typically fibers of the palmaris brevis muscle, which is innervated by a branch of the ulnar nerve.

V. After the skin has been incised, spread down to the palmar fascia using tenotomy scissors.

VI. Insert a small, self-retaining retractor. The palmar fascia is incised and two small right-angle retractors are used to retract the fatty tissue to visualize the flexor retinaculum. Further blunt dissection is needed to visualize the distal edge of the ligament.

VII. Next, carefully incise the flexor retinaculum from distally to proximally along its ulnar side using a 15-blade.

VIII. Using tenotomy scissors, release the most proximal portion of the flexor retinaculum and the antebrachial fascia.

IX. Under direct visualization, confirm that the flexor retinaculum has been completely released. Gently explore the carpal canal to rule out any extrinsic compression on the median nerve, such as a space-occupying lesion (Fig. 10-6).

X. Achieve meticulous hemostasis using bipolar electrocautery.

XI. Close the incision with 5-0 nylon using simple or horizontal mattress knots (Fig. 10-7).

Wound Dressing and Postoperative Care

I. Dress the wound in standard fashion with a soft dressing (Fig. 10-8).

II. Leave the digits free and encourage early finger motion.

III. Limit simultaneous wrist and finger flexion to prevent volar subluxation of the median nerve and flexor tendons.

IV. Suture removal typically occurs 5 to 10 days postoperatively.

Have your attending explain the significance of Kaplan's cardinal line. What landmarks does he or she use to plan the surgical incision?

Often, small branches of the palmar cutaneous branch of the median and ulnar nerves are encountered at this level and are protected.

Blunt dissection is taken between the palmar fascia and transverse carpal ligament to prevent injury to a potential transligamentous motor branch of the median nerve.

AVOID MAKING THE RETINACULAR INCISION TOO RADIAL TO PROTECT THE MEDIAN NERVE AND ITS BRANCHES. AVOID MAKING THE INCISION TOO ULNAR TO PROTECT THE CONTENTS OF GUYON'S CANAL (THE ULNAR NERVE AND ARTERY). A SMALL RIM OF LIGAMENT IS LEFT ON THE HOOK OF THE HAMATE TO LIMIT SUBLUXATION OF THE CANAL CONTENTS.

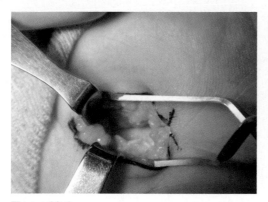

Figure 10-6
Carpal tunnel after release with median nerve visible.

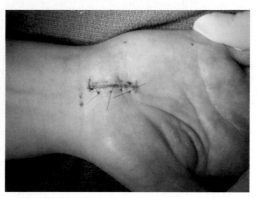

Figure 10-7
Wound closure.

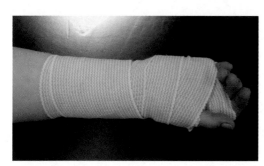

Figure 10-8
Postoperative dressing.

POSTOPERATIVE REHABILITATION

I. Patients are encouraged to increase use of the operative hand as tolerated in the postoperative period.

II. Patients are sent to formal occupational therapy, if needed, to increase wrist range of motion and improve intrinsic hand and grip strengthening.

COMPLICATIONS

I. The most common complication is incomplete release of the transverse carpal ligament.

II. Rarely, nerve (median, ulnar) or vascular (superficial arch) injury can occur.

III. Repeat surgical release of the carpal tunnel is generally associated with poor results.

> **THE RETINACULUM MUST BE INCISED VERY GENTLY BECAUSE THE MEDIAN NERVE CAN LIE DIRECTLY UNDERNEATH, AND ANY INADVERTENT DAMAGE TO THE NERVE CAN HAVE DEVASTATING CONSEQUENCES FOR THE PATIENT.**

SUGGESTED READINGS

Cranford CS, Ho JY, Kalainov DM, Hartigan BJ: Carpal tunnel syndrome. J Am Acad Orthop Surg 15:537–548, 2007.

Mackinnon SE, Novak CB: Compression neuropathies. In Green DP, Hotchkiss RN, Pederson WC, Wolfe SW (eds): Green's Operative Hand Surgery, 5th ed. Philadelphia, Churchill Livingstone, 2005.

Ranjan G: Nerve. In Beredjiklian PK, Bozentka DJ (eds): Review of Hand Surgery. Philadelphia, Saunders, 2004, pp 84–87.

Szabo RM, Steinberg DR: Nerve entrapment syndromes at the wrist. J Am Acad Orthop Surg 2:115–123, 1994.

Hand

Open Reduction and Internal Fixation of Distal Radius Fractures

Jonas L. Matzon and Pedro Beredjiklian

Case Study

A 74-year-old, left hand–dominant retired female presents to the emergency department with a painful and deformed left wrist. The patient was walking when she tripped over a curb and fell onto her outstretched left hand. She experienced immediate pain and deformity of her left wrist and was taken directly to the hospital by her husband. On arrival, she was complaining only of pain in her left wrist. She denied any loss of consciousness. She is neurovascularly intact and has only minor skin abrasions on her left elbow. Radiographs taken in the emergency department are shown in Figure 11-1.

BACKGROUND

    I. Distal radius fractures represent approximately one sixth of all fractures treated in the emergency department.

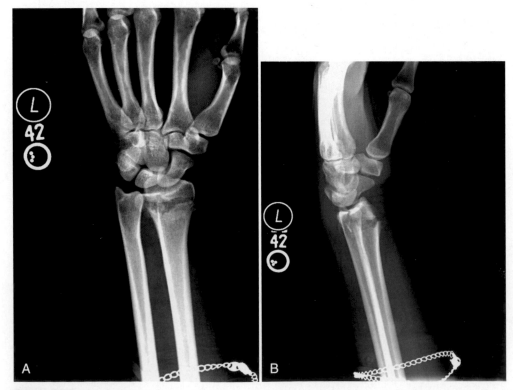

Figure 11-1
Posteroanterior (**A**) and lateral (**B**) radiographs demonstrating a left distal radius fracture.

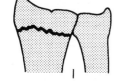
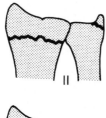
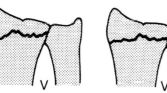
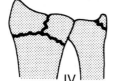
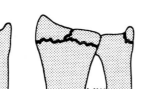

Figure 11-2

Frykman classification of distal radius fractures. *(From Fernandez DL, Wolfe SW: Distal radius fractures. In Green DP, Hotchkiss RN, Pederson WC, Wolfe SW [eds]: Green's Operative Hand Surgery, 5th ed. Philadelphia, Churchill Livingstone, 2005.)*

II. There are three peak age distributions for distal radius fractures:
   A. Children 5 to 14 years: usually secondary to trauma
   B. Males younger than 50 years of age: usually secondary to trauma
   C. Females older than 40 years of age: usually insufficiency fractures
III. Risk factors for distal radius fractures in the elderly include female gender, decreased bone mineral density, early menopause, ethnicity, and heredity.
IV. Fractures are best classified in terms of displacement, angulation, articular involvement, and comminution.
   A. Many eponyms have been used to describe specific fracture patterns.
      1. Colles': dorsally angulated extra-articular fracture
      2. Smith's: volarly angulated extra-articular fracture
      3. Barton's: articular shear fracture (dorsal or volar)
      4. Chauffeur's/Hutchinson's: radial styloid fracture
   B. Many classification systems are used to categorize distal radius fractures.
      1. Frykman's, shown in Figure 11-2
      2. Melone's, shown in Table 11-1

Table 11-1 Melone Classification	
I	Minimally displaced
II	Comminuted/stable Displaced medial complex Dorsal: die-punch, Barton
III	Displaced medial complex as a unit Displaced radial shaft fragments
IV	Wide separation or rotation of medial fragments Extensive soft tissue and periarticular damage

From Beredjiklian P, Bozentka D (eds): Review of Hand Surgery. Philadelphia, Saunders, 2004.

TREATMENT PROTOCOLS

I. **Treatment Considerations**
   A. Fracture classification and severity
   B. Neurovascular status
   C. Condition of soft tissue envelope
   D. Associated injuries

II. **Initial Treatment**
   A. Obtain a thorough history, including mechanism, patient age, occupation, and hand dominance.
   B. Perform a detailed physical examination.
      1. Visually evaluate the soft tissues around the wrist. Look for abrasions and determine if the fracture is open or closed.
      2. Examine the neurovascular function of the extremity.
         a. Assess the vascular status by palpating the radial pulse and checking for capillary refill.
         b. Test anterior interosseous nerve function by asking the patient to flex the thumb interphalangeal joint.
         c. Test posterior interosseous nerve function by asking the patient to extend the thumb.
         d. Test ulnar nerve function by having the patient cross the index and middle fingers or spread the fingers apart widely against resistance.
         e. Check sensation to light touch and two-point discrimination in the radial, ulnar, and median nerve distributions.
      3. Assess the patient's ability to contract the extensor pollicis longus muscle.
      4. Evaluate the forearm for possible compartment syndrome.
      5. Check ipsilateral shoulder, elbow, and carpal bones for associated injuries.
      6. Perform a total body trauma assessment, including contralateral upper extremity, bilateral lower extremities, and spine.
   C. Obtain adequate radiographs.
      1. Wrist: posteroanterior, lateral, and oblique views
      2. Forearm (including elbow): anteroposterior and lateral views
   D. Perform fracture reduction (closed).
      1. Under sterile conditions, provide anesthesia with 1% lidocaine without epinephrine via a hematoma block.
      2. Hang the arm from finger traps for approximately 5 to 10 minutes.
      3. Manipulate the distal fragment into better alignment using traction and then thumb pressure over the distal fragment.
   E. Immobilization
      1. Maintain the reduction while applying a sugar-tong splint with the wrist in neutral position
      2. Check postreduction radiographs for adequate length and alignment.
      3. Recheck the status of the neurovascular examination following fracture reduction.
   F. The patient may be discharged home and asked to follow up with a hand surgeon on an outpatient basis.

III. **Nonoperative Treatment**
   A. Historically, conservative management has been the mainstay of treatment.
   B. Indications
      1. Nondisplaced fractures
      2. Low-demand elderly patients with significant comorbidities
      3. Stable fractures that meet the following criteria:
         a. Volar tilt: less than 10-degree change
         b. Radial inclination: less than 5-degree change
         c. Radial length: less than 2-mm change
         d. Articular step-off: less than 2 mm

ALWAYS CHECK FOR SNUFFBOX PAIN TO EVALUATE FOR ASSOCIATED SCAPHOID FRACTURE.

If the fracture is intra-articular, consider obtaining a computed tomography scan to assist in preoperative planning.

NEUROLOGIC DETERIORATION OF MEDIAN NERVE FUNCTION AFTER FRACTURE REDUCTION SUGGESTS ACUTE CARPAL TUNNEL SYNDROME, WHICH IS A SURGICAL EMERGENCY. REMOVE THE SPLINT AND REASSESS THE NEUROLOGIC EXAMINATION. IF THERE IS NO IMPROVEMENT, PERFORM ACUTE SURGICAL DECOMPRESSION OF THE CARPAL TUNNEL IN THE OPERATING ROOM.

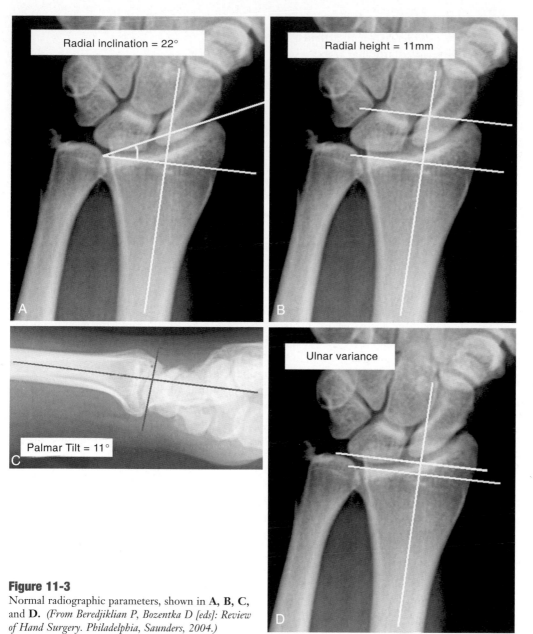

Figure 11-3
Normal radiographic parameters, shown in **A, B, C,** and **D.** *(From Beredjiklian P, Bozentka D [eds]: Review of Hand Surgery. Philadelphia, Saunders, 2004.)*

C. A sugar-tong splint should be maintained until swelling has decreased. It is then converted to a long-arm cast for 3 weeks, which is finally converted to a short-arm cast for an additional 3 weeks.

D. Nondisplaced and stable fractures may be treated in a short cast alone.

E. Close radiographic follow-up is required to monitor alignment and fracture displacement. Inadequate reduction may lead to fracture malunion (Fig. 11-3).

> Normal radiographic parameters: volar tilt = 11 degrees, radial inclination = 22 degrees, radial length = 11 mm. These parameters are used to determine the adequacy of fracture reduction.

SURGICAL ALTERNATIVES AND INDICATIONS

I. **Operative Treatment**

   A. The goal is anatomic reduction of the distal radius.

   B. Surgery is the treatment of choice in unstable or comminuted fractures due to difficulty maintaining reduction nonoperatively. Operative treatment also allows for earlier mobilization.

II. **Indications**
   A. Unstable/displaced articular fractures
   B. Impacted articular fractures
   C. Open fractures
   D. Radiocarpal fracture dislocations
   E. Failed closed reductions

III. **Surgical Options**
   A. Closed reduction and percutaneous pinning
      1. Considered for reducible extra-articular fractures and simple intra-articular fractures without metaphyseal comminution
      2. Requires good bone quality, so it is generally reserved for younger patients
   B. External fixation or hybrid fixation: relies on ligamentotaxis to indirectly control fracture fragments
   C. Open reduction and internal fixation (ORIF)

IV. **ORIF Approaches**
   A. Dorsal
      1. Advantages
         a. Avoids neurovascular structures
         b. Dorsal plates to provide buttress against fracture displacement and collapse
      2. Disadvantages
         a. Potential for hardware prominence
         b. Extensor tendon irritation and potential rupture
   B. Volar
      1. Advantages
         a. Fixed volar plating that transfers the load stress from the articular surface to the intact radial shaft
         b. Anatomic reduction of volar cortex that restores radial length, radial inclination, and volar tilt
      2. Disadvantages
         a. Increased risk of neurovascular injury
         b. Flexor tendon irritation and potential rupture

> Ask your attending to discuss the concept of ligamentotaxis and how it applies to the reduction of distal radius fractures.

> Which approach does your attending prefer to use and how is the decision influenced by specific fracture patterns?

SURGICAL ALGORITHM

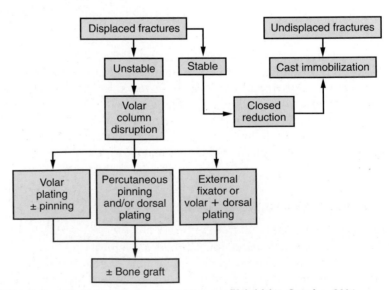

From Beredjiklian P, Bozentka D (eds): Review of Hand Surgery. Philadelphia, Saunders, 2004.

GENERAL PRINCIPLES OF DISTAL RADIUS FRACTURE FIXATION

I. The distal radius consists of three independent articular surfaces: scaphoid facet, lunate facet, and sigmoid notch.

II. The ulnar head articulates with the sigmoid notch and attaches to the triangular fibrocartilage complex.

III. The goal of operative treatment for distal radius fractures is to restore the articular surface and the normal anatomic relationships of the distal radius as well as to regain wrist mobility.

IV. The distal radius has a radial inclination averaging 22 degrees, a volar tilt averaging 11 degrees, and a radial length averaging 11 mm.

V. The fracture usually occurs due to the force exiting through the metaphyseal bone of the distal radius (path of least resistance). The approach used depends on the nature of the fracture.

VI. Because most of these injuries occur in older patients with poor quality bone, locking plate technology may be required.

VII. Bone grafting is often required if there is severe comminution, poor bone quality, or significant articular impaction.

VIII. Rigid internal fixation is required to allow for early mobilization and attainment of wrist range of motion.

COMPONENTS OF THE PROCEDURE

Positioning, Prepping, and Draping

I. The patient is placed supine on the operating room table.

II. A hand table is attached to the bed on the appropriate side.

III. A mini-fluoroscope machine is positioned to come in parallel to the hand table.

IV. The wrist is prepped and draped in standard fashion as outlined in Chapter 1 (Fig. 11-4).

V. Once the extremity is draped, a sterile marker is used to mark the incision.
   A. Volar approach: longitudinal incision directly over the distal aspect of the flexor carpi radialis (Fig. 11-5).
   B. Dorsal approach: longitudinal incision centered over the ulnar aspect of Lister's tubercle (Fig. 11-6)

VI. The arm is exsanguinated and the tourniquet is inflated prior to starting the case (see Chapter 1 for details).

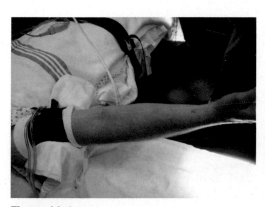

Figure 11-4
Tourniquet placement.

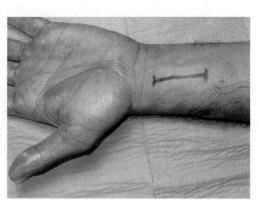

Figure 11-5
Volar incision.

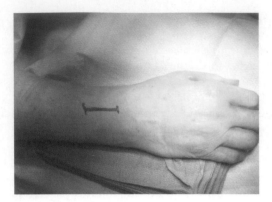

Figure 11-6
Dorsal incision.

Surgical Exposure

I. **Volar Approach**
   A. Make the skin incision using a 15-blade scalpel.
   B. Minimize any superficial bleeding using bipolar electrocautery.
   C. After the skin has been incised, dissect down to the flexor carpi radialis (FCR) using blunt tenotomy scissors. Spread longitudinally on the FCR tendon to avoid injuring the tendon.
   D. Develop the interval between the FCR (ulnar) and the radial artery (radial).
   E. Bluntly with right angle retractors, move the flexor pollicis longus and the deep flexors ulnarly to visualize the underlying pronator quadratus muscle.
   F. Insert a self-retaining retractor while taking care to protect the radial artery.
   G. With a 15-blade scalpel, make an L-shaped incision in the pronator quadratus along its radial and distal borders.
   H. Use a key elevator to subperiosteally elevate the pronator quadratus muscle from the surface of the volar radius.
   I. It is now possible to examine the fracture under direct visualization.

II. **Dorsal Approach**
   A. Make the previously defined skin incision using a 15-blade scalpel.
   B. Minimize any superficial bleeding using the bipolar electrocautery.
   C. Elevate small skin flaps, and then insert a self-retaining retractor.
   D. Identify the extensor retinaculum (Fig. 11-7) and then incise along the third dorsal extensor compartment (extensor pollicis longus).
   E. Retract the extensor pollicis longus tendon radially and cut down to bone.
   F. Subperiosteally using a 15-blade, elevate the deep layer of the dorsal compartments off the radius both radially and ulnarly (Fig. 11-8). Make sure not to enter the compartments or to visualize the tendons.

> **AVOID GOING TOO DISTALLY AND CUTTING THE WRIST CAPSULE/LIGAMENTS WHEN MAKING THE L-SHAPED INCISION.**

> Ask your attending about the advantages of the specific plates that are used to stabilize the distal radius.

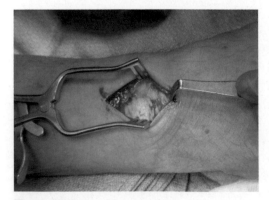

Figure 11-7
Superficial dissection with extensor retinaculum exposed.

Figure 11-8
Subperiosteal elevation of the dorsal compartments.

G. It is now possible to visualize the fracture directly.

H. Using an instrument such as a rongeur, remove Lister's tubercle.

Fracture Reduction and Fixation

I. Bring in the mini-fluoroscope machine to visualize the fracture radiographically.

II. Adequately reduce the fracture using standard fracture reduction techniques; confirm with fluoroscopy image.

III. Place the plate on the distal radius and once again verify its position using fluoroscopy (Fig. 11-9).

IV. When adequately positioned, fix the plate to the distal radius with screws.

Wound Closure and Dressing

I. **Deep Closure**

A. Volar approach. Repair the pronator quadratus with a nonabsorbable braided suture (e.g., 2-0 Vicryl).

B. Dorsal approach. Repair the extensor retinaculum with a nonabsorbable braided suture (e.g., 2-0 Vicryl). The extensor pollicis longus should be transposed subcutaneously to rest above the retinacular repair to prevent rupture.

II. Typically, close the incision with a smaller gauge monofilament suture (e.g., 5-0 nylon suture) using simple or horizontal mattress knots.

III. Dress the wound in standard fashion (see Chapter 1). A volar wrist splint is applied with the wrist in 30 degrees of extension. The dressing and splint stays on until the patient returns for a follow-up visit.

POSTOPERATIVE CARE

I. Typically, patients are admitted to the hospital overnight for pain control. It is important that they keep the extremity elevated above heart height to prevent excessive swelling.

II. The patient returns to the office approximately 7 to 10 days postoperatively, and sutures are removed at that time.

III. Physical therapy and activity depend on the fracture pattern and the stability achieved after fixation. Usually, after the first follow-up visit, active forearm and wrist motion is started. A removable thermoplastic wrist splint is used between therapy sessions.

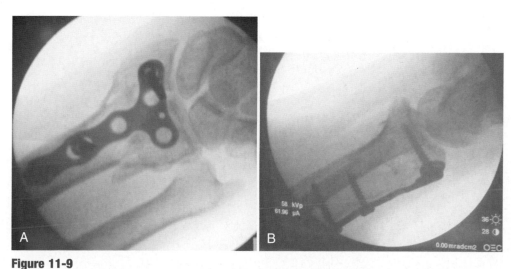

Figure 11-9
AP (**A**) and lateral (**B**) fluoroscopic views of a distal radius fracture following dorsal plate fixation.

IV. At 6 to 8 weeks postoperatively, the patient has usually regained most of his or her wrist motion.

RESULTS AND COMPLICATIONS

   I. Functional outcomes are correlated with comminution and associated carpal bone injuries.

  II. When complications occur after distal radius ORIF, they can be divided into early and late.

     A. Early

       1. Median nerve dysfunction

       2. Ulnar nerve injury

       3. Distal radioulnar joint instability

       4. Compartment syndrome

     B. Late

       1. Post-traumatic arthritis of the radiocarpal joint and/or the distal radioulnar joint

       2. Ulnocarpal abutment syndrome

       3. Extensor tendon rupture

       4. Malunion

       5. Nonunion

       6. Chronic regional pain syndrome (also known as reflex sympathetic dystrophy)

SUGGESTED READINGS

Chou KH, Sarris I, Papadimitriou NG, Sotereanos DG: Fractures of the hand, wrist, and forearm axis. In Beredjiklian PK, Bozentka DJ (eds): Review of Hand Surgery. Philadelphia, Saunders, 2004, pp 101–126.

Fernandez DL, Wolfe SW: Distal radius fractures. In Green DP, Hotchkiss RN, Pederson WC, Wolfe SW (eds): Green's Operative Hand Surgery, 5th ed. Philadelphia, Elsevier, 2005.

Nana AD, Joshi A, Lichtman DM: Plating of the distal radius. J Am Acad Orthop Surg 13:159–171, 2005.

Ruch DS: Fractures of the distal radius and ulna. In Bucholz RW, Heckman JD, Court-Brown (eds): Rockwood and Green's Fractures in Adults, 6th ed. Philadelphia, Lippincott Williams & Wilkins, 2006, pp 909–964.

Smith DW, Henry MH: Volar fixed-angle plating of the distal radius. J Am Acad Orthop Surg 13:28–36, 2005.

SPINE

CHAPTER 12

Anterior Cervical Diskectomy and Fusion

William Tally and **Scott A. Rushton**

Spine

Case Study

A 45-year-old woman with a 3-month history of left arm pain radiating into the thumb presents to clinic. She has had intermittent neck and left shoulder pain for approximately 1 year, which has also been insidiously worsening over the past 3 months. There is no history of trauma, and she works in an office setting. Currently, she is a nonsmoker, and her left arm pain is alleviated by placing her arm over her head. Recently she has noted some difficulty with using her left hand. The pain is worsening with lateral bending of her neck or quick rotational motions.

Detailed physical examination reveals decreased cervical range of motion. There is no evidence of shoulder girdle atrophy, and shoulder range of motion is within normal limits. Sensory examination reveals slight decrease in light touch and pin prick along the lateral forearm and thumb on the left. Motor examination demonstrates four fifths left wrist extensor strength and a decreased brachioradialis reflex. Tandem gait and Romberg testing are normal; Hoffman's sign is negative. An initial lateral cervical spine radiograph and an axial and sagittal magnetic resonance imaging scan are depicted in Figure 12-1.

BACKGROUND

I. Cervical degenerative disk disease (DDD) is highly prevalent in the aging population. Changes that occur over time in the intervertebral disks, posterior elements (e.g., facets joints, ligamentum flavum, spinal canal), and overall alignment of the cervical spine result in the entity known as cervical spondylosis.

II. The natural history of cervical spondylosis is a slowly progressive stepwise neurologic deterioration with long intervening periods of stable function. With severe degenerative changes, cervical alignment may also begin to worsen with loss of the natural cervical spine lordosis.

III. In general, patients with cervical spondylosis are initially treated conservatively and may present with a wide spectrum of symptoms, ranging from mild to severe. More severe cases may require surgical intervention to prevent irreversible progression of disease and functional deterioration.

IV. Anterior cervical diskectomy and fusion (ACDF) is considered the gold standard for the surgical treatment of cervical spondylosis. The three main pathologies encountered in candidates for ACDF are DDD with disk herniation, spondylosis, and myelopathy.

   A. DDD, also called a "soft disk" herniation, may result in radiculopathy or radiating pain down the upper extremity beyond the level of the elbow. This occurs due to chemical irritation or mechanical compression of a nerve root as it exits from a foramen. Radiculopathy often responds to physical therapy or transforaminal steroid injections. ACDF can be considered when there is progressive neurologic deficit due to nerve root compression.

   B. Spondylosis or degeneration of a spinal motion segment occurs throughout the cervical spine. When this degeneration leads to loss of the normal lordosis of the cervical spine or compromise of the space available for the spinal cord, surgical intervention may be required.

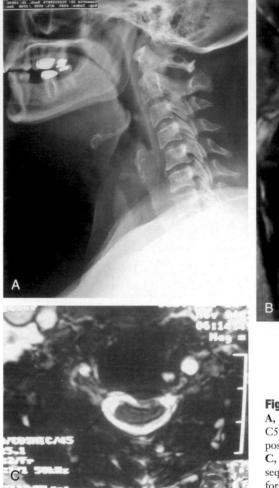
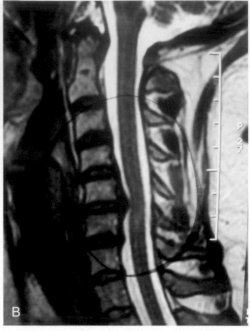

Figure 12-1
A, Lateral cervical spine film showing spondylosis at C5-C6. Note the disk-osteophyte complex at the posterior aspect of the vertebral bodies. **B,** Axial and **C,** sagittal T2 magnetic resonance imaging scan sequence showing the disk herniation with significant foraminal encroachment.

C. Myelopathy translates into pathology of the spinal cord. Severe spondylosis and/or large disk herniations can compromise the cross-sectional area of the spinal canal, leading to direct compression of the spinal cord. With spinal cord compression, patients typically present with clinical signs such as gait abnormalities (e.g., wide-based gait), hyperreflexia, upper motor neuron signs (e.g., positive Hoffman's sign), and complaints of hand clumsiness (e.g., difficulty buttoning a shirt).

D. In general, myelopathy is not responsive to conservative measures, and approximately one third of patients progress rapidly, one third progress slowly, and one third do not progress. There is no reliable means to predict which category any given patient will fall. ACDF is the procedure of choice if the compression is anterior and localized to the intervertebral disk space.

E. The initial evaluation begins with a detailed history. Information regarding the duration of symptoms as well as subjective complaints of upper extremity numbness, tingling, weakness, and difficulty with fine motor skills and gait must be obtained. Make sure to document if the patient has any bowel or bladder dysfunction, either retention or incontinence.

F. The physical examination should concentrate on observing the patient's gait, cervical range of motion, and documenting a thorough upper and lower extremity neurologic examination with a focus on muscle strength, sensation, and deep tendon reflexes. Upper motor neuron signs such as a Hoffman's sign may be indicative of spinal cord compression and myelopathy.

G. Initial imaging calls for anteroposterior, lateral, and oblique plain radiographs of the cervical spine. Radiographs are evaluated for disk height, osteophyte formation, foraminal narrowing/stenosis, and anterior or posterior vertebral

Hoffman's sign is elicited by flicking the tip of the long finger while the patient's hand is completely relaxed; a positive sign is elicited when the patient's thumb flexes at the interphalangeal joint.

Ask your attending what additional physical examination findings are indicative of cervical spondylosis and myelopathy.

body translation. If there is concern regarding cervical spine instability, flexion and extension radiographs should be obtained.

H. With a clinical picture of DDD and a high suspicion for disk herniation or cervical myelopathy, magnetic resonance imaging (MRI) is the study of choice. The MRI is assessed for disk desiccation, which is indicative of DDD and loss of disk height, disk herniation, spinal canal compromise, and spinal cord signal change or myelomalacia.

V. Risk Factors for Disease Progression

A. Genetic factors. These are being identified more and more as the leading risk for spondylosis and DDD.

B. Cervical spine injury

C. Environmental. The greatest risks are smoking, vibratory activities such as driving, and heavy lifting.

VI. Nonoperative Treatment

A. A soft disk herniation with radiculopathy is usually self-limited and, if the patient can tolerate the symptoms, usually completely resolves. Adjunctive physical therapy often helps relieve muscle spasm and stiffness as well as preventing disuse atrophy. Cervical collars have no role in this scenario. Transforaminal epidural steroid injection is a treatment option that may facilitate this process; however, these injections are not as innocuous or effective in the cervical spine as in the lumbar region.

B. Although cervical spondylosis is also often successfully treated with time and physical therapy, it is usually much more resistant to these measures. Again, cervical collars play no role, and transforaminal injections are controversial. In general, they are not usually effective in the short term and rarely is there long-term efficacy. Given their complication rate and lack of good results, most surgeons may not advocate injection therapy prior to surgery.

C. Myelopathy is somewhat more controversial with respect to conservative care. Some surgeons identify upper motor neuron signs as absolute indications for surgical intervention. Other surgeons are willing to observe the patient for signs of progression.

> Ask your attending about the role of conservative treatment in the management of cervical disk disease. At what point does he or she advocate the use of transforaminal steroid injections?

TREATMENT ALGORITHM

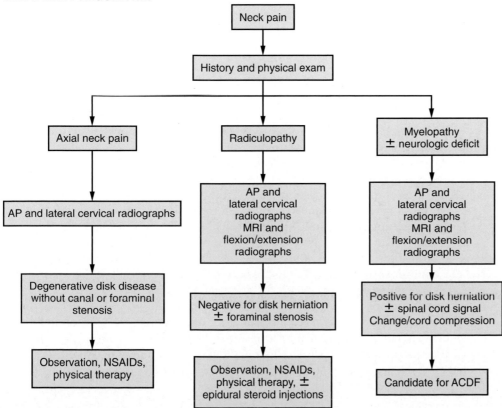

ALTERNATIVES, INDICATIONS, AND CONTRAINDICATIONS

I. **Surgical Alternatives to ACDF.** There are several surgical alternatives to ACDF that exist for treating the spectrum of cervical disc disease. The description of each of these options is beyond the scope of this text. The list below depicts the most common alternatives but is not meant to be an exhaustive list.

A. Anterior diskectomy

B. Posterior foraminotomy and microdiskectomy

C. Anterior uncinectomy and foraminotomy

D. Anterior corpectomy and fusion

E. Posterior laminectomy and fusion

F. Laminoplasty

G. Total disk arthroplasty

II. **Surgical Indications for ACDF**

A. Failed conservative treatment for at least 6 weeks

B. Large herniated nucleus pulposus

C. Persistent radicular symptoms

D. Disabling motor weakness (e.g., wrist drop)

E. Progressive neurologic deficit

F. Static neurologic deficit with associated radiculopathy or retractable pain

G. Cervical spine instability

H. MRI changes in spinal cord signal (myelomalacia)

I. Space available for the cord (small cross-sectional area)

III. **Contraindications to ACDF**

A. Current infection

B. Systemic infection

C. Cervical kyphotic deformity (requires additional posterior stabilization)

D. Three or more cervical levels involved

E. Inflammatory arthritis (may require additional posterior stabilization)

F. Instability (may require additional posterior stabilization)

G. Axial neck pain with no radiculopathy

H. Medical comorbidities (patient unable to safely tolerate stress of surgery)

I. Carotid stenosis (severe atherosclerotic disease)

J. Patients that smoke (relative contraindication)

> Ask your attending for which patient scenarios the surgical alternatives listed are typically used.

> Ask your attending if there are additional patient scenarios that should be considered as contraindications for anterior cervical diskectomy and fusion.

GENERAL PRINCIPLES OF ANTERIOR CERVICAL DISKECTOMY AND FUSION

I. The major goals of ACDF are as follows:

A. Decompression of neural elements (spinal cord or nerve roots)

B. Protection of the neural elements from injury and further deterioration

C. Restoration of cervical lordosis (restore sagittal balance of the cervical spine)

D. Alleviation of radicular symptoms

E. Alleviation of axial neck pain (contraindications to surgery if present without radiculopathy)

II. Adjacent level disease may be present at the time of office evaluation. In some situations, it may be prudent to address advanced degeneration at asymp-tomatic levels at the time of the index procedure. The patient should be counseled that this may result in pain postoperatively because these levels were previously asymptomatic.

III. The anterior surgical approach to the cervical spine is typically performed on the left side of the patient. The recurrent laryngeal nerve lies in the tracheoesophageal groove in a more predictable fashion on the left side.

IV. The superior and inferior end plates must be exposed to subchondral bone while maintaining a parallel relationship in both coronal and sagittal planes. Graft choices are autograft or allograft fibula or iliac crest, metallic cages, and bone substitutes such as poly-ethyl-ethyl-ketone (PEEK) spacers. Finally, correct graft sizing is critical to avoid kyphosis if undersized and overdistraction if too large. Overdistraction anteriorly puts significant stress on the posterior structures and usually results in facet joint pain.

V. All posterior osteophytes must be resected to accomplish central decompression. This may require removal of the posterior longitudinal ligament depending on the extent of the pathology.

VI. Anterior plating is almost routinely done during ACDF for graft stabilization. There are several plate options available. Statically locked plates have a mechanism in which the screw and plate act as a fixed angle device. This is a very rigid construct and allows minimal motion across the operative site. Regardless of the plate chosen, it is imperative that there is no impingement into the adjacent disk spaces as this will lead to rapid adjacent level degeneration.

VII. Intraoperative neuromonitoring is routinely done in most institutions when performing an ACDF. Baseline signals should be obtained during prepositioning and verified after each episode of patient manipulation. Currently the standard neuromonitoring modalities include free-run electromyography (EMG), transcutaneous motor evoked potential (tcMEP), and somatosensory evoked potential (SSEP).

VIII. Free-run EMG monitors muscle belly electrical activity in a continuous mode. This is an extremely sensitive modality that gives feedback on nerve irritation and stimulation during the procedure. It is critical to keep in mind that this modality is motor only and gives information regarding a nerve that is actively being injured. An acutely transected nerve does not result in EMG changes in the short term and thus such an injury cannot be reliably documented by this test alone.

IX. tcMEP is an evocative test in which the patient's motor cortex is electrically stimulated by scalp electrodes and the resulting muscle-evoked EMG is recorded. The amplitude and wave forms are analyzed against baseline and changes reported to the surgeon. This modality is an extremely sensitive marker for spinal cord injury; however, it is not very specific and is fraught with false-positive results.

X. SSEP monitors the posterior aspect of the spinal cord. This modality involves direct stimulation of a peripheral nerve while monitoring sensory cortex response via scalp electrodes. This modality has been found to be both sensitive and specific for clinically identifiable neurologic injury.

XI. The three modalities in concert are used to provide information on nerve root injury (EMG) and spinal cord function (tcMEP with SSEP). If neurologic monitoring detects a change in root or cord function during the case, the initial step is to reverse the maneuver previously accomplished. Additionally, the mean arterial pressure should be elevated to greater than 90 mm Hg. If the attending surgeon and the neurophysiologist believe that the neurologic change represents a real injury to the cord, an intravenous steroid protocol should be initiated.

> Ask your attending what steroid protocol is used in the event of an acute spinal cord injury in the operating room.

COMPONENTS OF THE PROCEDURE

Positioning, Prepping, and Draping

I. The patient is placed in the supine position on a radiolucent table.

II. A towel roll or inflatable A-line bag is placed perpendicularly under the shoulders. The roll and headboard should be adjusted to place the neck in slight extension.

III. The upper extremities are tucked and wrapped at the sides. Ensure that there is adequate ulnar nerve padding and that the forearms are in neutral supination/pronation (Fig. 12-2).

IV. Four-inch silk tape should be stretched from the lateral deltoids down to the foot of the bed. Adequate tension should hold the shoulders in the anatomically depressed position. Attempting to obtain more depression by increasing tension

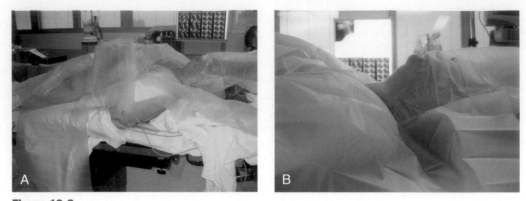

Figure 12-2
Pictures of patient positioned showing (**A**) extension and (**B**) patient tucked and taped.

only increases the risk to the brachial plexus while accomplishing little in the way of better exposure.
 V. The anterior neck and the iliac crest is prepped and draped in standard fashion (see Chapter 1 for details).

Surgical Approach

 I. Mark out the skin incision with a sterile marker prior to starting. The side of approach should be discussed with the attending surgeon. The incision should cross midline for 2 to 3 mm and extend approximately 4 cm laterally following Langer's lines (Fig. 12-3).
 II. Typically, a local anesthetic with epinephrine is injected along the length of the incision. This step helps with postoperative pain control while also decreasing skin and subcuticular bleeding, which can be considerable in the neck.
 III. Sharply incise the skin with a 15-blade. Continue with sharp dissection through the subcutaneous fat layer until the platysma muscle is visible (Fig. 12-4).
 IV. Next, develop the plane between the platysma and the overlying fat using blunt dissection. It is important to maintain hemostasis during every step.
 V. Sharply incise the platysma in line with the skin incision. Repeat the sweeping dissection using a Ray-Tec sponge and fingertip to develop the plane between the platysma and the underlying superficial cervical fascia.
 VI. Identify the interval between the sternocleidomastoid (SCM) muscle laterally and sternohyoid muscle medially. The anterior jugular vein usually lies in the depression. If the vein is small, it can be ligated; if it is large, it should be mobilized laterally with the SCM muscle. The SCM muscle is invested by the superficial

Figure 12-3
The neck with levels drawn over anatomic landmarks. The patient's head is oriented to the right.

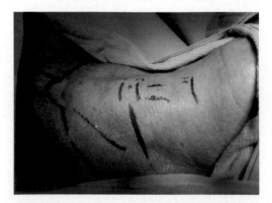

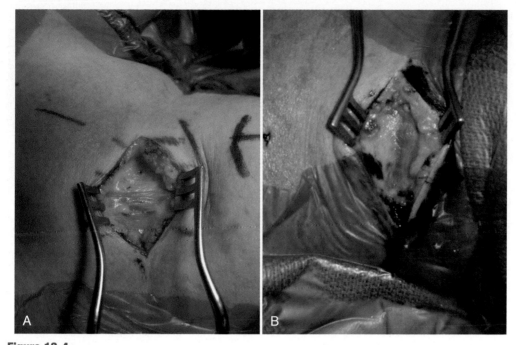

Figure 12-4
A, Superficial dissection through skin and subcutaneous tissue. **B,** The platysma is identified as the next layer.

cervical fascia. Dissection into deeper layers of the fascia allows for deeper access as well as superior/inferior extensile exposure.

VII. Using toothed forceps and Mayo scissors, lift the fascia anteriorly and begin to bluntly dissect. As the fascia becomes thinner, coagulate any small vessels that are identified. This is an extremely vascular area, so all dissection should be accomplished by spreading, not cutting. Once the fascia is penetrated, SCM muscle fibers should be identified laterally while the thicker fascial aponeurosis is visible medially. At this point, attention should be focused on extending the fascial release superiorly and inferiorly.

VIII. Once thorough release of the superficial cervical fascia is complete, the pretracheal fascia is encountered. This fascia surrounds the trachea and thyroid and does not need to be entered. During this mobilization, the goal is to develop the potential space between the pretracheal fascia medially and the carotid sheath laterally. By palpating the carotid pulse, and keeping these structures lateral, there are no worrisome structures in the plane of dissection.

IX. The posterior margin of this potential space is defined by the alar fascia, which is intimate with the prevertebral fascia. Bluntly dissect down to this level while being mindful of the location of the carotid sheath.

X. At this point, appendiceal retractors are placed over the SCM and carotid sheath laterally. A second appendiceal retractor is placed medially to retract the larynx, esophagus, and sternohyoid muscle medially.

XI. The anterior spine with its overlying longus colli muscles is now visible (Fig. 12-5). Identify the disk space of interest, which appears whiter than the vertebral bodies. Additionally, the disk bulges upward, and the bodies are recessed. Place a localizing spinal needle into the disk space, remove the retractors, and obtain a lateral fluoroscopic image. At the C6-C7 and C7-T1 levels, it may be necessary to mark a higher level due to the interference of the shoulders with obtaining a clear radiograph (Fig. 12-6).

XII. Once the level is confirmed, reinsert the appendiceal retractors and mark the disk space with Bovie cautery. Mobilize the longus muscles off the spine from the midbody above to the midbody below the level staying subperiosteal dissection. Care should be taken to stay below the muscle to avoid injury to the cervical

The three fascial layers encountered in the anterior cervical spine approach are the superficial cervical fascia, pretracheal fascia, and the prevertebral fascia.

BE CAUTIOUS WITH DISSECTION AROUND THE LONGUS COLLI MUSCLE DUE TO THE POTENTIAL FOR INJURY TO THE SYMPATHETIC CHAIN AND VERTEBRAL ARTERY. INJURY TO THE SYMPATHETIC CHAIN MAY LEAD TO HORNER'S SYNDROME, WHICH IS A CONSTELLATION OF PTOSIS, MIOSIS, AND ANHIDROSIS.

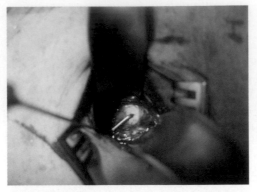

Figure 12-5
Exposed spine with a spinal needle in place within
the desired disk level.

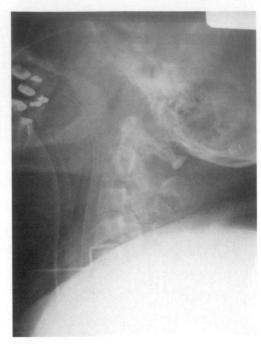

Figure 12-6
Marker film demonstrating the spinal needle in the
C4-C5 disk space.

sympathetics. Additionally, mobilization should only proceed laterally to the
margins of the vertebral body to avoid injury to the vertebral artery.

Diskectomy and Graft Placement

 I. Place a retractor with the smooth blade under the longus colli on the esophageal
    side and a toothed blade under the longus colli on the carotid side. Assemble the
    retractor, remove the appendiceals, and open the retractor. Ensure the blades stay
    below the longus muscles at all times during the procedure.

 II. Insert 14-mm Caspar pins into the waist of the superior and inferior vertebral
     bodies surrounding the disk of interest. Apply the grasshopper self-retaining
     retractor over the pins and open it until it is snug and then open two more clicks.
     Inform the neurophysiologist that the spine is distracted and motor testing should
     be checked (Fig. 12-7).

 III. Ask the anesthesiologist to deflate and repressurize the endotracheal tube
      cuff. With the retractors in place, it has been shown that tracheal endothelial
      pressures reach critical levels and that by repressuring the cuff, this risk is
      minimized.

Figure 12-7
Retractors in position.

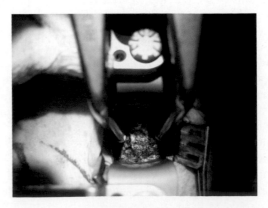

IV. Using a 15-blade on a long handle, incise along the superior and inferior end plate margins and vertically at the uncovertebral joints within the disk space. Always use the blade in a lateral to medial direction to minimize risk to surrounding structures.

V. Using a pituitary rongeur, remove as much disk material as is easily grasped through the defect created in the annulus fibrosus.

VI. The remaining disk and cartilaginous end plates are then mobilized using a 3-0 curette along the subchondral end plates. Continue until the bulk of the disk material is removed.

VII. In most cases, there is an overhanging osteophyte from the inferior lip of the superior endplate that interferes with clear visualization and access to the posterior disk space. Using a 2-mm Kerrison rongeur, resect this osteophyte back parallel to the endplate. Care should be taken not to violate the end plate during this maneuver (Fig. 12-8).

VIII. Once good visualization is obtained, remove any remaining disk until the posterior annulus and/or posterior osteophyte is reached.

IX. Using a curved 3-0 curette, work in a posterior to anterior and lateral to medial direction to completely expose clean subchondral bone along the entire slope of the joints.

X. Use a 5-mm acorn or round cutting burr to remove any posterior osteophytes. This allows for good surface contact for the graft (Fig. 12-9).

XI. Once the osteophyte has been thinned and the posterior longitudinal ligament is visible along the entire width of the disk space, remove the remaining osteophytes.

XII. Care should always be taken not to plunge posteriorly as the spinal cord is in intimate contact with the underlying posterior longitudinal ligament. By inserting the tip of the Kerrison rongeur parallel to the end plate and rotating the tip underneath the vertebral margin, a cleaner amputation of the posterior annulus and osteophyte is possible.

XIII. The central decompression is completed when a micronerve hook passes freely from lateral margin across to the contralateral margin under both the superior and inferior end plates.

XIV. At this time, attention should be directed toward the foramen on the symptomatic side. It is preferable to delay the foraminotomy until last because a dense vascular cuff surrounds the shoulder of the exiting nerve root and it is quite easy to injure this microvascular structure, causing significant bleeding.

XV. After thorough bony decompression, repeat palpation out along the nerve to ensure that there is no retained disk material along the nerve and that all osteophytic compression has been relieved. As you work further out along the nerve, keep in mind that the vertebral artery runs vertically just lateral to the exit of the foramen proper (Fig. 12-10). Therefore, the tip of the Kerrison rongeur must not

Ask your attending how and when he or she prefers to perform a foraminotomy.

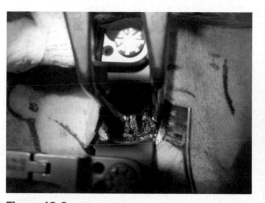

Figure 12-8
Partially removed overhanging osteophyte.

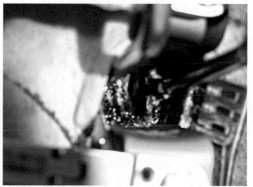

Figure 12-9
Pre and post posterior osteophyte resection.

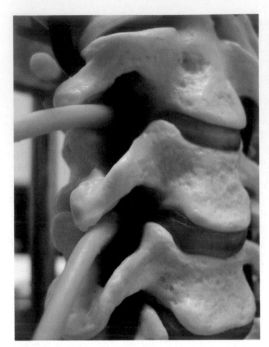

Figure 12-10
Depiction of artery and nerve anatomy.

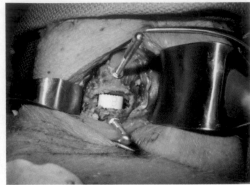

Figure 12-11
Graft recessed.

> Does your attending prefer autograft or allograft? Are there any patients that should receive autograft (e.g., smokers)? What technique does your attending physician prefer for harvesting autograft?

penetrate out the bony margin of the foramen, or vertebral artery injury is possible.

XVI. Trial spacers are available in various size intervals generally ranging from 5 up to 10 mm. The spacer is inserted using light taps with a mallet until the fit is snug, not tight. Once the size is chosen, autograft is harvested from the iliac crest.

XVII. Insert the graft with the same force as the spacer. If more effort is required, stop and recheck the sizing. Insertion is not complete until the anterior margin of the graft is countersunk below the anterior vertebral body (Fig. 12-11).

XVIII. Relax the Caspar pin distractor and ask the neurophysiologist to recheck motor signals. If there are any changes in the patient's neurologic status, remove the graft and re-evaluate the situation.

Plating/Stabilization

I. Remove the Caspar pins and distractor and back-fill the pin holes with bone wax.

II. Next, plane down any anterior osteophytes that prevent the plate from lying flat against the vertebral bodies. Remember that the esophagus is intimate with the plate and that any excessive anterior prominence will result in dysphagia.

III. Size the plate such that the screw holes are minimally covering the vertebral body above and below. Care should be taken to ensure that the plate does not override the margins of the adjacent disk spaces because this impingement leads to rapid adjacent level degeneration.

IV. Have an assistant hold the plate steady while you insert the screws. In some systems, pilot holes are necessary, whereas in others, the screws are self-drilling. In general, 14-mm screws are used, but different-sized screws may be necessary depending on patient anatomy. The screws should be angled slightly convergent toward, but not crossing, the midline. In addition, the superior screws are angled slightly upward, whereas the inferior screws are angled slightly downward (Fig. 12-12).

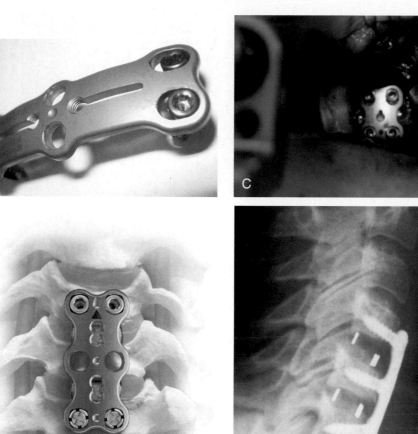

Figure 12-12
A, Anterior cervical plate. **B,** Spine model demonstrating proper placement of an anterior cervical plate.
C, Intraoperative view of plate placement. **D,** Postoperative lateral radiograph of an anterior cervical plate in proper position.

V. Re-evaluate the plate position with respect to the midline, superior, and inferior vertebral bodies. Secure all four screws if the position is adequate. Take a final fluoroscopic image and have the neurophysiologist obtain a final motor test.

Wound Closure

I. Ensure that all retractors are removed from the wound and that the wound is irrigated.
II. Make sure to achieve hemostasis prior to closing the wound. Most surgeons insert a Penrose or a small Jackson Pratt drain to minimize postoperative hematoma formation.
III. There is no distinct fascial layer that requires reapproximation. Close the subcutaneous layer and skin in a standard fashion, using a subcuticular closure for the skin (see Chapter 1 for details; Fig. 12-13).

POSTOPERATIVE CARE

I. Most patients are placed in a hard Philadelphia or Miami J collar prior to extubation. Following extubation, it is imperative that a detailed upper and lower extrem-

> Ask your attending how long the hard collar should stay in place.

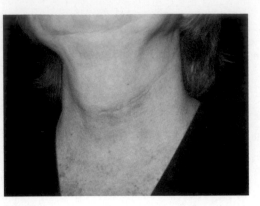

Figure 12-13
Healed anterior cervical wound.

ity neurologic examination be performed and documented in the patient's chart.

II. The patient is placed on appropriate postoperative antibiotics for 24 hours.

III. Deep venous thrombosis is rare, and sequential compression boots should be used while in bed. Pharmacologic anticoagulation is contraindicated following spine surgery due to the risk of an epidural hematoma.

IV. A liquid diet should be ordered for the next meal, and it can be advanced to house if the patient can tolerate swallowing. It is not uncommon for a mechanical soft diet to be needed for one or two meals postoperatively due to transient dysphagia.

COMPLICATIONS

I. Transient dysphagia is the most common complication and almost always resolves completely.

II. Dysphonia is a less common complication that also usually resolves, but not as quickly. In most cases, improvement is noted prior to hospital discharge. However, if the patient is still dysphonic at follow-up, a laryngoscopy is indicated to ascertain vocal cord paresis versus paralysis.

III. Postoperative hematoma is a rare but life-threatening complication. The evolution is usually slow, with the patient complaining of difficulty swallowing that is not improving and possibly worsening. This is followed by difficulty breathing. Unfortunately, there is often a rapid progression from difficulty breathing to airway compromise, so quick recognition and treatment is paramount. The airway should be protected by intubation on the floor followed by hematoma evacuation in the operating room. If intubation is not possible, it may be necessary to open the wound at bedside to relieve the pressure and allow intubation.

IV. Infection is a rare complication, but it can occur. Any infection is from an esophageal injury until proven otherwise. A swallowing study is indicated to evaluate for leaks.

V. Any neurological change in the postoperative period warrants repeat plain radiographs and an MRI.

SUGGESTED READINGS

Albert TJ, Murrell S: Surgical management of cervical radiculopathy. J Am Acad Orthop Surg 7:368–376, 1999.

Emery SE: Cervical spondylotic myelopathy: Diagnosis and treatment. J Am Acad Orthop Surg 9:376–388, 2001.

Rhee JM, Riew KD: Cervical spondylotic myelopathy: Including ossification of the posterior longitudinal ligament. In Orthopaedic Knowledge Update 3. Rosemont, IL, American Academy of Orthopaedic Surgeons, 2006, pp 235–251.

CHAPTER 13

Lumbar Microdiskectomy

Derek J. Donegan   and   Kingsley R. Chin

1

Case Study

A 44-year-old male presents to the clinic with an 8-week history of low back and left lateral leg pain. He complains of subjective leg weakness and numbness over the lateral malleolus, the lateral aspect of the foot, and the web space between his fourth and fifth toes. On presentation, his back pain has nearly resolved, and his weakness has markedly improved. His pain continues to be aggravated by activity and alleviated by rest. He describes the pain as a nagging, aching, and burning sensation with radiation from the left buttock to the outside part of the ankle and extending to the outside aspect of the left foot. He has participated in a low back stabilization program with physical therapy, taken nonsteroidal anti-inflammatory drugs daily, and received three epidural steroid injections. Axial and sagittal magnetic resonance imaging scans are presented in Figure 13-1.

BACKGROUND

I. Lumbar disk herniations are typically a result of a herniated disk fragment from the nucleus pulposus of the disk. In normal conditions, this nucleus is in the disk center secured by the surrounding annulus fibrosis. When this fragment of nucleus herniates, it irritates and/or compresses the adjacent nerve root and incites an inflammatory reaction. The inflammatory mediators and the mechanical compression lead to pain, weakness, and paresthesias along the dermatomal distribution of the involved nerve root and can be characterized by the term *radiculopathy*. This radicular pain syndrome in the distribution of the L4-S3 is also known as *sciatica*.

> Radiculopathy refers to the group of compressive symptoms occurring in a specific dermatomal distribution.

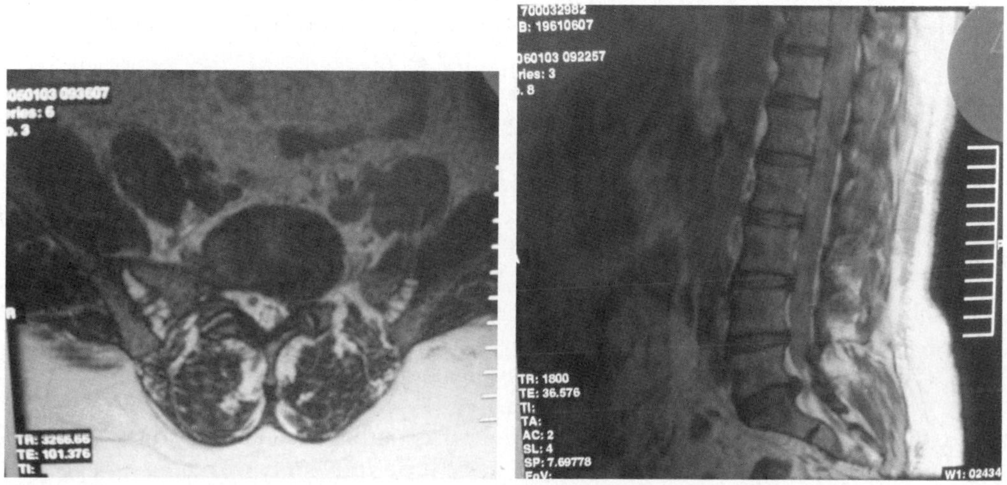

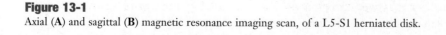

Figure 13-1

Axial (**A**) and sagittal (**B**) magnetic resonance imaging scan, of a L5-S1 herniated disk.

TABLE 13-1 Motor and Sensory Components of Posterolateral Disk Herniations

Disk Herniation	Nerve Root	Sensory Deficit	Motor Deficit	Reflex Changed
L3-L4	L4	Posterolateral thigh, anterior knee, and medial leg	Quadriceps Hip adductors	Decreased patellar tendon and tibialis anterior tendon
L4-L5	L5	Anterolateral leg, dorsum of foot, and great toe	Gluteus medius EHL EDL/EDB	Decreased tibialis posterior tendon
L5-S1	S1	Lateral malleolus, lateral foot, heel, and web of fourth and fifth toes	Gluteus maximus, peroneus longus and brevis, gastrocnemius-soleus complex	Decreased Achilles tendon

EDB, extensor digitorum brevis; EDL, extensor digitorum longus; EHL, extensor hallucis longus.

II. Most people experience back pain during their lifetime, but approximately 5% of males and 2.5% of females experience actual lumbar radiculopathy as a consequence of nerve root compression or irritation.

III. The typical history of lumbar disk herniation is of repetitive lower back and buttock pain that is relieved by rest. This pain is suddenly exacerbated by a flexion episode, with the sudden appearance of leg pain being much greater than back pain. Most radicular pain from nerve root compression caused by a herniated nucleus pulposus is evident by leg pain equal to or greater than the degree of back pain. The pain is usually intermittent and is exacerbated by activity, especially sitting, straining, sneezing, or coughing, and is relieved by rest. Other symptoms include weakness and paresthesias along the same myotome and dermatome, respectively.

> Lumbar disk herniation is characterized by leg pain greater than or equal to back pain.

IV. Physical examination findings in patients with lumbar disk herniations are characteristic to the level of disk herniation and nerve root involvement. A posterolateral disk herniation at the L4-L5 level typically causes impingement of the traversing nerve root, L5. Far lateral (foraminal or extraforaminal) disk herniations typically impinge on the exiting nerve root, L4. The patient may have a positive straight leg raise with hip flexion, keeping the knee extended. Patients may also exhibit objective weakness and paresthesias in the distribution of the involved nerve root. Table 13-1 summarizes the main motor and sensory components involved with posterolateral disk herniations at common lumbar disk levels.

V. More than 95% of the ruptures of the lumbar intervertebral disks occur at the L4-L5 level.

VI. When a herniated disk is suspected based on history and physical examination, magnetic resonance imaging is the imaging modality of choice for diagnosis. Plain lumbar radiographs have little utility.

> Magnetic resonance imaging is the imaging modality of choice for the diagnosis of a herniated disk.

VII. Herniated disks can be either contained or noncontained.
   A. A contained disk herniation occurs when the disk material herniates through the inner annulus but not the outer annulus. The disk material, although contained, can still distort the path of the nerve.
   B. A noncontained disk herniation occurs when the disk material penetrates both the inner and outer layers of the annulus. The material can therefore reside beneath the posterior longitudinal ligament, can penetrate through it, or can be sequestered as a free fragment.

VIII. Cauda equina syndrome consists of the combination of saddle anesthesia, bilateral ankle areflexia, loss of rectal tone, bilateral lower extremity weakness, and possible bowel and bladder dysfunction with retention or incontinence. Cauda equina can be caused by massive extrusion of a disk involving the entire diameter of the lumbar canal and is considered a surgical emergency.

> CAUDA EQUINA SYNDROME IS A SURGICAL EMERGENCY.

IX. The main goal of lumbar microdiskectomy is symptomatic relief of leg pain. Back pain is often not relieved and is not an indication for microdiskectomy.

TREATMENT ALGORITHM

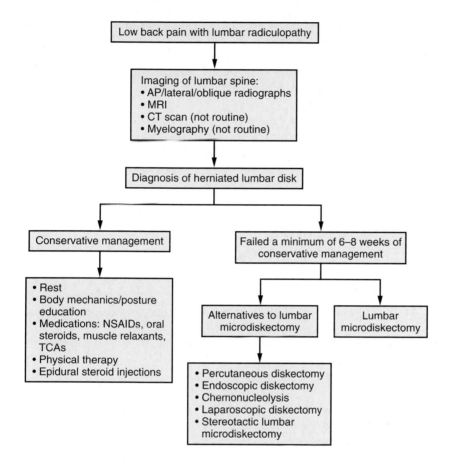

NONOPERATIVE TREATMENT OPTIONS

I. **Rest**
   A. Two days of rest have been shown to be better than longer periods in returning to work.
   B. Lying in the semi-Fowler position (lying with a pillow between both legs while flexing both the hips and knees) should relieve most of the pressure on the disk and nerve roots.
   C. As pain diminishes, the patient should be encouraged to begin nonstrenuous activities.

II. **Education in Proper Posture and Body Mechanics**
   A. "Back school" is a class regarding proper back ergonomics.
   B. This class is beneficial in decreasing the amount of time lost from work with acute exacerbations, but does little to decrease the incidence of recurrence of symptoms.

III. **Medications**
   A. Narcotics and muscle relaxants can help with the pain and paraspinal muscle spasms. However, these should be prescribed with caution, especially in the instances of chronic back and leg pain where drug addiction and increased depression are frequent.
   B. An oral steroid (methylprednisone—"steroid dose pack") taper may be prescribed acutely as a potent anti-inflammatory agent.

C. Nonsteroidal anti-inflammatory drugs are often a good adjunct to the conservative treatment approach.

D. Tricyclic antidepressant agents such as amitriptyline may be beneficial in reducing sleep disturbances and anxiety as well as providing pain relief without the need for narcotics.

IV. **Physical Therapy**

A. Exercises should be fitted for the individual symptoms and not forced as an absolute group of activities.

B. Patients whose pain is eased from passive extension can benefit from passive extension exercises rather than passive flexion, whereas patients whose pain is eased with passive flexion can benefit from passive flexion exercises rather than passive extension.

C. All exercises that exacerbate painful symptoms should be avoided.

D. Exercises should focus on strengthening the abdominal and lumbar paraspinal muscles and stretching the hamstrings. These modalities allow load transfer from the spinal column and intervertebral disks to the surrounding supporting structures.

E. The benefit of most physical therapy programs lies in the promotion of good posture and body mechanics.

V. **Epidural Steroid Injections**

> At which point in his or her treatment algorithm does your attending send patients for epidural injections? How successful have epidural injections been in his or her practice?

A. Injecting the combination of a long-acting steroid with an epidural anesthetic such as methylprednisone and lidocaine, bupivacaine, or procaine into the epidural space of the affected nerve root may provide pain relief for up to several months.

B. Most studies show a 60% to 85% short-term success rate but injections are most effective within 6 weeks of symptom onset.

C. Better results are found in patients with subacute or chronic leg pain with no prior surgery.

D. Epidural steroid injections tend to offer prolonged pain relief without excessive narcotic use.

E. The complication rate is approximately 5% and consists of failure to inject into the epidural space, intrathecal injections with inadvertent spinal anesthesia, transient hypotension, difficulties voiding, severe paresthesias, cardiac angina, headache, retinal hemorrhage, facial flushing, generalized erythema, and bacterial meningitis.

F. Contraindications include presence of current infection, neurological disease, hemorrhagic of bleeding diathesis, cauda equina syndrome, and a rapidly progressing neurologic deficit.

G. Typical protocols involve a series of three injections each at 7- to 10-day intervals.

SURGICAL ALTERNATIVES TO LUMBAR MICRODISKECTOMY

> Ask your attending about alternatives to microdiskectomy.

I. **Percutaneous Diskectomy**

A. Automated percutaneous diskectomy

1. Through an incision 8 to 12 cm from the midline, an automated percutaneous diskectomy device is placed through a cannula inserted in the center of the symptomatic disk under fluoroscopic guidance and uses suction and cutting to remove the appropriate disk material.

2. Indications are similar to those for a lumbar microdiskectomy (discussed later).

3. Contraindications include lumbar stenosis, lateral recess stenosis, or synovial joint cysts.

B. Percutaneous laser diskectomy

1. This technique is identical to the automated percutaneous diskectomy technique. Once there is access to the disk space, a laser is used to remove the appropriate disk material.

2. Indications are similar to those for lumbar microdiskectomy (discussed later).
3. Contraindications include previous history of lumbar surgery, lumbar stenosis, facet hypertrophy, and a free disk fragment.

II. **Percutaneous Endoscopic Diskectomy**
   A. This technique is similar to the automated percutaneous diskectomy technique. However, direct visualization is obtained with the use of an angled rigid endoscope, and the disk can be removed using forceps.
   B. Indications are similar to those for lumbar microdiskectomy and include contained or small noncontained disk herniations.
   C. Contraindications include severe motor deficits, rapidly progressive neurologic deficits, cauda equina, segmental instability, previous history of lumbar surgery, large noncontained disk herniations, sequestered disks, spinal stenosis, spondylolisthesis, tumors, and post-traumatic root compression.

III. **Lumbar Chymopapain Chemonucleolysis**
   A. This procedure is typically performed under local anesthesia and sedation with the patient in the prone or lateral decubitus position. An 18-gauge needle is inserted 8 to 11 cm from the midline and directed toward the affected disk space. Needle placement is confirmed with the use of fluoroscopy. Once the needle position is confirmed, chymopapain is injected over approximately a 4-minute period.
   B. Indications are similar to those for microdiskectomy and include contained and noncontained disk herniations.
   C. Contraindications include an allergy to papain or papaya, cauda equina syndrome, disk migration, central or lateral recess stenosis, severe spondylolisthesis, history of diskitis, peripheral neuropathy, pregnancy, and previous diskectomy at the same level.

IV. **Laparoscopic Diskectomy**
   A. The procedure is performed by either a transperitoneal approach or a retroperitoneal approach. Each type involves the use of laparoscopic ports that are used to insert instruments and visualizes the affected disk space. Once the disk space is visualized, the disk is removed under direct visualization.
   B. Transperitoneal laparoscopy is performed with the patient in the supine position, and the retroperitoneal approach is performed with the patient in the lateral decubitus position.
   C. Indications are similar to those for microdiskectomy and include leg pain greater than back pain, radicular signs and symptoms, and 6 weeks of failed conservative management,
   D. Contraindications include disk fragments that have completely migrated below the level of the disk space.

V. **Stereotactic Lumbar Microdiskectomy**
   A. This procedure is typically performed with the patient in the prone position on a computed tomography scan table under local anesthesia and sedation. The stereotactic system is used with computed tomography guidance to mark the target and entry points. Once confirmed, a trocar is placed along the target path. The position of the trocar tip is confirmed via computed tomography imaging and the procedure continues with the use of a nucleotome to aspirate the appropriate disk material.
   B. Indications are similar to those for microdiskectomy and include radicular signs and symptoms with corresponding imaging, as well as symptoms of diskogenic back pain without significant radicular symptoms.
   C. Contraindications include spondylosis, spondylolisthesis, spinal stenosis, and marked facet hypertrophy.

SURGICAL INDICATIONS FOR LUMBAR MICRODISKECTOMY

I. Indications for surgical treatment are not clearly delineated, because long-term results greater than 2 years between nonoperative and operative treatment are equivalent with surgery being more favorable for short-term outcomes. Therefore, surgery is an elective choice except in cases of cauda equina syndrome.

II. Relative indications include:

A. Patients demonstrating progressive neurologic deficit during a period of observation.

B. Patients with persistent bothersome lumbar radiculopathy despite conservative management for a period of 6 to 8 weeks.

RELATIVE CONTRAINDICATIONS FOR LUMBAR MICRODISKECTOMY

I. Patients who have back pain after their lumbar radiculopathy has resolved are not good surgical candidates for operative treatment. Surgical intervention is not geared toward curing a patient's back pain.

II. It is of utmost importance to ensure a complete workup is done prior to proceeding with surgery to ensure the diagnosis of a lumbar herniated disk is accurate and an alternative pathology has not been missed.

III. Patients that have undergone an inadequate period of conservative treatment are not considered to be good surgical candidates. The natural history demonstrates that 85% of patients with a herniated disk have resolution of their symptoms within 3 months.

GENERAL PRINCIPLES OF LUMBAR MICRODISKECTOMY

I. **Anatomy**

A. Vertebrae (Fig. 13-2)

1. Posteriorly, the bony arches encircle the spinal canal and consist of the transverse processes, facet joints, two pedicles, two laminae, and the spinous process.

2. The facet joints are composed of the superior and inferior articulating surfaces of the vertebrae below and above, respectively.

> Patients must fail conservative management before exploring surgical options.

> What duration of conservative management does your attending prefer before proceeding with surgical intervention?

> Back pain as the primary symptom is a relative contraindication for lumbar microdiskectomy unless the patient has substantial leg symptoms correlating with a single lumbar herniated disk and understands that microdiskectomy may not help the back pain.

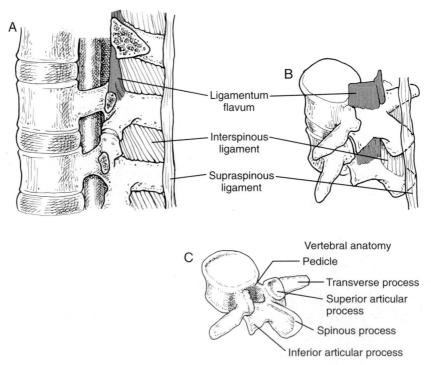

Figure 13-2
Vertebral anatomy. **A,** Sagittal view. **B,** Oblique view of the lumbar vertebrae, showing ligamentum flavum thickening in the caudad extent of intervertebral space and in the midline. **C,** Oblique view of single lumbar vertebra. *(From Miller R: Miller's Anesthesia, 6th ed. Philadelphia, Churchill Livingstone, 2005.)*

3. The neural foramen is adjacent to the pedicles and the facet joints and marks the exit of the corresponding nerve root.

B. Intervertebral disk

1. The disk provides support and allows for movement while resisting excessive movement.

2. The disk is composed of the nucleus pulposus, which is typically soft and surrounded by the annulus fibrosis, which is tough and fibrous.

3. Each disk is bonded to the vertebral body above and below by a thin cartilaginous bridge referred to as the *end plate*. This end plate is vascular and is responsible for disk nutrition. The end plate also supports the disk and decreases the risk of disk herniation and maintains its shape.

C. Ligaments

1. Each disk is reinforced anteriorly and posteriorly by the anterior and posterior longitudinal ligaments, respectively.

2. The laminae are connected by the ligamentum flavum, and the spinous processes are connected by the interspinous ligament and the supraspinous ligament.

D. Nerves

1. The cauda equina is the fanning bundle of the lumbar and sacral nerve roots exiting the spinal cord.

2. The cord typically terminates at the level of L1 or L2, which is termed the *conus medullaris*.

3. The exiting nerve root in the lumbar spine is numbered according to the pedicle above (i.e., the L4 nerve root passes below the L4 pedicle between the L4-L5 disk space).

II. **General Principles**

A. Lumbar microdiskectomy is considered the gold standard for surgical treatment of a herniated lumbar disk.

B. Microdiskectomy requires an operating microscope with a 400-mm lens, special retractors, a variety of small-angled rongeurs, and microinstruments.

C. The patient is placed in the prone position typically on an Andrews table.

D. The patient position allows the abdomen to hang free, which minimizes epidural venous dilation and bleeding.

E. Fluoroscopy is used to confirm the appropriate disk space.

F. The procedure is typically performed on an outpatient basis.

G. There is less postoperative pain secondary to the limited dissection utilized.

In the lumbar spine, the corresponding nerve exits below its vertebral body; therefore the L4 nerve root exits below L4 at the L4-L5 disk space.

An Andrews table allows for decreased bleeding due to minimizing epidural venous engorgement and opens the interlaminar space, making decompression easier.

ALWAYS CONFIRM THAT THE APPROPRIATE DISK SPACE IS BEING EXPOSED.

COMPONENTS OF THE PROCEDURE

Positioning, Prepping, and Draping

I. After induction of general anesthesia, the patient is placed in the prone position on an Andrews table with all bony prominences well padded (Fig. 13-3).

II. The lumbar spine is prepped and draped in standard fashion (see Chapter 1).

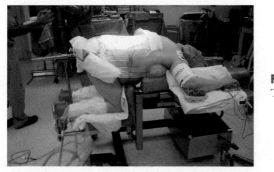

Figure 13-3
The patient is shown prone on an Andrew's table.

Surgical Approach

I. Using a 22-gauge spinal needle and fluoroscopy, the affected disk space is localized. The iliac crest can be used to correlate to the spinous process of the fourth lumbar vertebra.

II. The skin and soft tissues are then infiltrated with 20 mL of 1% lidocaine and 1:200,000 epinephrine.

III. Next an incision, approximating the width of the surgeon's index finger, is made approximately 1 cm lateral to the midline of the spine on the side toward the herniated disk at the appropriate level.

IV. Using a Cobb elevator, the subcutaneous layers are elevated off the lumbodorsal fascia.

V. Then an incision 0.5 mm lateral to the spinous process and in line with the skin incision is created through the lumbodorsal fascia.

VI. Using the Cobb elevator, the erector spinae muscles are elevated off the associated laminae and spinous processes.

VII. A speculum retractor system is then placed in the wound using the leading edge of the beveled side of the speculum. The instrument is positioned using a back-and-forth clockwise and counterclockwise rotation while slowly advancing it through the soft tissue planes (Fig. 13-4).

VIII. Once docked against the facet and lamina, using the assistance of a microscope and pituitary rongeur, the intervening soft tissue inside the cannula is removed until the interlaminar space is identified.

IX. A lateral fluoroscopic view is then taken with the speculum in place to confirm the location relative to the desired disk space.

X. If necessary, a laminotomy is performed to allow access to the disk space. At the L5-S1 level, bone resection is rare due to the large interlaminar space.

Disk Excision

I. Extraforaminal disks are then excised from outside the spine.

II. The dura and nerve roots are then exposed and retracted away from the herniated disk.

III. A probe is used to locate the annular defect, and a pituitary rongeur is used to remove any loose fragments. It is important to remove all of the loose disk fragments to minimize the recurrent disk herniation.

IV. The canal space beneath the nerve root and dura are then explored for loose disk fragments, and the foramen is probed to ensure adequate space for the nerve root.

V. Forced irrigation is then placed into the disk space through the annular defect to remove any additional loose disk fragment.

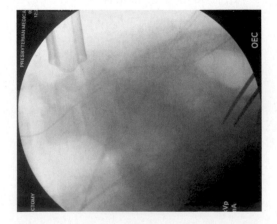

Figure 13-4
Intraoperative lateral fluoroscopy image demonstrating a speculum retractor in place and marking the appropriate disk space.

Wound Closure

I. The wound is then copiously irrigated and hemostasis is achieved.

II. The lumbodorsal fascia is then closed in standard fashion (see Chapter 1) to achieve a watertight closure.

III. The subcutaneous layer is closed in standard fashion and the skin edges are opposed with a subcutaneous closure (see Chapter 1). The lesion is covered with a sterile dressing.

IV. Toradol 30 mg is typically administered intravenously for postoperative pain.

POSTOPERATIVE CARE AND REHABILITATION

I. Mobilization is started immediately after surgery.

II. Pain is controlled with oral narcotics and muscle relaxants.

III. Anticoagulation for deep venous thrombosis prophylaxis is contraindicated.

IV. Isometric abdominal and lower extremity exercises are started.

V. Patients are instructed to minimize sitting and riding in a vehicle initially and increase as pain permits.

VI. The patient is advised to return to "back school" at postoperative week 4 to 6.

VII. Lifting, bending, and stooping are prohibited for the first several weeks but are gradually restarted after postoperative week 6.

VIII. Lower extremity strengthening exercises can be instituted postoperative weeks 8 to 12.

IX. Return to work mostly depends on the work requirements for each individual, but range anywhere from 2 to 3 weeks up to 3 months.

> **ANTICOAGULATION FOLLOWING SPINE SURGERY IS CONTRAINDICATED DUE TO THE RISK OF DEVELOPING AN EPIDURAL HEMATOMA, AND STUDIES HAVE SHOWN THAT LEG COMPRESSION DEVICES PROVIDE ENOUGH PROTECTION AGAINST DVT.**

> Ask your attending about his or her postoperative rehabilitation protocol.

COMMON COMPLICATIONS OF LUMBAR MICRODISKECTOMY

I. Wound infection

II. Postoperative diskitis

III. Dural tears

IV. Thrombophlebitis

V. Nerve root injury

VI. Pulmonary embolism

VII. Cauda equina syndrome

VIII. Pyogenic spondylitis

IX. Injury to abdominal blood vessels

X. Injury to abdominal viscera

> Symptoms of a dural tear include a headache that is worse when upright and alleviated by lying flat.

SUGGESTED READINGS

Chin KR, Adams SB, Khoury L, Zurakowski D: Patient behavior patterns if given access to their surgeon's cellular telephone. Clin Orthop 439:260–268, 2005.

Chin KR, Michener TA: Prospective of a 3-blade speculum cannula for minimally invasive lumbar microdiscectomy. J Spinal Disord Tech 19:257–261, 2006.

Chin KR, Sundram H, Marcotte P: Bleeding risk with ketorolac after lumbar microdiscectomy. J Spinal Disord Tech 20:123–126, 2007.

Williams KD, Park AL: Lower back pain and disorders of intervertebral discs. In Canale ST (ed): Campbell's Operative Orthopaedics, 10th ed. Philadelphia, Mosby, 2003, pp 1955–2028.

Spine

CHAPTER 14

Posterior Lumbar Fusion for Degenerative Spondylolisthesis/Stenosis

Safdar N. Khan and Eric O. Klineberg

Case Study

A 69-year-old female dance instructor with a 3-year history of back and leg pain presents to the clinic. She complains predominantly of leg pain, which is greater than the back pain. She has some radicular symptoms with burning and numbness and "shooting pains" down the back of her legs to the soles of the feet. She is, however, able to find a position of comfort. When sitting in a chair at home, she has minimal back symptoms and no leg pain. On sitting up or standing, she has worsening of her back pain, and her leg pain begins after standing or walking for only a few moments. She is able to walk farther when leaning forward or holding onto a shopping cart. She denies any bowel or bladder dysfunction. The patient has had physical therapy and lumbar epidural steroid injections, which initially relieved the pain, but the past few injections have led to no significant relief. Anteroposterior and lateral radiographs of the lumbar spine are presented in Figure 14-1.

BACKGROUND

I. The term spondylosis is defined as nonspecific degenerative changes in the architecture of the spine and surrounding soft tissues. These degenerative changes may lead to anterior or posterior movement of one vertebral body on the subsequent, lower vertebral body. This is known as spondylolisthesis. With long-standing disease, the degenerative process may result in stenosis or narrowing of the spinal canal.

II. Degenerative spondylolisthesis is extremely common at the L4-L5 level, with 1 to 3 mm of vertebral body translation occurring in nearly 40% of asymptomatic patients. The pathogenesis is primarily related to chronic intervertebral disk degeneration and segmental and rotational instability with facet joint arthrosis. As the disk degenerates, the spinal segment loses some of its stability and is able to translate both anterior and posterior with flexion and extension. This eventually results in mechanical back pain, with relief of symptoms while sitting or lying down, but exacerbation of pain with sitting up or walking (spinal segment moves to a new position).

> The L4-L5 level is the most common level for degenerative spondylolisthesis.

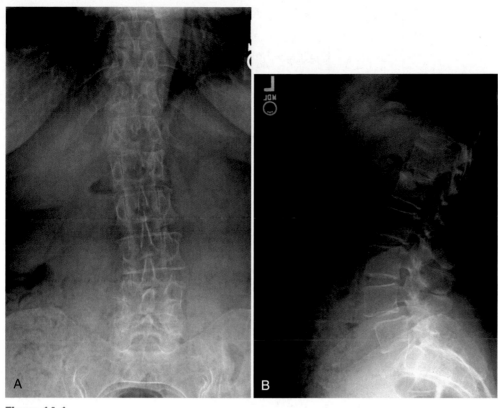

Figure 14-1
Anteroposterior (**A**) and lateral (**B**) radiographs of the lumbar spine show degenerative spondylolisthesis of L4 over L5.

III. Degenerative spondylolisthesis rarely progresses beyond 25% anterolisthesis due to intact posterior elements in contrast to congenital spondylolisthesis.

IV. The degenerative process rarely becomes symptomatic before 50 years of age and disproportionately affects women, especially black women, with a male-to-female ratio of 1:6.

V. Degenerative spondylolisthesis is generally asymptomatic; however, it can be associated with symptomatic spinal stenosis, which is the most common reason for lumbar surgery in patients older than 65 years of age.

VI. Patients typically complain of low back pain and radicular or referred leg pain, and it may produce symptoms of classic neurogenic claudication.

VII. In central stenosis with resulting neuroclaudication, patients detail activity-related lower extremity pain or heaviness, which diminishes with spinal flexion. These patients usually note increased activity tolerance when ambulating in a flexed position (e.g., walking with a cane or shopping cart).

VIII. Lateral recess stenosis usually heralds itself with monoradicular symptoms. The nerve root most commonly involved is L5. These monoradicular symptoms may or may not be related to activity or positional changes.

Remember to take a thorough history and ask questions specifically directed toward differentiating vascular claudication from neurogenic claudication.

A complete physical examination should include evaluation for myelopathy (clinical signs demonstrating spinal cord impingement).
Remember to have all patients tandem walk and ask them specifically about difficulty in performing fine motor tasks such as buttoning shirts, and so on.

TREATMENT ALGORITHM

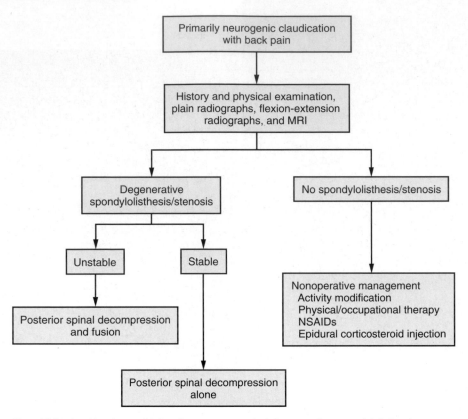

Note: This algorithm is a guideline for management of degenerative spondylolisthesis with stenosis.

What is your attending's treatment algorithm for axial back pain without any leg pain?

TREATMENT PROTOCOLS

I. **Treatment Considerations.** All of these considerations play an important role in the decision-making process of treating patients with degenerative spondylolisthesis/stenosis.
  A. Patient age
  B. Activity level
  C. Overall health
  D. Amount of leg pain compared with back pain
  E. Patient expectations
  F. Sagittal and coronal imbalance

II. Patients with leg pain, minimal back pain, and a stable spondylolisthesis may only need decompressive surgery. Relief can be dramatic in patients with primarily lower extremity claudication symptoms. Similarly, the operative approach may vary. Younger patients may benefit with reconstruction of the anterior column and restoration of the lumbar lordosis, whereas older patients usually benefit with faster posterior-only procedures.

III. **Imaging Modalities**
  A. Plain radiographs should be assessed for the following features:
    1. Global lumbar lordosis, soft tissue shadows, fractures of the pars interarticularis, and tumors
    2. Sagittal and coronal alignment
    3. Evidence and extent of spondylolisthesis as classified by the Meyerding classification

a. Grade I: less than 25% anterolisthesis
b. Grade II: 25% to 50% anterolisthesis
c. Grade III: 50% to 75% anterolisthesis
d. Grade IV: 75% to 100% anterolisthesis
e. Grade V: more than 100% anterolisthesis (spondyloptosis)
4. Pedicle morphology (e.g., size, orientation)
B. Flexion-extension radiographs. Standing lumbar flexion-extension radiographs reveal the extent of listhesis (translation) and correlate to the degree of posterior element incompetence. The listhesis may also be stable in older patients. In these patients, the anterior column has gone on to fuse with the degeneration of the anterior disc.
C. Computed tomography (CT) scan with or without myelography
1. Useful when additional bony detail is needed to assess the degree of stenosis and facet joint involvement joints.
2. CT myelography is used in revision cases to evaluate stenosis proximal and distal to the previously fused segment when instrumentation scatter makes using magnetic resonance imaging (MRI) difficult.
D. MRI
1. MRI is the imaging modality of choice to evaluate the disc space, intervertebral disk morphology, and spinal nerves relative to their foramina.
2. Axial MRI scans linked to the sagittal views reveal areas of intervertebral disk herniation and stenosis (central vs. lateral vs. foraminal vs. far lateral).

> Do not forget to assess active adolescent patients with back pain for pars interarticularis fractures with 30-degree oblique radiographs ("Scottie dog" view) and/or bone scans (Fig. 14-2).

Spine

Superior articular process   Pars fracture

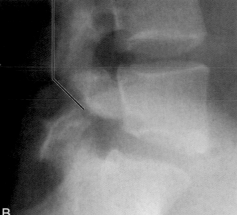

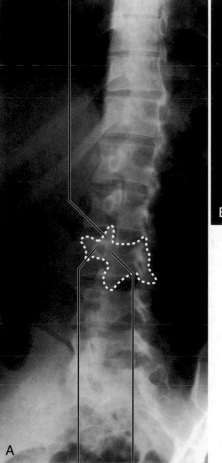

Figure 14-2
Radiograph of lumbar region of vertebral column, oblique view ("Scottie dog"). **A,** Normal. **B,** Fracture of pars interarticularis. *(From Drake RL, Vogl W, Mitchell AWM: Gray's Anatomy for Students. Philadelphia, Churchill Livingstone, 2005.)*

Pedicle   Pars interarticularis

Ask your attending to explain the different types of spinal stenosis and their clinical presentations.

ALWAYS QUESTION PATIENTS FOR A HISTORY OF A PACEMAKER, METAL IN THE EYE, ANEURYSM CLIPS, OR OTHER METAL IMPLANTS IN THE BODY PRIOR TO OBTAINING A MAGNETIC RESONANCE IMAGING SCAN.

3. Facet signal changes can be seen on T2-weighted scans, and this correlates with unstable spondylolisthesis.
4. Note: MRI scans are taken with patients supine; the actual amount of spinal compression may be worse as the patient stands and the listhesis becomes more evident. Also, reduction of the spondylolisthesis in the MRI scanner may suggest that simple patient positioning in physiologic lordosis on the operating table may reduce the listhesis.

IV. **Nonoperative Treatment Options**
  A. Initial treatment strategy
   1. Nonsteroidal anti-inflammatory drugs or acetaminophen
   2. Activity modification (i.e., participating in low-impact activity, avoiding offending motions)
   3. Heat and cold therapy, modalities such as iontophoresis, and ultrasound
   4. Physical and occupational therapy
     a. Physical therapy should focus on eliminating stiffness and strengthening the paraspinal muscles.
       (1) Typically a home exercise program can be taught.
       (2) Aqua therapy can be used for exercises and decreasing stress across muscles and joints due to the buoyant effects of water.
     b. Occupational therapy is aimed at teaching alternative ways of accomplishing activities of daily living that may be impaired or elicit symptoms.
  B. Epidural corticosteroid injection
   1. Injections are considered if adequate progress has not been made after 4 to 6 weeks of physical therapy.
     a. Steroids are typically injected in combination with a local anesthetic (lidocaine and/or bupivacaine).
     b. Targeted steroid injections can be performed at various foramina, which may be both therapeutic (relieve pain) and diagnostic (differentiates between L5 and S1 intervertebral disk involvement) in patients with back and leg pain and multilevel stenosis. This may aid in determining future levels of decompression/fusion.
   2. Steroids can decrease pain that may be limiting a patient's ability to perform exercises.
   3. An injection can be repeated after several months if it gives symptomatic relief, but no more than three injections per year should be administered.
   4. Although prolonged relief may not be possible with epidural injections, they can give patients some short-term relief and better define the disease process and prognosis for any surgical intervention.

Radicular leg pain is typically the principal indication for surgery in patients who fail nonoperative management. Surgical intervention has a more predictable outcome regarding relief of leg than relief of isolated axial back pain.

SURGICAL INDICATIONS FOR LUMBAR DECOMPRESSION/FUSION FOR DEGENERATIVE LUMBAR SPONDYLOLISTHESIS/STENOSIS

  I. Failed nonoperative treatment (minimum 3 to 6 months)
 II. Prominent or progressive lower extremity weakness
III. Acute foot drop due to massive disk herniation in young, active patients (see Chapter 13 for details on treatment of acute disk herniations)

RELATIVE CONTRAINDICATIONS TO LUMBAR DECOMPRESSION/FUSION FOR DEGENERATIVE LUMBAR SPONDYLOLISTHESIS/STENOSIS

  I. Current or recent infection (e.g., diskitis or osteomyelitis)
 II. Local skin problems (e.g., decubitus ulcers)
III. Medical instability. Patient is unable to safely tolerate the stress of surgery.

GENERAL PRINCIPLES OF LUMBAR DECOMPRESSION/FUSION FOR DEGENERATIVE LUMBAR SPONDYLOLISTHESIS/STENOSIS

I. Decompressive lumbar laminectomy with posterolateral fusion with pedicle screw instrumentation for degenerative spondylolisthesis/spinal stenosis usually results in significant relief of neurogenic claudication. The key portion of the procedure is decompression of the neural elements; fusion prevents continued motion or worsening of motion once the posterior elements have been removed.

II. Preoperative imaging with CT scans, MRI, or CT myelograms (revision cases) is mandatory to visualize the degree and location of the spinal stenosis. Imaging studies must correlate with the patient's symptoms.

III. The goals of lumbosacral segmental instrumentation are to reduce deformity and to provide stability, thus increasing the chances for successful posterolateral fusion. The pedicle is the strongest portion of the vertebra; thus, it is the ideal anatomic structure for three-column spinal fixation.

IV. Intraoperative radiographs are mandatory to confirm appropriate levels for decompression and fusion. Sacralization of the lowest lumbar segment can lead to confusion with regard to determining the correct level of surgery.

V. Pedicle screw pullout strength is a function of bone mineral density; a preoperative dual-energy x-ray absorptiometry scan indicating less than 0.45 g/cm^2 of bone density predicts pedicle screw loosening. Screw purchase may be increased with triangulated (convergent) placement of bilateral pedicle screws at a single level.

VI. Because the pedicle is the strongest part of the vertebral body where screw purchase is optimal, adding long screws do not promote greater stability. It is advisable to stay 0.5 cm from the anterior cortex to avoid perforation. Screw length and vertebral body depth can be measured on preoperative CT scans.

> **DO NOT ASSUME THAT ALL PATIENTS HAVE FIVE LUMBAR VERTEBRAE. SOME PATIENTS MAY HAVE SACRALIZATION OF A LUMBAR VERTEBRA.**

Spine

COMPONENTS OF THE DECOMPRESSIVE LAMINECTOMY AND POSTEROLATERAL FUSION WITH PEDICLE SCREW PLACEMENT

Positioning, Prepping, and Draping

I. The patient is typically placed in the prone position on a Jackson table (Fig. 14-3) with the abdomen hanging free and decompressed. This position

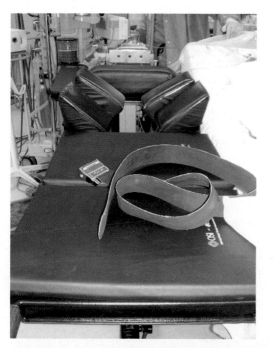

Figure 14-3
Jackson spine table for prone patient positioning.

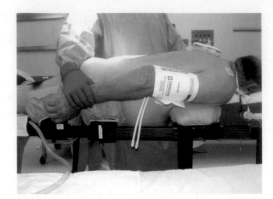

Figure 14-4
Patient in the prone position prior to prepping and draping.

The iliac crests correspond to the L4-L5 disc space. This surface anatomic landmark aids in determining the appropriate incision level.

decreases the mean central venous pressure, leading to decreased engorgement of the epidural veins and diminished intraoperative blood loss.

II. The patient may also be placed in a kneeling position, but this position should be avoided if considering fusion because this will decrease lumbar lordosis.

III. Patients are typically placed under general anesthesia for the procedure. Care must be taken to ensure that no pressure is on the orbits because postoperative vision loss is a catastrophic complication.

IV. The skin should be shaved over the surgical site and the iliac crests palpated.

V. All bony prominences are well padded, including the knees and the ankles. Remember to place padding in the axilla as well as the elbows. Ideally, the arms should be placed with the shoulders and elbows at less than 90 degrees of flexion to prevent an axillary or ulnar nerve neurapraxia (Fig. 14-4).

VI. Neuromonitoring is often used when spine fusion is planned with pedicle screw fixation. Make sure that the neurophysiologist has adequately placed the appropriate leads prior to prepping the patient. (See Chapter 34 for details on nerve monitoring and spine surgery.)

VII. Once adequately positioned, the surgical field is prepped and draped in standard fashion according to the surgical principles outlined in Chapter 1.

VIII. Next mark the skin incision using a sterile marker utilizing the iliac crests as an anatomic landmark.

Surgical Approach

I. An incision is made over the midline, most frequently over L4-L5 and extending the length of the area to be decompressed.

II. The dissection is carried down to the fascia, and self-retaining retractors are positioned. Using a Cobb elevator and Bovie cautery, the fascia is incised on either side of the midline and reflected laterally to the facet joints. Care must be taken not to violate the capsules of the facets not involved in the final fusion levels.

III. A Kocher clamp is placed on a preselected spinous process and a Woodson probe placed on the undersurface of the corresponding lamina. Once this is done, an intraoperative lateral radiograph is taken to delineate the exact fusion level.

IV. Once the fusion level is confirmed, a far lateral dissection then ensues with stripping of the posterior spinous musculature, including the multifidus muscles from the appropriate transverse processes.

V. The muscles are stripped from medial to lateral using a Cobb to assist in retracting. The Bovie tip is kept visualized at all times and stay on bone to avoid plunging into the spinal canal. Steady, sweeping motions are used to peel the musculofascial layers off the spine. The spinous process, lamina, pars interarticularis, facet joints, and transverse process are exposed at each lumbar level requiring fusion.

VI. Once adequate exposure has been accomplished, the spinal canal can be decompressed.

Decompression and Pedicle Screw Placement

I. Decompression is initiated with removal of the interspinous ligament using a heavy rongeur. Use a large Leksell to remove the superior spinous process and half of the inferior spinous process for adequate exposure.

II. Begin thinning the lamina on both sides with a high-speed burr. Then, begin decompressing the central stenosis with a Kerrison rongeur. Leave the ligamentum flavum as a temporary shield over the dura.

III. Decompression with a Kerrison rongeur is done in a caudal to cephalad manner. Be mindful of the pars interarticularis on each side to avoid fractures.

IV. A medial facetectomy aids in lateral recess decompression. The medial aspect of the inferior facet may be removed with a sharp ¼-inch osteotome, and the underlying superior facet may be removed with a Kerrison rongeur. Remove the ligamentum flavum and bone bilaterally out to the level of the pedicle.

V. A Woodson probe is used to feel the pedicle from within the canal. Adequate decompression should allow the tip of the probe to pass into the foramina.

VI. Once the decompression has been completed, pedicle screw fixation and posterolateral spine fusion can be attempted.

VII. Classically, the entry point to the pedicle is defined by the intersection of a horizontal line in the midline of the transverse process and a vertical line in the inferior lateral facet margin. The horizontal line is 1 to 2 mm below the facet joint line and the vertical line should be 2 to 3 mm lateral to the lateral pars and must be angulated laterally as one moves caudally in the lumbar spine.

VIII. A 4-0 burr is then used to decorticate the entry point. A pedicle probe is used to proceed through the pedicle and the vertebral body. The screw path may be tapped, and a ball-tipped probe is used to feel the inferior, medial and lateral walls for cortical cutout.

IX. Screws can then be inserted. If there is any doubt to the nature of the interpedicular tract, fluoroscopic guidance can be used.

X. Alternatively, a "canoe technique" may be used to place pedicle screws. In this technique, a rongeur is used to bite off the facet osteophytes at its junction with its corresponding pars interarticularis. Then, a unicortical bite ("canoe") is carefully made with a rongeur on the exposed dorsal surface of the transverse process. A curette is then used to decorticate the transverse process from lateral to medial, taking care not to break the transverse process. Continuing medially, at the junction of the transverse process, pars interarticularis, and the facet joint, the pedicle entry site is carefully breached. A ball-tipped probe is then used to feel for cortical cutout followed by pedicle screw placement.

XI. Intraoperative electromyographic potentials measured by neuromonitoring are used to ensure appropriate position of the pedicle screws. Threshold value normative data is as follows:
A. 0 to 4 mA: high likelihood of pedicle wall breach
B. 4 to 8 mA: possible pedicle wall breach
C. More than 8 mA: no pedicle wall breach

XII. The wound is thoroughly irrigated with a pulse irrigator.

XIII. The next step is rod placement. The pedicle screw head may be monoaxial (uniplanar) or polyaxial (multiplanar) depending on the instrumentation system used. Similarly, precontoured rods or intraoperatively contoured rods may be used.

XIV. Short rods are placed between two adjacent pedicle screws. The rod is secured to the pedicle screw with the use of an end cap. The end caps are tightened using a torque wrench.

REMEMBER FOR LUMBAR PEDICLE SCREW PLACEMENT, MEDIAL ANGULATION INCREASES BY 10 DEGREES PER LEVEL, FROM 0 DEGREES AT THE UPPER LUMBAR LEVEL TO 30 DEGREES AT L5.

Note that lateral recess decompression is best performed by the surgeon from the opposite side of the table.

ONCE PEDICLE SCREW PLACEMENT AND DECOMPRESSION IS COMPLETE, MAKE SURE TO OBTAIN ANOTHER SET OF INTRAOPERATIVE POSTEROANTERIOR AND LATERAL RADIOGRAPHS. YOU MAY CHANGE THE ORIENTATION OF YOUR PEDICLE SCREWS BASED ON THESE FINAL RADIOGRAPHS (Fig. 14-5).

Spine

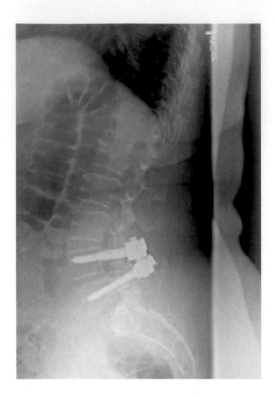

Figure 14-5
Lateral postoperative radiograph of a posterolateral fusion at the L4-L5 level.

XV. The transverse processes of the fused levels are decorticated with a 4-0 burr. Be careful not to fracture the transverse processes.

XVI. Bone graft (iliac crest bone graft vs. bone morphogenetic protein) is placed in the lateral gutter over the decorticated transverse processes.

Wound Closure

I. After thorough irrigation with a pulse irrigator, adequate hemostasis is achieved and a subfascial drain is placed prior to closing the wound.

II. The wound is closed in standard fashion with a Biosyn subcuticular closure used for reapproximating the skin, and a sterile dressing is applied (see Chapter 1 for details).

POSTOPERATIVE CARE

I. The drain is removed on postoperative day 2 or when the drain output is less than 30 mL per shift.

II. Postoperatively, patients are encouraged to ambulate with help as soon as possible.

III. Remember to order standing radiographs (AP and lateral) when able.

IV. The use of a postoperative orthosis is arguable. A lumbar corset for comfort may be given to the patient when out of bed.

V. Deep venous thrombosis chemoprophylaxis is not required due to the risk of epidural hematoma formation. Sequential compression devices are placed on both lower extremities while the patient is in the hospital.

VI. Follow-up in 4 weeks with repeat anteroposterior and lateral standing lumbar spine radiographs. In the interim, tell patients that they should not do any bending, twisting, or lifting more than 5 pounds.

COMPLICATIONS

I. Nerve/spinal cord injury

II. Inadequate decompression

III. Infection

IV. Iatrogenic durotomy

V. Incidental durotomy. If this occurs, a watertight seal should be obtained either primarily with a 6-0 Prolene suture or with a facial graft. Fibrin glue (cryoprecipitate, thrombin, and calcium) can be placed over the defect. The patient should be on complete bed rest for 24 hours after the procedure and monitored for a dural leak. If there is a dural leak, the patient typically presents with a headache when sitting up. If in doubt, whether intraoperatively or in the postoperative period, a neurosurgical consult should be obtained.

SUGGESTED READINGS

Bell G: Orthopaedic Knowledge Update: Spine 2. Rosemont, IL, American Academy of Orthopaedic Surgeons, 2002.

Weinstein JN, Lurie JD, Tosteson TD, et al: Surgical versus nonsurgical treatment for lumbar degenerative spondylolisthesis. N Engl J Med 356:2257–2270, 2007.

SECTION IV

PELVIS AND ACETABULUM

CHAPTER 15

Open Reduction and Internal Fixation of Posterior Wall Fractures

Keith D. Baldwin,   Jaimo Ahn,   and   Samir Mehta

Case Study

A 23-year-old man presents to the trauma center after being involved in a motor vehicle collision. When he arrived in the resuscitation bay, airway, breathing, circulation, disability, and exposure were assessed according to the Advanced Trauma Life Support (ATLS) protocol. The patient is tachycardic but normotensive, warm, and well perfused. There is no stridor or wheezing, and the respiratory rate is slightly tachypneic. A detailed secondary survey is conducted and is significant for hip and groin pain, obvious deformity of the left lower extremity compared to the right (shortened and internally rotated), and visible discomfort with attempted range of motion of the left hip. Two large-bore intravenous catheters are placed, intravenous fluid is started, and laboratory studies are obtained. Radiographs of the chest and pelvis are taken. A dislocated left hip is noted on the anteroposterior (AP) pelvic radiograph. Sedation is given and the hip is reduced in the resuscitation bay. The patient is taken to computed tomography for evaluation, and postreduction images (Fig. 15-1) are obtained. A distal femoral traction pin is placed. The patient has no additional operative injuries and is admitted for definitive stabilization of the posterior wall fracture within 24 to 72 hours based on his medical progress.

Pelvis and Acetabulum

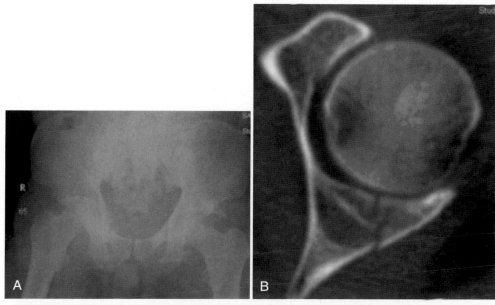

Figure 15-1

A, Anteroposterior radiograph of the pelvis demonstrating a left hip dislocation with a posterior wall fragment. **B,** A postreduction computed tomography scan depicts a concentrically reduced hip joint with a minimally displaced posterior wall fracture.

The Judet-Letournel classification for acetabular fractures is divided into elementary and associated fracture patterns. Elementary fracture patterns include the following: posterior wall, posterior column, anterior wall, anterior column, and transverse. Associated fracture patterns consist of the following: T-type, posterior column/posterior wall, transverse/posterior wall, anterior column/posterior hemitransverse, and associated both column.

Sciatic nerve injury is present in as many as 30% of posterior hip dislocations.

IF RADIOGRAPHS REVEAL A FRACTURE-DISLOCATION OF THE FEMORAL HEAD WITH AN ASSOCIATED POSTERIOR WALL FRACTURE, THEN AN IMMEDIATE ATTEMPT AT A CLOSED REDUCTION IS WARRANTED.

BACKGROUND

I. Posterior wall fractures are the most common type of acetabular fractures and comprise approximately 50% of all acetabular fractures (associated and elementary patterns) in most published series.

II. The amount of injury to the posterior wall is typically dictated by such factors as mechanism of injury, position of the femoral head within the acetabulum, position of the lower extremity at time of impact, patient age, bone quality, and energy imparted to the patient.

III. Posterior wall fractures are sometimes colloquially referred to as "dashboard injuries."

IV. Posterior wall fractures are associated with posterior dislocations of the hip joint between 40% and 70% of the time in various series.

V. An isolated posterior wall fracture can be classified as an "elementary" fracture pattern in the Judet-Letournel classification of acetabular fractures.

VI. Posterior wall fractures can also occur as a part of more complex fracture patterns, so when a posterior wall fracture is detected, the entire pelvic ring should be assessed.

VII. A low threshold should be maintained to assess the entire pelvic ring and acetabulum.

VIII. The posterior wall can be best visualized on an obturator oblique radiograph of the pelvis.

IX. An isolated femoral head dislocation without an associated fracture of the posterior wall is a rare occurrence (10% in the highest series). More often, dislocation of the femoral head results in a fracture of the posterior wall (tension-type failure).

X. Post-traumatic injury to the sciatic nerve can occur up to 30% of the time with a posterior wall fracture-dislocation.

INITIAL TREATMENT

I. **Treatment Considerations**
   A. Energy imparted to the patient
   B. General trauma survey including standard ATLS protocol
   C. Thorough secondary survey, including detailed neurovascular examination
   D. Evaluation and documentation of rectal tone
   E. Vaginal examination to rule out open fractures of the pelvic ring
   F. Urgent reduction and maintaining reduction of a dislocated femoral head

II. **Initial Approach**
   A. General trauma survey
      1. ATLS protocol
         a. Adequate resuscitation
         b. Maintain hemodynamic stability
         c. Circumferential sheet or commercial pelvic binder to reduce pelvic volume
      2. Evaluate soft tissue
      3. Ultrasound examination or other visceral/abdominal organ system evaluation
      4. Standard radiographs (lateral cervical spine, anteroposterior chest, anteroposterior pelvis)
      5. Dislocated femoral head should be addressed urgently with reduction
   B. Neurovascular evaluation
      1. Vascular assessment by palpation or Doppler
         a. Dorsalis pedis artery
         b. Posterior tibial artery
         c. Popliteal artery
         d. Have a low threshold for performing ankle brachial indices in light of a dislocated hip or other abnormal physical examination finding

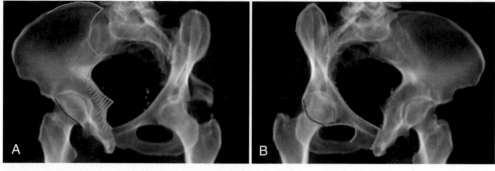

Figure 15-2
Iliac oblique (**A**) best demonstrates the posterior column (*light blue*) and anterior wall (*purple*). Obturator oblique (**B**) best demonstrates the anterior column (*green*) and posterior wall (*red*).

     2. Neurological assessment: sciatic nerve
        a. Motor: foot dorsiflexion for anterior tibialis muscle
        b. Sensation: webspace between the first and second toe
  C. Additional imaging
     1. AP pelvis radiograph (if not obtained with initial trauma workup)
     2. Judet radiographs
        a. Iliac oblique (45-degree external rotation) radiograph to visualize the following structures:
           (1) Posterior column
           (2) Anterior wall
        b. Obturator oblique (45-degree internal rotation) radiograph to visualize the following structures (Fig. 15-2):
           (1) Anterior column
           (2) Posterior wall
     3. Computed tomography (CT)
        a. Should be obtained with the femoral head reduced in the acetabulum
        b. Fine-cut CT scan (usually 1.5 3 mm) is recommended through the region of concern
        c. Demonstrates complexity of fracture
        d. Allows for assessment of marginal fracture impaction (Fig. 15-3)
        e. Identifies presence of intra-articular fragments (Fig. 15-4)
        f. Helps rule out associated femoral head or neck fractures

> **A THOROUGH NEUROLOGICAL EXAMINATION OF THE INVOLVED EXTREMITY IS MANDATORY, WITH DOCUMENTATION OF SCIATIC NERVE FUNCTION, BECAUSE THE NERVE IS AT RISK FOR IATROGENIC INJURY AS WELL.**

> **CONSIDER OTHER DASHBOARD INJURIES SUCH AS POSTERIOR CRUCIATE LIGAMENT RUPTURE.**

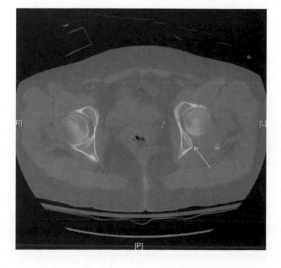

Figure 15-3
Axial computed tomography scan demonstrating marginal impaction (*arrow*). The marginal impaction needs to be reduced, similar to opening a door along its hinges, before reduction of the posterior wall component. The void left by impaction of the subchondral surface into the soft cancellous bone may need to be filled with allograft or autograft. Marginal impaction often indicates the region where the anterior femoral head was in contact with the posterior wall. There may be a corresponding defect of the femoral head.

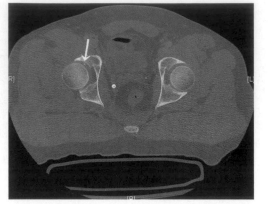

Figure 15-4
Axial computed tomography scan demonstrating an
incarcerated fragment with nonconcentric reduction
(*arrow*). Debris within the articulation of the femoral
head with the acetabulum can prevent accurate and
concentric reduction of the femoral head.

TREATMENT ALGORITHM

> RADIOGRAPHICALLY,
> INVOLVEMENT OF BETWEEN
> 25% AND 40% OF THE
> POSTERIOR WALL IMPLIES AN
> UNSTABLE POSTERIOR WALL
> FRACTURE.

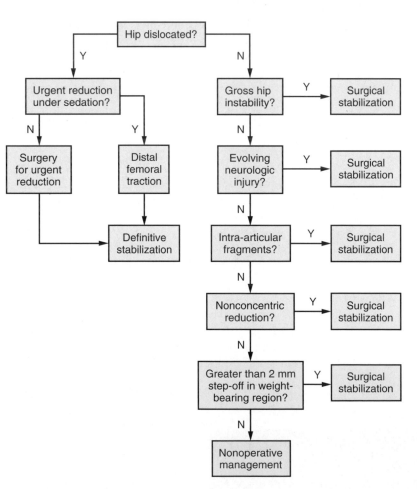

NONOPERATIVE TREATMENT

I. **Indications**

A. Small posterior wall fracture with no history of dislocation or instability

B. Examination under anesthesia (with fluoroscopy) that reveals a stable hip joint
with no subluxation or dislocation

C. Stable neurologic examination

D. Radiographic criteria

1. Concentric reduction

2. No intra-articular or incarcerated fracture fragments

3. Less than 2 mm of articular weight-bearing surface displacement

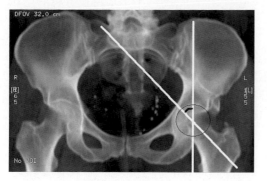

Figure 15-5
The roof arc angle is constructed by a vertical line through the rotational center of the acetabulum and a second line through the point where the fracture crosses the radiographic dome. The roof arc angle is the angle formed by the intersection of these lines.

    4. Roof arc angle greater than 45 degrees on three radiographic views (Fig. 15-5)

    5. Subchondral arc of 10 mm by CT

II. **Management**

  A. Unstable posterior wall fractures

    1. Distal femoral traction can be considered in patients who are not surgical candidates.

    2. Usually approximately 10 to 15 pounds of traction is needed.

    3. Duration is 3 to 4 weeks.

    4. Progressive weight bearing is typically started at 6 weeks.

    5. Frequent radiographic assessment is required to assess for fracture displacement.

  B. Stable posterior wall fractures

    1. Touch-down weight bearing is appropriate.

    2. Sixty-degree hip flexion precautions should be taken.

    3. Weekly radiographic assessment for loss of reduction is necessary.

    4. Progress the patient to full weight bearing at 6 to 12 weeks following the injury.

    5. Physical therapy for abdominal strengthening, low back exercises, and quadriceps training of involved limb are usually helpful adjuncts in obtaining an optimal functional outcome.

OPERATIVE TREATMENT

  I. **Indications**

    A. Irreducible fracture-dislocation

    B. Unstable hip

      1. Gross instability

      2. Inability to maintain reduction

      3. Greater than 25% to 40% of posterior wall involvement on CT (Fig. 15-6)

    C. Incarcerated fragments

    D. Evolving neurologic injury

    E. Greater than 2 mm of articular surface displacement

  II. **Relative Contraindications to Surgical Treatment**

    A. Severe soft tissue injury (Morel-Lavalle lesion)

    B. Visceral injury

    C. Local or systemic infection

    D. Severe osteoporosis

    E. Medical comorbidities

  III. **Timing**

    A. Surgical emergency

      1. Open acetabular fracture

      2. Evolving neurologic injury

      3. Vascular compromise

      4. Irreducible dislocation

Pelvis and Acetabulum

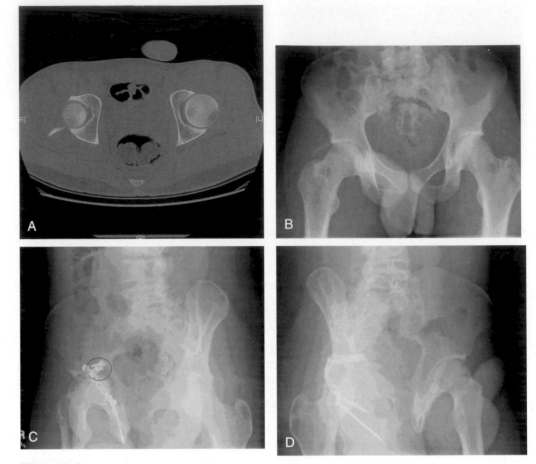

Figure 15-6

An atypical unstable posterior wall fracture. The computed tomography scan (**A**) shows less than 25% of the posterior wall involved. However, the patient had a history of femoral head dislocation acutely reduced and unstable hip on fluoroscopic examination in the operating room. **B** is a preoperative anteroposterior pelvis radiograph. The postoperative Judet view radiographs (**C** and **D**) reveal a small fragment fixation contoured and balanced over the small posterior wall piece. However, given the size and peripheral nature of the fragment, an additional spring plate (*circle*) was used to enhance fixation.

   B. Delayed surgical stabilization
      1. Open reduction and internal fixation performed within 24 to 96 hours of presentation if stable
      2. Optimize operating room environment
      3. Preoperative planning
      4. Soft tissue management

RELEVANT SURGICAL ANATOMY

   I. **Palpable Surface Landmarks**
      A. Posterior superior iliac spine
      B. Greater trochanter
      C. Femoral shaft
   II. **Superficial Surgical Anatomy**
      A. Gluteus maximus
      B. Tensor fascia lata
      C. Trochanteric bursa
      D. Inferior gluteal nerve
   III. **Deep Surgical Anatomy**
      A. Retraction of the gluteus medius reveals the gluteus minimus and the short external rotators (including the quadratus femoris).

B. Overlying the quadratus femoris is the sciatic nerve.

C. Sciatic nerve and the piriformis are intimate. Aberrant muscle bellies of the piriformis or anatomic variants of the sciatic nerve need to be taken into account when performing the piriformis tendon tenotomy.

IV. **Vascular Anatomy**

A. The medial femoral circumflex artery provides the major blood supply to the femoral head.

B. This artery is at risk with dissection or resection of the quadratus femoris.

COMPONENTS OF THE PROCEDURE

Positioning, Prepping, and Draping

I. The patient can be positioned in either the prone or lateral position on a radiolucent table.

A. The lateral position is more familiar to most surgeons.

B. Prone positioning often helps facilitate reduction and plate application.

C. In this chapter, the authors describe prone positioning (Fig. 15-7).

II. The involved limb should be draped free into the sterile field.

III. Fluoroscopic imaging should be used to confirm that appropriate views can be obtained intraoperatively prior to starting the case. The surgical field should be prepped and draped in standard fashion according to the surgical principles outlined in Chapter 1.

Surgical Exposure

I. In a Kocher-Langenbach approach exposure for isolated posterior wall fractures, an 8- to 10-cm skin incision is made from the tip of the greater trochanter distally along the shaft of the femur. A second incision (approximately 12 to 18 cm) is made from the posterior sacroiliac spine to the tip of the greater trochanter. The two incisions should meet (Fig. 15-8).

II. The tensor fascia lata is split to the level of the tip of the greater trochanter. The superior skin incision is then carried down to the fascia of the gluteus maximus,

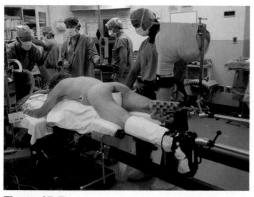

Figure 15-7

Prone positioning for the Kocher-Langenbach approach to the acetabulum. The patient is being positioned on a special operating table (Profx, OSI Medical, California) designed in particular for pelvic and acetabular surgery. The involved limb is on the patient's right side. The table allows for control of the limb and can flex the knee and extend the hip to take tension off of the sciatic nerve. Furthermore, the table is radiolucent. Alternatively, and more commonly, the procedure can be performed on a radiolucent table (e.g., Jackson table).

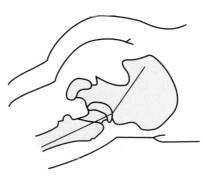

Figure 15-8

An 8- to 10-cm skin incision is made from the tip of the greater trochanter distally along the shaft of the femur. The second incision (approximately 12 to 18 cm) is made from the posterior sacroiliac spine to the tip of the greater trochanter. The two incisions should meet at the area indicated. The incision line above is shown.

which is incised in line with the superficial skin incision. The gluteus maximus muscle belly is then bluntly divided, maintaining hemostasis.

III. The trochanteric bursa is excised, and the hematoma that is typically present is removed.

IV. The gluteus medius is retracted superiorly, revealing the gluteus minimus and the short external rotators. The gluteus minimus is débrided to the level of the superior gluteal neurovascular bundle.

V. The sciatic nerve is identified and its course followed to assess any anomalous anatomy. The sciatic nerve rests on the quadratus femoris muscle, which should be identified. Iatrogenic injury to this muscle may damage the medial femoral circumflex artery.

VI. The piriformis tendon and conjoint tendon (superior gemellus, obturator internus, and inferior gemellus) are tenotomized and tagged for later repair.

VII. The knee is bent to 90 degrees and the hip is extended, which minimizes tension on the sciatic nerve. A retractor can be placed anterior to the sciatic nerve, but with great care.

VIII. After subperiosteal elevation of the greater sciatic notch and quadrilateral surface, the posterior wall fracture is exposed. The fracture should then be débrided. Be cautious not to devascularize the fracture fragments by disrupting their capsular blood supply.

IX. If intra-articular fragments are present that need to be removed, traction on the leg along with pharmacologic relaxation (paralysis) allows access to the joint.

Fracture Reduction

I. The fracture should be reduced under direct visualization, with the assistance of a ball-spike pusher and K-wires for provisional stabilization. Prior to definitive reduction, any marginal fracture impaction should be addressed.

II. Lag screws may be placed perpendicular to the fracture plane if necessary to maintain reduction.

III. A buttress plate is the mainstay of fixation. One or two 3.5-mm pelvic reconstruction plates may be necessary. The plates are usually between six to eight holes in length, and the plates need to be undercountered prior to application. As the screws are placed into the plate, it contours to the bone and provides the desired buttress effect. It is important to balance the plate well along the posterior wall fragment so that it is well contained by the force of the plate.

IV. The screws placed should be directed away from the joint. Two screws in the proximal portion of the plate and two screws in the distal portion of the plate are usually sufficient in terms of fixation.

V. Once the posterior wall fragment is reduced, the limb should be taken through a range of motion to assess any restrictions. Fluoroscopic imaging should also be used to confirm the extra-articular placement of the screws.

VI. The wound should be thoroughly irrigated at this point. Any necrotic muscle should be débrided as this is a potential source of heterotopic ossification. The tenotomized tendons, piriformis, and conjoint tendons are repaired using a large-caliber, nonabsorbable, braided suture. A layered closure in standard fashion over drains should be performed (see Chapter 1 for details).

POSTOPERATIVE CARE AND COMMON COMPLICATIONS

I. **Postoperative Evaluation**
   A. Assess sciatic nerve function.
   B. Assess neurovascular status.
   C. Obtain postoperative hemoglobin and manage drain output.

II. **Surgical Wound Infection**
   A. Higher risk when postoperative hematoma occurs
   B. Higher risk with coexisting abdominal and or visceral organ damage
   C. Higher risk when local soft tissue compromised

III. **Heterotopic Ossification**
   A. Occurs in approximately 20% of cases where no prophylaxis is initiated
   B. Prophylaxis
      1. Indomethacin 25 mg three times daily PO for 6 to 8 weeks
      2. Radiation therapy (1 dose 700 cGy within 48 hours of surgery)
   C. Most commonly occurs with extended iliofemoral exposure; Kocher-Langenbach is the second most common.

IV. **Post-traumatic Arthritis**
   A. Up to 20% occurrence in anatomically reduced posterior wall fractures
   B. Risk factors
      1. Greater than 2 mm of articular step-off
      2. Marginal impaction
      3. Femoral head impaction
      4. Cartilage necrosis
      5. Posterior wall resorption
   C. Aseptic necrosis (osteonecrosis)
      1. Between 5% and 10% of posterior wall fractures
      2. Limited association between surgical approach and development of avascular necrosis

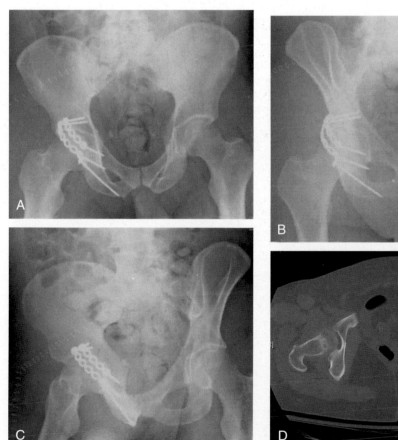
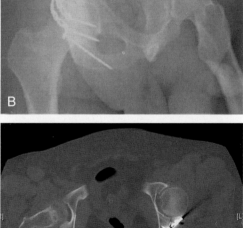

Figure 15-9
A to **C**, Postoperative anteroposterior and Judet radiographs following fixation of an unstable posterior wall fracture. Due to the size of the posterior wall component, an atypical construct with two small fragment plates was used in this case. **D**, The axial computed tomography scan reveals reduction of the posterior wall articular surface with less than 2 mm of step-off and a concentric reduction of the femoral head.

3. Often related to energy imparted at time of injury (e.g., impaction of femoral head or dislocation)

V. **Thromboembolitis**
   A. Mechanotherapy and pharmacotherapy
   B. Early mobilization

REHABILITATION

I. Touch-down weight bearing begins immediately postoperatively. If there is bilateral lower extremity involvement, it may be necessary to consider wheelchair transfers or a pressure unloading seating system.

II. No hip flexion precautions are necessary.

III. Pharmacologic thromboprophylaxis is mandatory.

IV. Lower extremity strengthening exercises are essential for obtaining an optimal functional outcome.

V. At 6 weeks postoperatively:
   A. Assess radiographs (Fig. 15-9).
   B. Progress from touch-down weight bearing to full weight bearing over the course of the subsequent 6 weeks.

VI. The patient should be transitioned to full weight bearing by 12 weeks postoperatively.

VII. Physical therapy, including abdominal strengthening and low back programs along with aquatic therapy, is also useful adjunct treatment in the postoperative period.

SUGGESTED READINGS

Buchholz RW, Heckman JD, Court-Brown CM (eds): Rockwood and Green's Fractures in Adults, 6th ed. Philadelphia, Lippincott Williams & Wilkins, 2006.

Koval KJ, Zuckerman JD: Handbook of Fractures, 3rd ed. Philadelphia, Lippincott Williams & Wilkins, 2006.

Thompson JC: Netter's Concise Atlas of Orthopaedic Anatomy. Teterboro, NJ, Medimedia USA, 2002.

Tile M, Helfet D, Kellam J: Fractures of the Pelvis and Acetabulum. Philadelphia, Lippincott Williams & Wilkins, 2003.

CHAPTER 16

External and Internal Fixation of Symphysis Pubis Widening

Nirav H. Amin, Jaimo Ahn, and Samir Mehta

Case Study

A 35-year-old male involved in a motor vehicle collision is taken to an emergency department and evaluated in the resuscitation bay. Following a general trauma survey utilizing the Advanced Trauma Life Support (ATLS) protocol, the patient is hemodynamically stable but isolated orthopedic injuries are noted. On physical examination, the patient complains of pain through the anterior aspect of the pelvis along with pain on palpation. There are no open injures and both lower extremities are neurovascularly intact. An anteroposterior (AP) pelvis radiograph demonstrates a pubic symphysis disruption (Fig. 16-1).

BACKGROUND

I. The incidence of pelvic ring injuries is approximately 20/100,000 to 37/100,000 and represents 0.3% to 6% of all fractures; 20% occur in patients with polytrauma. Pelvic fractures are often the result of high-energy, blunt forces such as motor vehicle collisions or falls from a height. Therefore, patients with these fractures require an emergent and thorough evaluation.

II. Treatment can be surgical or nonsurgical, but emphasis should be placed on reconstituting a stable pelvic ring that allows appropriate transfer of weight from the axial skeleton (lower extremities) to the appendicular skeleton (spine and pelvis).

III. As compared with the extremities, the pelvis has greater soft tissue constraints and protects vital nonmusculoskeletal organs. Therefore, treatment of pelvic ring injuries often requires techniques that differ from those used in the extremities.

> Approximately 40% of patients who have a pelvic fracture have an intra-abdominal source of bleeding.

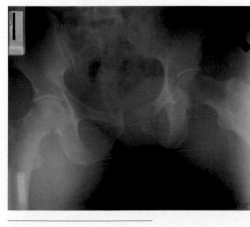

Figure 16-1
Pelvis anteroposterior radiograph with increased widening of the pubic symphysis consistent with an injury of the anterior pelvic ring given the patient's mechanism of injury. The right sacroiliac joint also shows some potential widening. The remainder of the pelvic ring, including the sacrum, the acetabuli, and the proximal femora, show no fractures or dislocations. A computed tomography scan would further evaluate these regions of interest.

Pelvis and Acetabulum

IV. Some basic mechanisms of injury include an anteroposterior directed force, which can cause external rotation of a hemipelvis relative to the sacrum; a laterally directed force, which can cause internal rotation; and a cephalad or caudad force vector, which can cause a "vertical shear" of the injured hemipelvis. All these mechanisms may cause disruption of the posterior, anterior, or both portions of the pelvic ring.

ANATOMY

I. **Bony Anatomy.** The pelvis is composed of three bones: one sacrum and two innominate bones, which in turn form from the fusion of the immature ischium (posteroinferior); ilium (superior); and pubis (anteroinferior). The acetabulum forms at the junction of these three bones. Important bony prominences and landmarks include the anterior superior iliac spine, anterior inferior iliac spine, iliac crest and fossa, posterior superior iliac spine, ischial spine, ischial tuberosity, inferior and superior pubic rami, pectineal eminence, and pubic tubercle (Fig. 16-2).

II. **Ring Stability.** The bony pelvis is stabilized primarily by the pubic symphyseal ligaments anteriorly and the posterior and interosseous ligaments posteriorly. The pubic symphysis is composed of a complex of hyaline cartilage, fibrocartilage, and fibrous tissues. The sacroiliac (SI) joints are composed of both hyaline and fibrocartilage. The SI joints are stabilized by anterior, posterior, and interosseous ligaments; the latter are the strongest ligaments in the body. The anterior and posterior elements of the pelvis are further stabilized relative to each other through sacrospinous (AP and rotational vectors) and long and short sacrotuberous (vertical vector) ligaments. From an inlet view, the sacrum forms an inverted keystone or suspension bridge (Fig. 16-3) that has inherent stability when the surrounding structures are in continuity; with loss of bony or ligamentous constraints, the sacrum tends to displace anteriorly (the bridge will fall). From an outlet view (Fig. 16-4), the sacrum forms the keystone of an arch that transfers weight from the spine to the acetabuli.

III. **Nonmusculoskeletal Structures.** The pelvis has an intimate and constrained relationship with a number of structures including branches of the lumbosacral plexus, main and terminal branches of the iliac vascular system, lower gastrointestinal tract, and genitourologic structures including the bladder and urethra. Knowledge of this anatomy is critical to the complete evaluation of the patient, as well as for surgical management.

THE MOST COMMON NERVE INJURED IS L5, AND THE SECOND MOST COMMON IS S1.

Absence of intra-abdominal or intrathoracic bleeding in a patient with shock indicates the pelvis as a likely source.

ANGIOGRAPHY SHOULD BE CONSIDERED IF HEMORRHAGE CONTINUES DESPITE A REDUCTION OF THE PELVIC VOLUME.

INITIAL MANAGEMENT

I. **General Trauma Survey**
   A. ATLS protocol, general resuscitation, and attendance to life-threatening issues
   B. Initial evaluation of head/neck and thoracoabdominal injuries typically before extremities
   C. Application of sheet or pelvic binder to stabilize pelvis if injury is suspected
   D. Further evaluation and workup of noted or suspected injuries. The hemodynamically unstable patient represents a complex clinical scenario requiring multiple points of evaluation and decision-making (see Treatment Algorithm).

II. **Pelvic and Related Musculoskeletal Physical Examination**
   A. Inspect the skin for open wounds or bruising
   B. Assess AP and lateral pelvic stability by gentle compression. Gross instability should not be further exacerbated by forceful examination; equivocal stability may be additionally assessed using image intensification.
   C. Inspect and palpate both hips and lower extremities to assess range of motion.

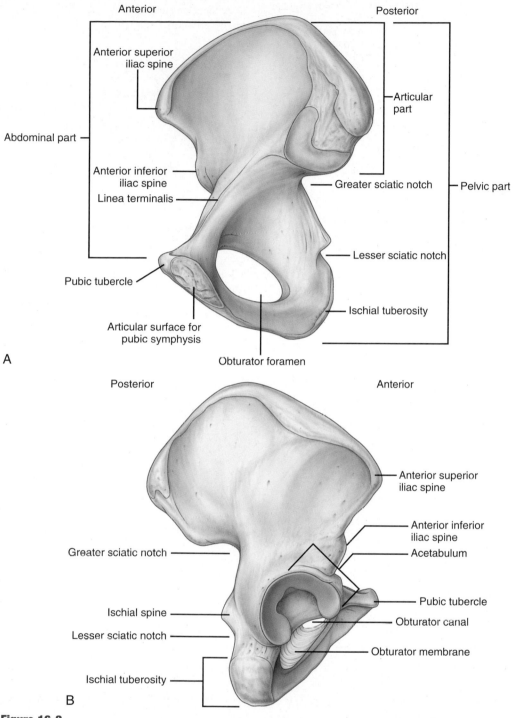

Anterior

Posterior

Anterior superior
iliac spine

Articular
part

Abdominal part

Anterior inferior
iliac spine

Linea terminalis

Greater sciatic notch

Pelvic part

Lesser sciatic notch

Pubic tubercle

Ischial tuberosity

Articular surface for
pubic symphysis

Obturator foramen

A

Posterior

Anterior

Anterior superior
iliac spine

Anterior inferior
iliac spine

Greater sciatic notch

Acetabulum

Ischial spine

Pubic tubercle

Lesser sciatic notch

Obturator canal

Obturator membrane

Ischial tuberosity

B

Figure 16-2
Right pelvic bone. **A,** Medial view. **B,** Lateral view. *(From Drake RL, Vogl W, Mitchell AWM: Gray's Anatomy for Students. Philadelphia, Churchill Livingstone, 2005.)*

Pelvis and Acetabulum

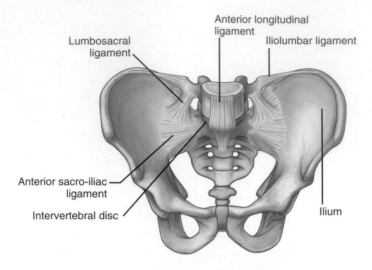

Figure 16-3
The posterior pelvic ring can be thought of as a suspension bridge in cross-section. The sacrum is an inverted keystone or represents a suspension bridge–like arrangement of the posterior pelvic ring. Loss of the ligamentous support allows the bridge to "fall" or results in an anterior displacement of the sacrum. *(From Drake RL, Vogl W, Mitchell AWM: Gray's Anatomy for Students. Philadelphia, Churchill Livingstone, 2005.)*

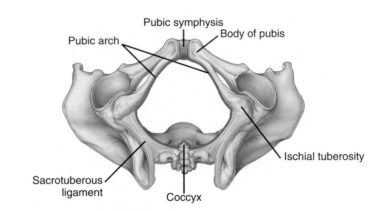

Figure 16-4
An outlet view of the pelvis depicting the sacrum as the keystone of the pelvis. *(From Drake RL, Vogl W, Mitchell AWM: Gray's Anatomy for Students. Philadelphia, Churchill Livingstone, 2005.)*

Large ecchymoses over the thigh, buttocks, or sacrum may suggest Morel-Lavalle lesion (internal degloving injury with shearing of the skin from the subcutaneous fat). The high risk of infection associated with operating through this lesion can have an impact on both surgical timing and exposure options.

Significant blood loss from pelvic trauma is more likely to be venous rather than arterial.

IN INJURIES REQUIRING PLACEMENT OF A SUPRAPUBIC CATHETER, ENCOURAGE UROLOGISTS OR TRAUMATOLOGISTS TO MAINTAIN A SAFE DISTANCE FROM POTENTIAL SURGICAL INCISIONS FOR RING FIXATION. THE SAME IS TRUE IF THE PATIENT REQUIRES A DIVERSION (COLOSTOMY) OF THE GASTROINTESTINAL TRACT SECONDARY TO INTRA-ABDOMINAL INJURY.

Displaced rami fractures and sacroiliac joint disruptions are at higher risk for urethral injuries.

    D. Perform careful pelvic and lower extremity neurologic assessment because lumbar and sacral plexus injuries are not uncommon.

    E. Difficulty in palpating peripheral pulses in the lower extremities or abnormal Doppler signals necessitate obtaining ankle brachial index measurements.

III. **Assessment of Associated Structures**

    A. In men, blood at the urethral meatus, a boggy or high-riding prostate, or scrotal hematoma suggests urologic injury and may require cystography or urethrography prior to Foley catheter placement.

    B. In women, blood at the urethral meatus, vaginal tears, or difficulty with Foley catheter insertion suggests urologic injury.

    C. Vaginal bleeding associated with a pelvic fracture may indicate an open fracture. Gynecologic evaluation is a necessity in these patients.

    D. Evaluation and documentation of rectal tone is mandatory in patients with a pelvic ring injury.

TREATMENT ALGORITHM

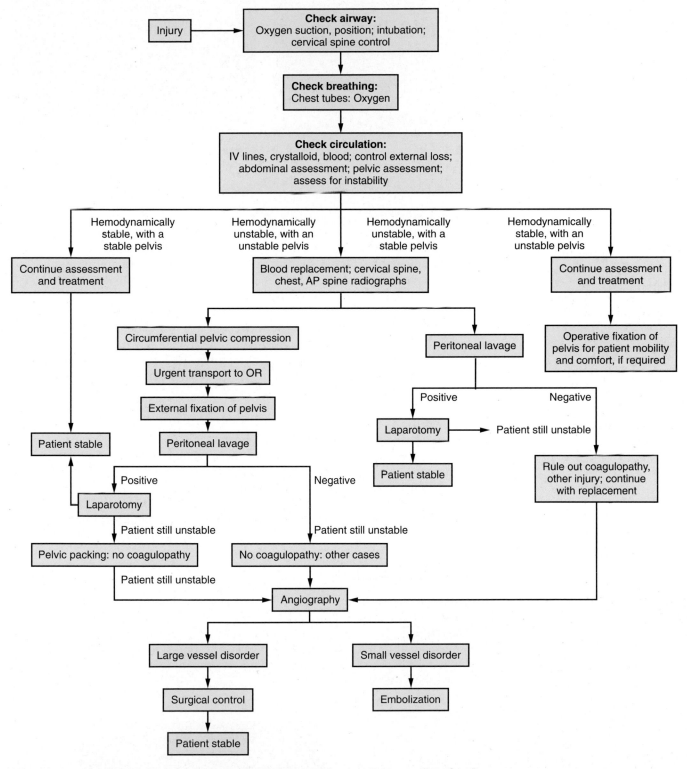

AP, anteroposterior; ED, emergency department; IV, intravenous; OR, operating room. *(Data from Browner BD, Levine AM, Jupiter JB, et al: Skeletal Trauma: Fractures, Dislocations, Ligamentous Injuries, 2nd ed. Philadelphia, Saunders, 1998.)*

Pelvis and Acetabulum

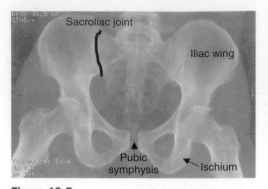

Figure 16-5
Anteroposterior view of the pelvis.

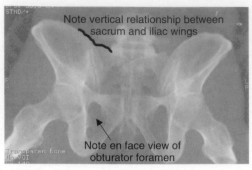

Figure 16-6
Outlet view of the pelvis.

IMAGING STUDIES

I. **Standard Radiographic Views**
   A. AP radiographs (Fig. 16-5). Anterior fractures, symphyseal injuries, significant SI displacement, and iliac wing injuries are readily seen; can demonstrate 90% of pelvic fractures. Sacral injuries can also be described but less frequently.
   B. The outlet view, or 40-degree cephalad view (Fig. 16-6), is useful for assessment of vertical displacement of the hemipelvis. A widened sacroiliac joint and fractures of the sacrum (including neural foramina) may be visualized.
   C. The inlet view, or 40-degree caudad view (Fig. 16-7), assesses AP displacement of the SI joint, sacrum, or iliac wing. Rotational deformities of the hemipelvis can also be evaluated.
   D. Judet views are used to evaluate acetabular fractures (see Chapter 15 for details).

II. **Cross-Sectional and Reconstructed Images**
   A. Computed tomography scans with fine cuts and reconstruction may reveal minimally displaced fractures especially of the posterior ring and may provide additional resolution regarding fracture fragments.
   B. Magnetic resonance imaging is largely reserved for assessment of ligamentous injuries or intrapelvic soft tissue structures and rarely indicated in acute traumatic injuries.

> Physiologic widening of the pubic symphysis that occurs normally and naturally during pregnancy should not be mistaken for an anterior ring injury.

FRACTURE CLASSIFICATION

I. **Anatomic.** The Letournel system is a descriptive system based on the location of the fracture.

II. **Mechanism**
   A. Penal first introduced a mechanistic classification system in 1961 composed of lateral compression (LC), anterior-posterior compression (APC), and the vertical shear (VS).

Figure 16-7
Inlet view of the pelvis.

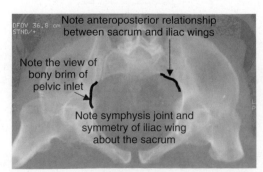

B. Young and Burgess (1986) further subdivided LC into the following three types.
   1. Pubic rami fractures with impaction of the SI joint
   2. Pubic rami fractures with internal rotation and posterior disruption (iliac wing fracture or varying degrees of anterior SI impaction and posterior SI disruption depending on location of impact on ilium)
   3. LC fracture on one side with an associated APC (external rotation) fracture on contralateral side
C. APC fractures were divided into three subtypes.
   1. Anterior ring widening with intact posterior elements.
   2. Anterior widening of the SI joint, external rotation of the ilium, and disruption of sacrotuberous and sacrospinous ligaments.
   3. Complete anterior and posterior SI joint disruption.
D. One of the strengths of this system is that it is predictive of associated injuries and may aid in the initial evaluation and stabilization of the patient.

III. **Stability**
A. Buchholz in 1981 and Tile in 1988 created a system based on stability.
B. The Tile classification is divided into three types (Fig. 16-8).
   1. Type A: stable
      a. 1: Avulsion
      b. 2: Minimally displaced ring
   2. Type B: rotationally unstable
   3. Type C: rotationally and vertically unstable
C. The OTA/AO scheme presents a variation where:
   1. Type A: stable
      a. 1: Avulsion
      b. 2: Impaction
      c. 3: Transverse sacral/coccygeal fracture

> Different Young and Burgess types appear to be associated with certain injury patterns: anterior-posterior compression with hemorrhage as well as thoracic, urologic, and head injuries; vertical shear with hemorrhage; and lateral compression with thoracic injuries.

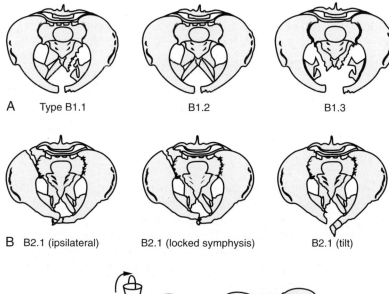

A   Type B1.1   B1.2   B1.3

B   B2.1 (ipsilateral)   B2.1 (locked symphysis)   B2.1 (tilt)

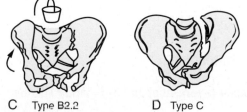

C   Type B2.2   D   Type C

Figure 16-8
Tile classification of pelvic ring disruptions. This classification system is potentially predictive of stability. *(From Koo H, Leeridge M, Bhandari M, et al: Interobserver reliability of the Young-Burgess and Tile classification systems of fractures of the pelvic ring. OTA [poster], 2002.)*

Pelvis and Acetabulum

2. Type B: partially stable
   a. 1: Unilateral/partial radiographic change in external or internal rotation
   b. 2: Bilateral/partial injury
3. Type C: unstable
   a. 1: Unilateral/complete
   b. 2: Bilateral/complete-incomplete
   c. 3: Bilateral/complete

D. One of the strengths of this system is that it helps guide treatment options.

SURGICAL ALTERNATIVE: EXTERNAL FIXATION

I. Three options exist for external fixation of the pelvis as either a temporizing solution until the patient is hemodynamically stable for definitive fixation or as a definitive solution based on the fracture pattern and type of surgery required.
  A. Anteriorly based external fixation constructs
     1. ASIS or iliac wing
     2. AIIS or supra-acetabular (author's preferred method)
  B. Posteriorly based external fixation constructs may be necessary in the AO/OTA type C injuries and are performed with a C-clamp or Hannover frame.

II. Goals
  A. Improve stability of pelvis by placing a frame referenced to the site of injury (anterior or posterior).
  B. Decrease pelvic volume and limit blood loss.
  C. Recreate "ring" structure to pelvis.
  D. Restore continuity of axial skeleton to appendicular skeleton.
  E. Maintain access to abdominal and urologic structures for operative treatment.
  F. Provide pain relief and assist in mobilization of patient for nursing care and physical therapy.
  G. Limit intrapelvic hardware in patients for future childbirth.

GENERAL PRINCIPLES OF PUBIC SYMPHYSIS INJURIES

I. Isolated pubic symphysis injuries are usually stable and rarely need operative management. Patients may bear weight as tolerated until the injury has healed and pain relief has reached a plateau.

II. Significantly displaced anterior injuries (e.g., disruption of the pubic symphysis) indicate potential concomitant posterior ring injury and may require stabilization and fixation.

III. Stable posterior ring injuries (minimal displacement or rotation, impaction type injuries) with mild anterior injuries (e.g., less than 2.5 cm of symphyseal diastasis) may also be considered for nonoperative treatment.

IV. Seemingly stable posterior ring injuries with significant anterior displacement (e.g., greater than 2.5 cm of symphyseal diastasis) or with unacceptable rotational displacement may be candidates for surgical stabilization.

V. Injuries with unstable posterior and anterior elements require anterior and/or posterior stabilization and fixation.

COMPONENTS OF THE PROCEDURE

Anterior Inferior Iliac Spine (Supra-Acetabular) External Fixation

I. The patient is placed in the supine position on a radiolucent operating room table. The abdomen and thorax are draped into the surgical field but the lower extremities are not. Laterally, the patient is prepped down to the table (to include the possibility of SI joint fixation).

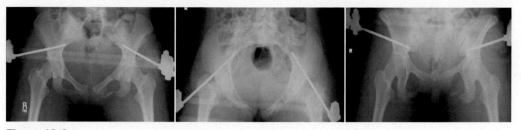

Figure 16-9
Anteroposterior, inlet, and outlet pelvic radiographs showing placement of supra-acetabular pins for anterior external fixation.

II. Fluoroscopic imaging is obtained prior to prepping and draping to ensure that Judet, inlet, and outlet views, as well as an AP image, can be obtained.

III. Once the patient is adequately positioned and fluoroscopic imaging is in place, the patient is prepped and draped in standard fashion according to the surgical principles outlined in Chapter 1.

IV. A roll-over modified outlet view is obtained to define the region of the supra-acetabulum. The supra-acetabular region is then localized with a K-wire.

V. The K-wire is then overdrilled with a cannulated drill (usually 3.5-mm in size) through the anterior cortex only.

VI. A roll-over–inlet view is obtained to confirm the direction of drilling toward the posterior inferior iliac spine.

VII. A 5-mm Schanz pin is slowly inserted by manual power. Multiple images are obtained to confirm the direction and location of the pin. Usually, the pin is inserted to a depth of at least 70 to 80 mm.

VIII. The same technique is repeated on the contralateral side.

IX. A carbon graphite bar is used to connect the two Schanz pins. The pelvis is reduced prior to tightening of the clamps.

X. If there is continued posterior widening of the sacroiliac joint, consideration for the placement of a percutaneous iliosacral screw is made.

XI. Postoperative radiographs are shown in Figure 16-9.

> **BE SURE TO DOCUMENT A DETAILED VASCULAR AND NEUROLOGIC STATUS BEFORE AND AFTER REDUCTION ATTEMPTS.**

Open Reduction and Internal Fixation

I. **Patient Positioning, Prepping, and Draping**

   A. The patient is placed in a supine position on a radiolucent table with the chest, abdomen, and lateral flanks prepped into the field. The extremities do not need to be prepped into the field, but traction should be maintained with a traction pin in patients with cephalad displacement of the hemipelvis.

   B. Fluoroscopic imaging is obtained prior to prepping and draping to ensure that inlet, outlet, and AP images can be obtained.

   C. Once the patient is adequately positioned and fluoroscopic imaging is in proper place, the patient is prepped and draped in standard fashion according to the surgical principles outlined in Chapter 1.

II. **Surgical Exposure (Modified Pfannenstiel Approach)**

   A. With a 15-blade, a transverse incision is made approximately 1 cm proximal to the superior border of the pubic symphysis centered with respect to the umbilicus. The length of the incision is approximately 5 to 6 cm.

   B. The incision can be carried laterally just past the external inguinal ring.

   C. Dissection through the subcutaneous tissue yields identification of the aponeurotic fibers of the external oblique and anterior rectus fascia.

   D. The spermatic cord/round ligament (females) is identified. Pay careful attention to the spermatic cord/round ligament during the surgical approach to avoid injury to these structures.

   E. Next, an incision is made along the linea alba (between the heads of the rectus abdominis), extending distally onto the symphysis pubis.

F. The posterior rectus sheath is carefully incised so as to not injure the prostatic venous plexus and bladder (typically identified by overlying fat).

G. The bladder is protected by interposing a lap sponge, malleable retractor, or both between the surgeon and the structure.

H. The symphyseal ligament is débrided where it is torn, and the margins of the ligament are defined sharply.

I. The pubic rami are exposed lateral to the symphysis via subperiosteal dissection along the posterosuperior and posterior surface. During this dissection, anterior attachment of both heads of the rectus is maintained (traumatic disruptions of the rectus attachment are sometimes seen and should be repaired after fixation of the symphysis).

J. If a corona mortis is present, it should be addressed prior to extending the dissection further or beginning reduction maneuvers. It can be ligated or coagulated.

III. **Reduction**

A. Once adequately exposed, a sharp Weber clamp may be applied anteriorly engaging the pubic tubercles.

1. Predrilling small pilot holes (with a 2.5- or 2.0-mm bit) may aid in secure application of the clamp.

2. Both rotational and flexion-extension deformities may be corrected in this manner.

3. If greater force is required or the bone is osteoporotic, a Farabeuf or Jungbluth clamp may be applied anteriorly and secured with 3.5-mm screws (details of this technique are beyond the scope of this discussion).

4. The larger screw-assisted clamps are often required if there is posterior displacement of the hemipelvis or if the fracture is being reduced after some healing has occurred (delayed fixation).

B. Reduction is assessed by fluoroscopic AP, inlet, and outlet views using both anterior and posterior anatomy to gauge reduction quality and restoration of ring structure.

IV. **Fixation**

A. Fixation is typically performed with a single six- or eight-hole 3.5-mm pelvic reconstruction plate. The plate may need to be slightly contoured to fit the symphysis.

B. The plate is placed superiorly and slightly posteriorly. Four to six screws are placed in the plate. The goal with screw fixation is to use the longest screws possible as screw fixation is, in part, dependent on screw length. This requires screws to be angled to reach the most bone (Fig. 16-10). Care should be taken not to extrude the screws through the anterior or posterior aspects of the anterior ring.

C. A second plate may be applied anteriorly if the patient is felt to be unstable. Usually, this anterior plate is two or three holes. However, this is often only utilized for revision situations.

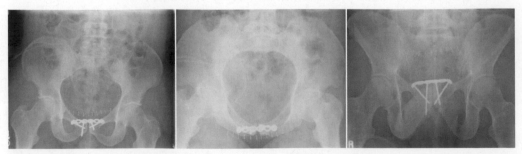

Figure 16-10

Anteroposterior, inlet, and outlet radiographs after open reduction and internal fixation of a pubic symphyseal injury. Note the contour of the plate as well as the length of the screws utilized for fixation.

V. **Closure**
   A. The wound is irrigated and drains are placed deep and superficial to the rectus abdominis muscle.
   B. The wound is closed in standard fashion according to the surgical principles outlined in Chapter 1.
   C. Bladder injuries should be addressed prior to definitive closure of the incision.
   D. It is important to repair the heads of the rectus muscle to their distal attachments if a surgical or traumatic detachment is recognized.

POSTOPERATIVE CONSIDERATIONS

I. **Postoperative Care**
   A. Careful monitoring of neurovascular status
   B. Obtaining postoperative radiographs including AP, inlet, and outlet views. If there is a concern for secondary injury, then a computed tomography scan should be obtained.
   C. Postoperative resuscitation as necessary
   D. Deep venous thrombosis prophylaxis with consideration of preoperative vena-caval filter if indicated (particularly in those patients with an associated long bone fracture)
   E. Early mobilization
   F. Physical therapy for range of motion, strengthening, and gait training, including an abdominal and low back program

II. **Weight-bearing Status**
   A. Uninvolved lower extremity may be weight bearing as tolerated.
   B. Involved lower extremity is touch-down weight bearing for at least 6 weeks.
   C. Progress from touch down to full weight bearing from 6 to 12 weeks assuming radiographic and clinical signs of healing.
   D. If bilateral unstable pelvic fractures have been fixed, patients should not be mobilized until radiographic evidence of fracture healing is noted. Once there is evidence of fracture healing, the less injured side is advanced to partial weight bearing by the 8th to 12th week.

COMPLICATIONS

I. Increased infection risk with the following:
   A. Associated abdominal and pelvic visceral injuries
   B. Contusion or shear injury to soft tissues
   C. Postoperative hematoma formation
II. Abnormal or continuous bleeding from fracture and/or subsequent surgical procedures
III. Deep vein thrombosis or thrombophlebitis
IV. Intrapelvic or intra-abdominal compartment syndrome
V. Thromboembolic events due to disruption of the pelvic venous vasculature and prolonged immobilization
VI. Dyspareunia
VII. Malunion: chronic pain, gait instability, limb length equalities, sitting difficulties, pelvic outlet obstruction, and low back pain
VIII. Nonunion, which is rare, but occurs more frequently in patients younger than 35 years of age. Chronic pain, gait instability, and nerve root irritation may occur. Further surgery using bone graft and alternative fixation constructs may be needed for union.
IX. Hardware failure, which is common. When the symphyseal ligament heals and the fractures unite, there is some motion (normal) at the pubic symphysis. This motion can lead to either screw loosening or plate breakage. Patients should be warned of this preoperatively. If this does occur after the patient heals, it is usually not a surgical emergency and can be addressed only if symptomatic.

Pelvis and Acetabulum

SUGGESTED READINGS

Browner B, Jupiter J, Levine A, Trafton P: Skeletal Trauma: Fractures, Dislocations, Ligamentous Injuries, 3rd ed. Philadelphia, Saunders, 2002.

Bucholz RW, Heckman JD, Court-Brown CM (eds): Rockwood and Green's Fractures in Adults, 6th ed. Philadelphia, Lippincott Williams & Wilkins, 2006.

Koval KJ, Zuckerman JD: Handbook of Fractures, 3rd ed. Philadelphia, Lippincott Williams & Wilkins, 2006.

Thompson JC: Netter's Concise Atlas of Orthopaedic Anatomy. Medimedia USA, 2002.

Tile M, Helfet DL, Kellam JF (eds): Fractures of the Pelvis and Acetabulum, 3rd ed. Philadelphia, Lippincott Williams & Wilkins, 2003.

HIP

CHAPTER 17

Hip Decompression and Grafting

Gregory K. Deirmengian and Jonathan P. Garino

Case Study

A 45-year-old male is referred to the office by his primary physician with an insidious onset of right groin pain of 2 months' duration. He explains that the pain is moderate in severity and aching in nature, and it radiates to the anteromedial thigh. It has not responded to a 3-week trial of nonsteroidal anti-inflammatory drugs (NSAIDs). The pain seems to be exacerbated by activity and improves but is not completely resolved with rest. The patient is normally active and plays tennis twice a week but has not been able to participate since the pain began. The patient has a past medical history significant only for Crohn's disease, which has led to hospital admission and administration of intravenous and oral steroids multiple times in the past, most recently 3 months ago. The patient lives with his wife and two children, and he drinks four beers per day on average. Physical examination is significant for an antalgic limp and concordant pain with flexion and internal rotation. Laboratory studies are within normal limits. Figure 17-1 shows an anteroposterior (AP) radiograph and a magnetic resonance imaging scan of the right hip.

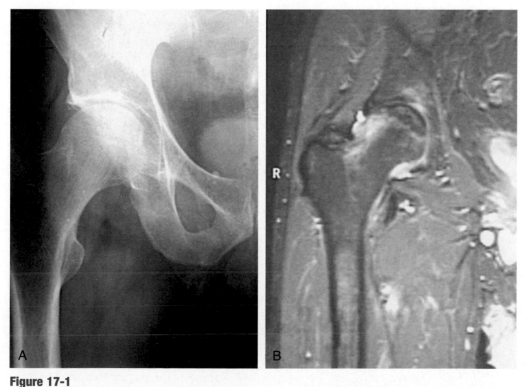

Figure 17-1

Plain anteroposterior (**A**) and coronal (**B**) magnetic resonance imaging scan of the right hip. *(Modified from Wiesel SW, Delahay JN: Principles of Orthopaedic Medicine and Surgery. Philadelphia, Saunders, 2001.)*

BACKGROUND

I. Osteonecrosis of the femoral head is a pathologic process characterized by osteocyte death that results in a decline in structural bone integrity. When a sufficient degree and duration of force beyond the threshold of the weakened subchondral bone is applied, femoral head collapse occurs. With time, motion and force applied to the incongruent joint surface leads to osteoarthritis.

II. Osteonecrosis of the femoral head is relatively common, with 20,000 new cases diagnosed each year. The diagnosis accounts for 5% to 10% of total hip replacements per year in the United States. The male-to-female distribution is 4:1 and the mean age of onset is in the 30s. Bilateral disease has been reported in as many as 80% of atraumatic cases. It is relatively common for a patient to present with symptomatic osteonecrosis of one hip and asymptomatic osteonecrosis of the contralateral hip that is diagnosed based on a high level of suspicion.

III. The natural history of osteonecrosis of the femoral head demonstrates clinical and radiographic progression to collapse and possible degenerative joint disease requiring surgery. The typical time frame is 2 to 3 years from the onset of symptoms. There are no clear factors associated with more rapid progression.

IV. **Etiology**

   A. Traumatic
   1. Hip dislocation. The incidence of osteonecrosis is 10% to 25%. Negative predictors include severe injury, associated femoral neck and acetabular fractures, and delayed reduction (>12 hours).
   2. Femoral neck fracture. The incidence of osteonecrosis is 15% to 50%. Negative predictors include severity of initial displacement and malreduction after open reduction and internal fixation.
   3. Minor contusive trauma. This risk factor is not as common but has been reported.

   B. Atraumatic
   1. Corticosteroids. These account for 10% to 30% of cases. Trends suggest that higher doses in short durations pose a higher risk of osteonecrosis than lower doses administered for a longer time period. It is likely that the risk of osteonecrosis increases once the aggregate amount of corticosteroids over a patient's lifetime exceeds 2.0 grams.
   2. Alcohol. This accounts for 10% to 40% of cases. Consumption of more than 400 mL of alcohol per day is associated with a 10-fold increased risk of osteonecrosis.
   3. Hemoglobinopathies. Associated disorders include sickle cell disease, hemoglobin SC disease, and thalassemias.
   4. Dysbarism (Caisson's disease), which affects tunnel workers and deep sea divers
   5. Pregnancy
   6. Hyperlipidemia
   7. Gaucher's disease
   8. Systemic lupus erythematosus
   9. Idiopathic

V. **Vascular Anatomy, Pathophysiology, and Pathogenesis**

   A. Vascular anatomy (Fig. 17-2)
   1. The extracapsular arterial ring is formed posteriorly by a large branch of the medial circumflex femoral artery and anteriorly by branches of the lateral circumflex femoral artery.
   2. The ascending cervical arteries, also known as the retinacular arteries, arise from the extracapsular arterial ring. They penetrate beneath the hip capsule

> How does your attending manage the asymptomatic hip in cases of bilateral osteonecrosis with a symptomatic contralateral hip?

> The two most common atraumatic causes of osteonecrosis are steroid use and alcohol consumption.

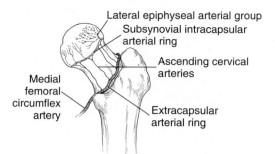

Lateral epiphyseal arterial group
Subsynovial intracapsular
arterial ring
Medial
femoral
circumflex
artery
Ascending cervical
arteries
Extracapsular
arterial ring

Figure 17-2
Blood supply of the femoral head and neck. *(From Canale ST [ed]: Campbell's Operative Orthopaedics, 10th ed. Philadelphia, Mosby, 2003.)*

and travel along the femoral neck, where they send branches into the metaphysis. The superior retinacular arteries are the main source of blood supply to the femoral head.

    3. The subsynovial intra-articular ring is formed by the ascending cervical arteries at the junction of the femoral neck and articular cartilage of the femoral head. They sprout epiphyseal branches, which enter the femoral head.

    4. The artery of the ligamentum teres is a branch of the obturator artery and a minor contributor to femoral head blood supply in adults.

  B. Pathophysiology
    1. The microcirculation of the femoral head is tenuous and vulnerable.
    2. Diminution or disruption of the extraosseous or intraosseous sources of blood leads to bone ischemia and eventual necrosis.
    3. The level and extent of occlusion determines the number, size, and location of femoral head zones involved in the necrosis.

  C. Pathogenesis. Vascular occlusion leads to ischemia and osteocyte necrosis by one of three mechanisms.
    1. Vascular disruption occurs with fractures and dislocations.
    2. Extravascular compression is due to marrow adipose deposition and lipocyte hypertrophy, leading to an increase in the extravascular intraosseous pressure with resulting decreased blood flow and venous drainage. Adipose deposition results from the use of alcohol and corticosteroids, hyperlipidemia, and Gaucher's disease.
    3. Intravascular congestion is due to thrombotic occlusion and fat emboli resulting from hypercoagulability, hemoglobinopathies, and pregnancy.

VI. **Imaging and Classification**
  A. Radiographs
    1. Early stages are characterized by heterogeneous areas of mottled sclerosis and lucency, usually in the anterosuperior femoral head.
    2. Later stages are characterized by subchondral fracture and collapse (crescent sign).
    3. End-stage disease is characterized by signs of secondary osteoarthritis.
  B. Bone scan
    1. In the acute infarction phase, the ischemic segment shows photopenia.
    2. In the repair phase, the diseased segment shows a signal "hot spot."
  C. Magnetic resonance imaging
    1. Early stages show low signal intensity on both T1-weighted and T2-weighted images.
    2. More advanced stages show low signal intensity on T1-weighted images and alternating "ribbons" of low and high signal intensity on T2-weighted images.
  D. The University of Pennsylvania system for staging osteonecrosis is given in Box 17-1.

VII. **Differential Diagnosis**
  A. Synovitis. Presentation can resemble stage 0 osteonecrosis.
  B. Trochanteric bursitis. Presentation can resemble stage 0 osteonecrosis.
  C. Labral tear. Presentation can resemble stage 0 osteonecrosis.

Specific bones that have a tenuous blood supply include the talar body, proximal pole of the scaphoid, odontoid process, and femoral head.

Hip

BOX 17-1. University of Pennsylvania System for Staging Osteonecrosis

Stage Criteria
  0. Normal radiographs and magnetic resonance imaging (MRI) scan
  I. Normal radiographs and abnormal MRI
     A. <15% of the femoral head affected
     B. 15% to 30% of the femoral head affected
     C. >30% of the femoral head affected
  II. Cystic and sclerotic radiographic changes
     A. <15% of the femoral head affected
     B. 15% to 30% of the femoral head affected
     C. >30% of the femoral head affected
  III. Crescent sign on radiographs, with no articular flattening
     A. <15% of the articular surface
     B. 15% to 30% of the articular surface
     C. >30% of the articular surface
  IV. Femoral head flattening
     A. <15% of the articular surface and <2 mm depression
     B. 15% to 30% of the articular surface or 2 to 4 mm depression
     C. >30% of the articular surface or >4 mm depression
  V. Joint narrowing or acetabular changes
     A. Mild
     B. Moderate
     C. Severe
  VI. Advanced degenerative changes

    D. Transient osteoporosis. Magnetic resonance imaging changes are more diffuse, and typically a homogeneous high signal is seen acutely on T2-weighted images.
    E. Femoral neck stress fracture
    F. Metastatic disease

TREATMENT PROTOCOLS, ALTERNATIVES, INDICATIONS, AND CONTRAINDICATIONS

   I. **Conservative Treatment.** Indications include early-stage to middle-stage I lesions and absence of medical clearance for surgery.
      A. Limited weight bearing, pain control, and close clinical follow-up with radiographic imaging and magnetic resonance imaging are necessary.
      B. Risk factors, including steroids (when medically possible) and alcohol, should be avoided.
      C. Medications such as those in the bisphosphonate and statin classes may help delay disease progression.
      D. Late stage I lesions and beyond are less likely to be successfully treated by this method.
   II. **Core Decompression with and without Bone Grafting**
      A. Core decompression is a technique that involves drilling the medullary bone of the femoral head to decrease pressure and improve circulation.
      B. When successful, the technique provides pain relief and prevents disease progression.

C. Under most circumstances, it is necessary to remove necrotic bone and replace it with nonvascularized or vascularized bone graft to improve the chances of a successful clinical outcome. As a general guideline, core decompression without bone grafting should only be considered for the smallest lesions.

D. Examples of nonvascularized bone graft include cancellous allograft chips, structural allograft, iliac crest autograft, and femoral head allograft (as described below). Examples of vascularized bone graft include a vascularized free fibula bone graft.

E. The success rate of the technique varies widely in the literature, but the best estimate of success rate is approximately 66%.

F. Indications include stage IA, IB, IIA, and IIB (pre-subchondral collapse lesions). Vascularized free fibula bone grafting should be considered in younger patients with extensive disease in an attempt to maximize the chances for success and to avoid a total hip arthroplasty (THA).

G. Contraindications include any degree of collapse and stage III to VI, which are predictors of poor outcome after treatment by core decompression. Larger lesions (stage IC and IIC) are more difficult to manage with core decompression alone and require bone grafting.

III. **Osteotomy**

A. Several osteotomy procedures have been attempted with varying degrees of success. Specifics are beyond the scope of this chapter.

B. The goal of such procedures is to reorient the joint surface such that the line of force through the joint is redirected across healthy bone.

C. Examples include intertrochanteric osteotomy and transtrochanteric rotational osteotomies.

D. Indications include late presubchondral collapse and early postsubchondral collapse lesions.

E. Contraindications. Less invasive options are available for disease stages less severe than late presubchondral collapse. Osteotomy techniques are not successful if a significant degree of collapse or arthritic changes are present.

IV. **Resurfacing Arthroplasty**

A. This technique is an option for younger patients with disease that precludes an attempt to preserve native bone but lacks acetabular involvement requiring THA.

B. The potential advantage is the ability to save bone stock for future revision as well as preservation of more native anatomy and hip biomechanics.

C. Specific complications include femoral neck fracture and loss of prosthetic fixation.

D. Indications include young patients with stage III and IV and early stage V osteonecrosis of the femoral head.

E. Contraindications include middle to late stage V and stage VI with acetabular involvement, active infection, concomitant osteoporosis, and insufficient femoral head bone stock due to collapse or cystic degeneration that would compromise fixation.

V. **THA**

A. Although it is the least bone-sparing option, THA represents a reliable means of treating the pathology and reproducibly reducing hip pain.

B. THA also serves as an excellent salvage option for other failed attempts at treatment, such as core decompression and resurfacing arthroplasty.

C. Indications include stage III to VI osteonecrosis. At this time, THA is likely the best option for patients with stage VI osteonecrosis.

D. Contraindications include stage I and II osteonecrosis, which should be treated with other nonarthroplasty options. Lack of medical clearance also precludes patients from management with THA.

> The success rate of core decompression for femoral head osteonecrosis can be quoted to patients as 66%.

> Acetabular and femoral resurfacing arthroplasty has more recently re-emerged as bone-conserving means of managing osteonecrosis of the hip, although long-term outcomes of these new designs are not yet available.

Hip

TREATMENT ALGORITHM

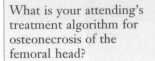

What is your attending's treatment algorithm for osteonecrosis of the femoral head?

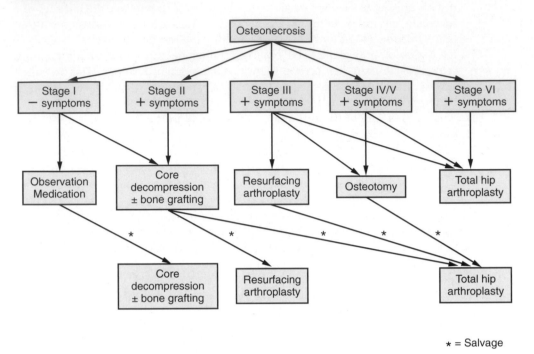

★ = Salvage

GENERAL PRINCIPLES OF CORE DECOMPRESSION

I. Preoperatively, it must be ensured that signs of femoral head collapse, representing advanced disease, are absent.

II. In combination with elimination of risk factors such as alcohol and steroids, core decompression serves to reverse the cycle of decreased vascularity and increased pressure within the femoral head.

III. The least invasive and most common means of accessing the center of the femoral head is laterally, through a small skin incision and an osteotomy of the lateral cortex of the proximal femur, just large enough to accommodate the trephine.

IV. Under anteroposterior (AP) and lateral fluoroscopic guidance, the most appropriately sized trephine is advanced to the lesion under multiple passes, and the contents of the cores are removed and examined on a back table. Bone that appears pathologic (hard, dense, and homogeneous) is sent to pathology, and bone that is medullary in appearance is saved and later reintroduced into the femoral head void as bone graft.

V. Postoperatively, patients' weight bearing must be restricted for several months to avoid a proximal femur fracture through the iatrogenic stress riser.

VI. Postoperatively, some patients experience immediate relief due to the decreased pressure within the femoral head.

COMPONENTS OF THE PROCEDURE

Positioning, Prepping, and Draping

I. The patient is placed in the supine position on a fracture table (Fig. 17-3). The fracture table is used to ease fluoroscopy and positioning of the hip in space. The traction device of the fracture table is not needed for the procedure. The orientation of personnel and equipment is of great importance in making sure the procedure runs smoothly (Fig. 17-4).

II. Prior to transferring the patient to the fracture table, a perineal post is properly placed and the patient is shifted inferiorly until the perineum is up

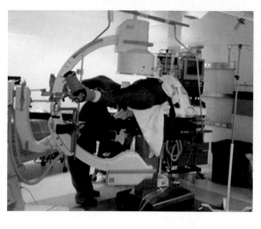

Figure 17-3
Operative setup with fluoroscopy on a fracture table.

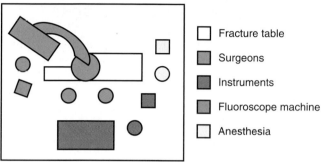

☐ Fracture table

▨ Surgeons

▨ Instruments

▨ Fluoroscope machine

☐ Anesthesia

Figure 17-4
Diagram of the operative setup.

against the post. The feet are padded well with Webril and secured in the foot holders.

III. The nonoperative leg is positioned in a flexed, abducted, and externally rotated position to accommodate the fluoroscope machine between the patient's legs. The operative leg is positioned in line with the axis of the body and internally rotated 15 degrees to make the femoral neck parallel to the ground. The internal rotation accounts for the natural anteversion of the femoral neck and allows for a true AP radiograph of the hip to be taken during the procedure.

IV. The upper extremity on the ipsilateral side of the hip lesion is well padded and secured over the patient's chest (see Fig. 17-3). At this point, the fluoroscope is properly positioned and images are obtained to make sure that an AP and lateral view of the hip is well visualized (Fig. 17-5).

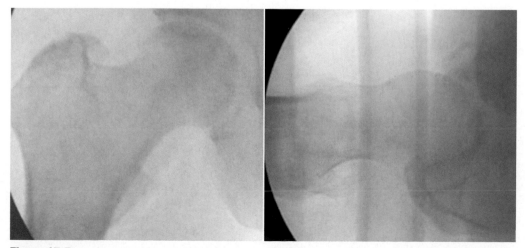

Figure 17-5
Fluoroscopic hip images after operative setup.

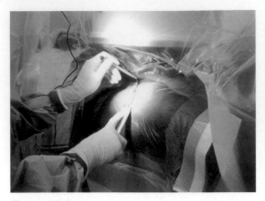

Figure 17-6
Shower curtain setup.

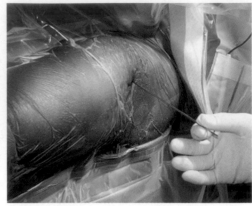

Figure 17-7
Percutaneous Steinmann pin insertion site.

PLACING THE NONOPERATIVE LEG IN A HYPERFLEXED/ HYPERABDUCTED/EXTERNALLY ROTATED POSITION PUTS IT AT RISK FOR THIGH COMPARTMENT SYNDROME.

EXCESSIVE PRESSURE ON THE PERINEUM FROM THE PERINEAL POST MAY RESULT IN A PUDENDAL NERVE PALSY POSTOPERATIVELY.

PLACING THE STARTING POINT TOO LOW IN THE DIAPHYSEAL CORTEX CAUSES A STRESS RISER THAT MAY LEAD TO A SUBTROCHANTERIC FRACTURE EITHER INTRAOPERATIVELY OR POSTOPERATIVELY.

V. A shower curtain drape is typically used to maintain a sterile field. Two poles positioned at both ends of the patient are positioned prior to the start of the case.

VI. The operative field is defined with 1010 drapes, taking care to maintain a wide surgical field, and then sterilized.

VII. Draping is performed by securing sterile blue towels to the inner borders of the 10 × 10 drapes. The blue towels and sterile field are now covered with Ioban, and the entire field is then covered with the shower curtain drape, which is then secured to the shower curtain poles. (Fig. 17-6).

Surgical Exposure

I. The lateral femoral starting point is localized through percutaneous insertion of a $\frac{1}{8}$-inch Steinmann pin under fluoroscopic guidance (Fig. 17-7). The starting point should be superior to the diaphyseal femoral cortex. The angle of the Steinmann pin should aim toward the lesion, as determined by preoperative imaging. AP and lateral fluoroscopic views verify the correct starting point and angle of approach (Fig. 17-8).

II. A 2- to 3-cm skin incision is centered around the Steinmann pin entry site. The pin can be removed at this point to ease the surgical approach. While obtaining hemostasis, the subcutaneous soft tissues are sharply dissected to the level of the fascia using a scalpel. The fascia can be clearly identified by removal of soft tissue using a Cobb elevator. This is helpful at the conclusion of the procedure when

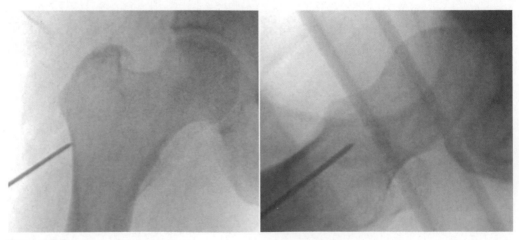

Figure 17-8
Fluoroscopic images demonstrating the Steinmann pin starting point and angle.

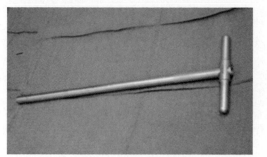

Figure 17-9
Trephine.

closing the wound. It is important to avoid overdissection, which may lead to fascia devitalization.

III. A small longitudinal incision is made in the fascia in line with the fibers, and it is extended proximally and distally as needed. Just deep to the fascia is the vastus lateralis muscle. A Cobb elevator is used to separate the vastus lateralis muscle in line with its fibers. This minimizes the degree of trauma to the muscle and allows access to the base of the greater trochanter and lateral femoral cortex.

Osteonecrosis Lesion Localization, Decompression, and Grafting

I. The Steinmann pin is reintroduced into the wound and repositioned on the lateral femoral cortex. A wire driver is used to advance the Steinmann pin into the femoral head lesion under fluoroscopic guidance. Try to avoid breaching the chondral surface of the femoral head and allowing the pin to violate the hip joint.

II. A 9- to 10-mm cannulated anterior cruciate ligament drill is used over the Steinmann pin to create an opening in the lateral femoral cortex to allow other instruments to easily traverse the path to the lesion. A trephine (Fig. 17-9) is introduced over the guidewire, through the lateral cortical opening, and advanced by hand to the lesion. The first trephine used is typically a smaller size instrument (e.g., 8 mm). A second, larger trephine (9 mm) is advanced by hand through the lesion in a controlled manner, taking care to prevent breaching the chondral surface into the hip joint (Fig. 17-10).

III. The contents of the first trephine are removed and examined. The bone removed from this trephine is typically viable cancellous bone. This bone is placed in saline on the back table and maintained for insertion into the lesion.

IV. After the second trephine has traversed the lesion, it is removed from the wound, and the contents are examined on the back table (Fig. 17-11). The extracted bone consists of dense necrotic bone that is secured from the osteonecrosis lesion. This bone is removed from the trephine and sent to pathology for analysis.

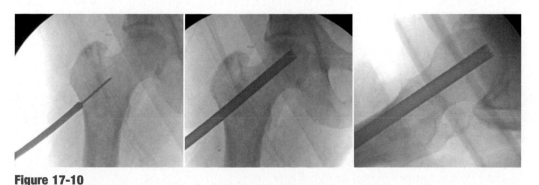

Figure 17-10
Fluoroscopic images demonstrating femoral head lesion trephinization.

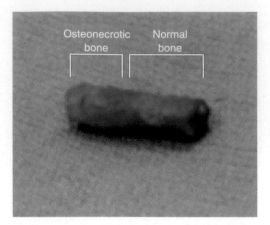

Figure 17-11
Trephinization contents.

V. The smaller trephine (8 mm) is reintroduced into the tunnel created from the lateral femoral cortex to the osteonecrosis lesion. A cannula is placed into the trephine, and pressure is maintained on the bone graft with the cannula while the trephine is slowly removed. This allows the bone graft to fill the femoral head defect.

Wound Closure

A wheatlander (self-retaining retractor) is placed in the subcutaneous soft tissue to expose the fascia. The fascial layer, the subcutaneous soft tissue, and dermal layer are closed in standard fashion (see Chapter 1). The skin edges are approximated with staples and then secured with a sterile dressing and a Tegaderm.

POSTOPERATIVE CARE AND REHABILITATION

I. Patients are routinely admitted to the hospital overnight for pain control and physical therapy clearance, but they are typically discharged home on the first postoperative day.
II. Patients with bilateral surgery and elderly patients with unilateral surgery may require a short stay at a rehabilitation facility.
III. Patients are made 50% weight bearing for 6 weeks to protect the vulnerable subchondral bone, after which their weight-bearing is advanced. Patients who receive bilateral core decompressions are made 50% weight bearing bilaterally or are required to exhibit "four-point gait" for 6 weeks.
IV. The pathology specimen is followed to confirm the suspected diagnosis of osteonecrosis.
V. Patients are followed in the office setting both clinically and radiographically for disease progression, and salvage procedures are considered if the disease process progresses despite the core decompression.

COMPLICATIONS

I. Infection
II. Hematoma
III. Persistent pain (due to preexisting arthritis, persistent osteonecrosis, occult fracture)
IV. Postoperative trochanteric bursitis
V. Postoperative/intraoperative fracture
VI. Postoperative femoral head collapse

SUGGESTED READINGS

Barrack RL, Rosenberg AG: Master Techniques in Orthopaedic Surgery: The Hip, 2nd ed. Philadelphia, Lippincott Williams & Wilkins, 2006.

Callaghan JJ, Rosenberg AG, Rubash HE: The Adult Hip. Philadelphia, Lippincott Williams & Wilkins, 2007.

Wiesel SW, Delahay JN: Principles of Orthopaedic Medicine and Surgery. Philadelphia, Saunders, 2004.

CHAPTER 18

Total Hip Arthroplasty

Kristofer J. Jones, Stephan G. Pill, and Charles L. Nelson

Case Study

A 58-year-old obese female presents with right hip pain that has gradually developed over the past 5 years. She reports that the pain wraps around the right hip, "shoots into the groin," and occasionally radiates down the thigh to the inside part of the knee. The pain has significantly limited her from activities of daily living. The pain disrupts her sleep most nights, and now she reports increasing difficulty getting into and out of her car and putting on her shoes. Prolonged standing and walking also exacerbate the pain. She is now limited to ambulating four blocks due to hip pain and started using a cane in the contralateral hand 1 month ago. She denies morning stiffness or pain in other joints. She cannot recall any preceding traumatic injury to the area and states that she has been taking up to six ibuprofen tablets per day, which has provided mild relief. Her right hip has 70 degrees of flexion, 10 degrees of internal rotation, and a 10-degree flexion contracture. The right leg is 2 cm shorter than the left but is otherwise neurovascularly intact. An effort at weight loss, physical therapy, and over-the-counter supplements has failed to provide relief. She presents to your office desperate for a solution to her problems. An anteroposterior (AP) radiograph of the right hip is presented in Figure 18-1.

BACKGROUND

I. Osteoarthritis (OA), also known as degenerative joint disease, is the most prevalent form of arthritis, and it is a leading cause of physical disability worldwide. Approximately 16 million people in the United States have osteoarthritis and 1 in 3 people older than 60 years of age suffer from the disease.

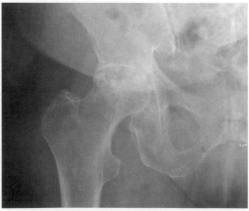

Figure 18-1
Anteroposterior view of the right hip.

II. OA of the hip is characterized by focal articular cartilage degeneration, most often in the weight-bearing portion of the joint. As localized areas of hyaline articular cartilage degenerate, resultant forces experienced at these particular sites increase across the hip. Ultimately, joint failure occurs when progressive cartilage loss leads to bony remodeling and significant alterations in stress forces across the joint.

III. Patients with OA of the hip classically present with insidious pain, typically characterized as a dull ache that is elicited with activity and relieved by rest. This pain can be localized to the groin or inguinal region, and in some cases, on the side of the buttock or upper thigh. Patients typically experience decreased range of motion as well as joint instability.

IV. OA of the hip is one of the leading causes of patients presenting with a painful hip; however, it is important to rule out inflammatory arthritic conditions (rheumatoid and psoriatic arthritis), tumors, infection, crystalline arthropathies (gout and pseudogout), and osteonecrosis, because the treatment protocol largely varies according to the diagnosis.

V. Total hip arthroplasty (THA) is indicated in patients suffering from hip joint degeneration from any number of causes. Persistent joint pain and physical disability following a trial of conservative treatment (weight reduction, low-impact aerobic exercise, aquatic therapy, pharmacologic therapy) are the primary reasons for performing the procedure. Approximately 250,000 THA procedures are performed in the United States on an annual basis, with long-term follow-up studies demonstrating 96% success rates at 10 years.

VI. Several important factors determine the appropriateness of THA. The overall goals of surgical intervention are to relieve pain and improve function through the restoration of joint stability and anatomic alignment of the lower extremity.

VII. The presence of significant medical comorbidities may preclude surgical intervention. Ultimately, the risks of perioperative mortality must be weighed against the expected functional gains following THA.

TREATMENT ALGORITHM

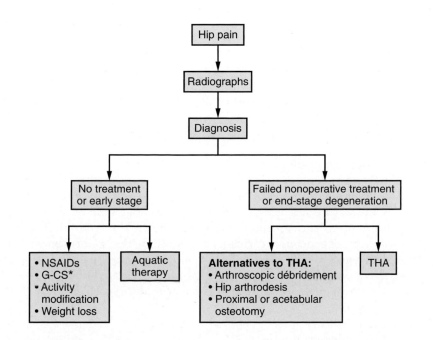

*Glucosamine–chondroitin sulfate

TREATMENT PROTOCOLS

I. **Treatment Considerations.** The following factors should be weighed when determining whether surgical intervention is in the best interest of the patient.
   A. Patient age
   B. Presence/absence of medical comorbidities
   C. Symptom severity (pain, decreased range of motion, instability, muscle weakness)
   D. Limitation in functional ability
   E. Extent of arthritic changes/deformity
   F. Expected activity level

II. **Nonoperative Treatment Options**
   A. Weight reduction. Nonpharmacologic therapy remains a mainstay of OA of the hip. Given the association between obesity and the development and progression of OA, weight loss should be emphasized from the first office visit.
   B. Low-impact exercise. A low-impact exercise program has the potential to increase aerobic capacity, muscle strength, and endurance, thereby optimizing hip function and facilitating weight loss.
   C. Aquatic therapy. In patients with symptomatic arthritis, formal aquatic therapy programs can improve symptoms and functional range of motion.
   D. Pharmacologic therapy. Pharmacologic intervention can be used to augment exercise and physical therapy regimens. Drug treatment should be individualized according to symptom severity, medical comorbidities, drug side effects, therapeutic cost, and patient preferences.
      1. Acetaminophen
      2. Nonsteroidal anti-inflammatory drugs (NSAIDs). Clinicians may use conventional NSAIDs or cyclooxygenase-II inhibitors for patients who are at risk for developing gastrointestinal toxicity or bleeding.
   E. Glucosamine and chondroitin sulfate oral supplementation. These dietary supplements are derivatives of glycosaminoglycans, which are naturally occurring compounds found in articular cartilage. Recent meta-analyses have demonstrated that these dietary supplements may have a small analgesic in mild OA.
   F. Intra-articular glucocorticoid injections. Intra-articular steroid injections of the hip have not been studied extensively, so there is no clear consensus on the benefit of this procedure. When combined with local anesthetics, an injection may be of benefit in localizing the pain to the hip joint in patients who may have pain referred from other sites (e.g., lumbar spine).
   G. Intra-articular hyaluronic acid (viscosupplementation) injections. Although viscosupplementation has proven to be useful for patients with early to moderate arthritic changes of the knee, these injections are not currently approved for the treatment of osteoarthritis of the hip.

SURGICAL ALTERNATIVES TO TOTAL HIP ARTHROPLASTY

I. **Arthroscopic Débridement**
   A. Initial arthroscopic examination can help the surgeon identify the precise location and extent of chondral degeneration and identify additional pathology that may not have been clearly observed with radiographic or advanced imaging. Arthroscopic débridement of the hip facilitates the removal of inflammatory mediators, degenerative cartilage, and loose bodies. Débridement with chondral abrasion, as well as loose body removal, is occasionally useful in the management of early to moderate arthritis, with associated mechanical symptoms, that is not suitable for more aggressive procedures such as THA.
   B. Indications
      1. Early arthritis
      2. Mechanical symptoms
      3. Duration of symptoms less than 1 year

II. **Hip Arthrodesis**
  A. Given the fact that current technologic advances in the field of THA have not been perfected to meet the everyday demands of young, active patients in need of surgical intervention, hip arthrodesis remains a feasible option for some patients. The limitations of THA in this patient population are largely due to the limited lifespan of the implants. The downfalls of hip arthrodesis include the potential for new onset of ipsilateral knee pain and back pain (up to 60% in one long-term study), as well as difficulties with various activities of daily living such as putting on socks and shoes.
  B. Indications. This operation is ideally suited for young, active laborers who are motivated to return to work.
    1. Unilateral hip arthritis
    2. Age younger than 35 years
    3. No evidence of degenerative changes or preexisting pain in the lumbar spine, ipsilateral knee, or contralateral hip
    4. Failed treatment for septic arthritis
  C. Contraindications
    1. Bilateral hip arthritis
    2. Ipsilateral knee instability
    3. Pain or radiographic abnormalities of the ipsilateral knee, contralateral hip, or lumbar spine
    4. Neurologic deficits (e.g., cerebral palsy)

III. **Osteotomy**
  A. There are several hip osteotomy options with the primary goal being to transfer loading forces from a degenerative area of the hip to a healthier region, preventing disease progression and preserving viable remaining articular cartilage. This goal is achieved through the repositioning of the femoral and/or acetabular articular surfaces, ultimately resulting in improved anatomic alignment of the hip and reconstitution of hip biomechanics.
  B. Two classes of hip osteotomies
    1. Reconstructive osteotomy: the operative correction of an existing hip deformity to prevent the formation of degenerative changes
    2. Salvage osteotomy: operative correction of a hip with preexisting pathology that can not yet be classified as end-stage degenerative disease
  C. Types of osteotomies
    1. Proximal femoral osteotomies
      a. Varus osteotomy
        (1) Goal of the procedure: to improve femoral head containment within the acetabulum to reduce femoral head extrusion and redirect forces medially
        (2) Indications
          (a) Hip instability
          (b) Proximal femoral deformity
      b. Valgus osteotomy
        (1) Goal of the procedure: to increase articular congruency between the femoral head and acetabulum, resulting in decreased stress forces at the superolateral aspect of the acetabulum
        (2) Indications
          (a) Degenerative changes in the superolateral or medial acetabulum
          (b) More than 60 degrees of hip flexion and more than 20 degrees of adduction
    2. Pelvic osteotomies. A number of pelvic osteotomies can be utilized to redirect abnormal forces at the hip and establish congruency between the femoral head and acetabulum. Young patients with a longstanding history of developmental dysplasia of the hip and resultant hip arthritis largely benefit from these procedures. The most common pelvic osteotomies include the Ganz periacetabular ostcotomy, Salter-single innominate,

> Optimal hip arthrodesis position is 20 to 30 degrees of hip flexion, neutral to 5 degrees of adduction, and neutral to 5 degrees of external rotation.

Hip

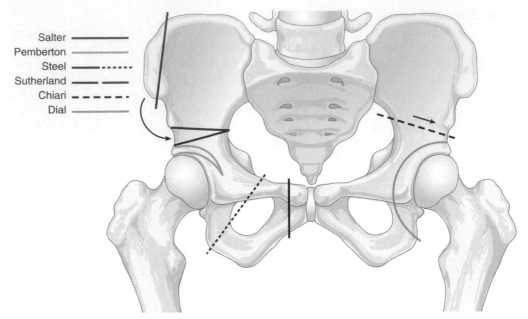

Figure 18-2

Several different pelvic osteotomies. *(From Garino JP, Beredjiklian P [eds]: Core Knowledge in Orthopaedics: Adult Reconstruction and Arthroplasty. Philadelphia, Mosby, 2007.)*

Sutherland-double innominate, and Steel-triple innominate osteotomies. A detailed discussion of these procedures is beyond the scope of this chapter (Fig. 18-2).

SURGICAL INDICATIONS FOR TOTAL HIP ARTHROPLASTY

I. **End-Stage Degenerative Joint Disease**
   A. Most common causes
      1. Osteoarthritis
      2. Rheumatoid arthritis
      3. Osteonecrosis
      4. Post-traumatic arthritis
   B. Other conditions that may result in end-stage joint deterioration
      1. Diseases leading to osteonecrosis of the femoral head
         a. Sickle cell disease
         b. Gaucher's disease
         c. Alcoholism
         d. Systemic lupus erythematosus
         e. Chronic steroid use
      2. Inflammatory arthritides
         a. Juvenile idiopathic arthritis
         b. Spondyloarthropathies
            (1) Ankylosing spondylitis
            (2) Reiter's syndrome
            (3) Psoriatic arthritis
            (4) Enteropathic arthritis
   C. Radiographic features and diagnostic criteria

OSTEOARTHRITIS	RHEUMATOID ARTHRITIS
1. Eccentric joint space narrowing	1. Symmetric joint space narrowing
2. Bony sclerosis	2. Periarticular osteopenia/osteoporosis
3. Subchondral cyst	3. Joint erosion
4. Osteophyte formation	4. Ankylosis

II. **Failed Nonoperative Treatment**
   A. Activity/behavioral modification
   B. Low-impact aerobic exercise
   C. Weight loss
   D. Physical therapy
   E. Ambulatory assistive devices (cane or walker)
   F. Pharmacologic therapy (NSAIDs, cyclooxygenase-II inhibitors)
   G. Dietary supplements (glucosamine–chondroitin sulfate)

CONTRAINDICATIONS TO TOTAL HIP ARTHROPLASTY

   I. **Absolute Contraindication:** active infection (local or systemic)
   II. **Relative Contraindications**
   A. Morbid obesity
   B. Neurologic dysfunction
   C. Severe medical comorbidities (patient unable to safely tolerate the stress of surgery)

GENERAL PRINCIPLES OF TOTAL HIP ARTHROPLASTY

   I. THA stability is a function of component positioning, component sizing/fit, abductor complex/soft tissue tension, and component fixation.
   II. Proper alignment of the acetabular and femoral components is typically 20 to 30 degrees of acetabular anteversion, 35 to 40 degrees of acetabular inclination (theta angle), and 10 to 15 degrees of femoral stem anteversion (Fig. 18-3).
   III. Improper alignment can lead to anterior instability (increased acetabular anteversion), posterior instability (retroverted cup or stem), trochanteric impingement (decreased theta), or superior instability (increased theta angle). The end point of instability is hip dislocation.
   IV. The primary arc range of motion of the hip contributes to stability and depends on the head-to-neck diameter ratio, as well as any modifications made to the neck

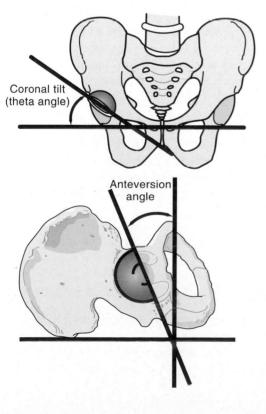

Coronal tilt
(theta angle)

Anteversion
angle

Figure 18-3
Acetabular cup position in coronal and sagittal plane. Coronal tilt (also known as theta angle) should be 35 to 40 degrees. In the sagittal plane, cup anteversion should be 20 to 30 degrees. *(From Miller MD: Review of Orthopaedics, 4th ed. Philadelphia, Saunders, 2004.)*

Hip

or cup (e.g., acetabular augmentation and neck collars). The greater the head-to-neck ratio, the greater the range of motion prior to neck impingement on the acetabular component.

V. The excursion distance is defined as the distance the head must travel to lever out once the neck impinges on the acetabular component. The excursion distance is typically half the diameter of the head. A larger diameter head has a larger excursion distance and thus confers greater hip stability.

VI. The hip abductor complex (gluteus medius and minimus) tension must be maintained for optimal hip stability.

VII. Any process that interferes with proper soft tissue function or coordination, such as stroke, dementia, delirium, or cerebellar dysfunction, can increase the risk of hip instability.

VIII. Obtaining optimum component fixation depends on the size and depth of the implants' pores, minimizing gaps between the bone and implants as well as the quality of the host bone (e.g., prior irradiation leads to an increased risk of loosening).

IX. The femoral and acetabular components can be cemented or noncemented. The disadvantage of cement is that it can fatigue and has no ability to remodel, leading to microfracture and failure. Cemented cups fail at a higher rate than cemented stems because cement is less able to resist shear and tension than compression. The bone ingrowth and remodeling in noncemented components is dynamic and life-lasting.

X. Current cementing technique is considered "third generation," which includes vacuum treatment for porosity reduction, pressurization, precoated stems, and centralization to avoid mantle defects. A mantle defect is a place in a cement column where the prosthesis touches the bone and serves as an area of concentrated stress associated with a higher loosening rate. A cement mantle of 2 mm around the entire prosthesis is generally recommended.

XI. A noncemented porous coated stem may be more appropriate in young active patients due to the risk of cement failing over time.

XII. There are two different techniques for implant fixation: press fit and line-to-line. In *press fit*, the implant is slightly larger than the reamed size, creating compression hoop stresses for temporary fixation. In line-to-line fit, the same diameter implant as the reamer is used and extensive porous coating provides the initial interference "scratch" fit. Screws provide initial fixation of the acetabular cup.

XIII. Safe acetabular screw placement is ensured by using quadrants based on the anterior superior iliac spine and center of the acetabulum. Posterior-superior is the safe zone; posterior-inferior is safe for screws less than 20 mm (sciatic nerve); anterior-inferior may injure the obturator nerve, artery, or vein; and anterior-superior is the "zone of death" (external iliac vessels) (Fig. 18-4).

XIV. One of the major problems facing THA today is osteolysis secondary to wear particles being generated at the articulating surface. Traditional articular bearings for THA are "hard on soft" (metal on polyethylene), although some newer bearings are "hard on hard" (metal on metal or ceramic on ceramic), which have better wear properties.

COMPONENTS OF THE PROCEDURE

Positioning, Prepping, and Draping

I. There are several approaches to the hip that dictate patient position. The following is a description of the posterolateral approach.

II. The patient is positioned in a lateral decubitus position with the operative hip up. Padded lateral holders are used against the sacrum and anterior superior iliac spine

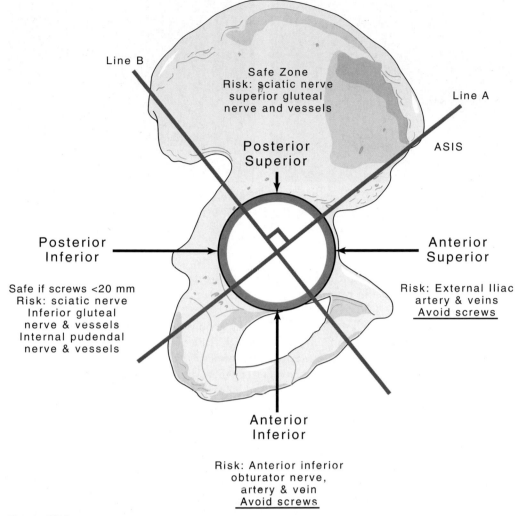

Line B

Safe Zone
Risk: sciatic nerve
superior gluteal
nerve and vessels

Line A

Posterior
Superior

ASIS

Posterior
Inferior

Anterior
Superior

Safe if screws <20 mm
Risk: sciatic nerve
Inferior gluteal
nerve & vessels
Internal pudendal
nerve & vessels

Risk: External Iliac
artery & veins
Avoid screws

Anterior
Inferior

Risk: Anterior inferior
obturator nerve,
artery & vein
Avoid screws

Figure 18-4

Acetabular zones for screw insertion. *Line A* is formed by drawing a line from the anterior superior iliac spine (ASIS) to the center of the acetabular socket. *Line B* is then drawn perpendicular to *A*, also passing through the center of the socket. The posterior-superior quadrant is the preferred zone for screw insertion. *(From Miller MD: Review of Orthopaedics, 4th ed. Philadelphia, Saunders, 2004.)*

to hold the patient in place. Make sure that the operative leg can be flexed to 90 degrees to enable intraoperative assessment of hip stability.

III. Place an axillary roll as well as padding under bony prominences of the contralateral lower extremity.

IV. The extremity is prepped and draped in standard fashion as outlined in Chapter 1 (Fig. 18-5).

> If an extremity holder is not available, hold the leg at the ankle in external rotation in a stable fashion to lock the extremity and help avoid contamination during prepping.

Surgical Approach and Applied Surgical Anatomy

I. Mark the borders of the greater trochanter (superior, anterior, and posterior), femoral shaft, and vastus ridge.

II. Draw an 8- to 10-cm line centered over the posterior one third of the greater trochanter and curve it posterosuperiorly at the level of the tip of the greater trochanter (the incision should be straight when the hip is flexed to 90 degrees) (Fig. 18-6). In most patients, approximately one third of the incision extends above and two thirds below the greater trochanter. Make sure to increase the length of the incision as necessary, based on patient size, deformity, and soft tissue tension.

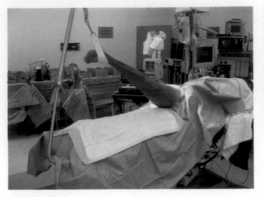

Figure 18-5
The right lower extremity suspended, with body in lateral decubitus position.

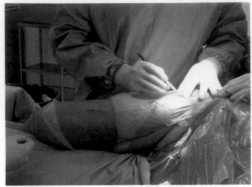

Figure 18-6
The incision is individualized according to the approach used.

III. Incise through skin and subcutaneous tissues with a 10-blade.

IV. Insert self-retaining retractors or rakes to assist in finding the level of the fascia lata.

V. Make small flaps with either a scalpel or a Cobb with a sponge to obtain a clear margin of fascia, which facilitates closure at the end of the case.

VI. Use the scalpel or Bovie to make a small puncture in the fascia lata over the bare area at the tip of the greater trochanter where there are no subfascial muscular attachments.

VII. Use a scalpel or Mayo scissors to split the fascia. Start by spreading under the fascia to clear its undersurface, and then push the scissors in a direction parallel to the orientation of the fascia. The decussating fibers of the underlying gluteus maximus proximally dictate the direction in which the fascial incision should be extended.

VIII. A Charnley retractor may be used at this point for improving visualization, and is placed under the split fascia. In this chapter, a Charnley retractor is not used, and a series of other retractors are used to gain adequate exposure.

IX. Split the gluteus maximus to expose the underlying trochanteric bursa over the trochanter.

X. Perform a bursectomy for better visualization if necessary.

XI. Palpate the piriformis tendon and then locate the gluteus medius. Internally rotate the leg to place the short external rotators on stretch and move the posterior trochanter further away from the sciatic nerve.

XII. Place a C-retractor or double-angle Hohmann retractor under the gluteus medius (over the gluteus minimus) and place it over the anterior lip of the acetabulum (may use a Cobb to help identify the correct plane).

XIII. Insert an Aufranc retractor distally, just proximal to the quadratus femoris muscle and under the inferior aspect of the femoral neck.

XIV. Use a Bovie to dissect the piriformis and conjoined tendon off of their insertions on the greater trochanter. Now define the plane between the piriformis and the gluteus minimus and reposition the C-retractor under the minimus and over the anterior lip of the acetabulum.

XV. Next, make a capsulotomy (trapezoidal or rectangular shaped) to gain access to the hip joint.

XVI. Tag the external rotators and capsule with heavy suture for later repair prior to closure. At this stage, release the posterior inferior capsule along the inferior femoral neck.

XVII. Now the hip can be dislocated by internally rotating and adducting the leg. It may be necessary to release some inferior capsule prior to dislocating the hip.

The conjoined tendon is the confluence of the superior and inferior gemellus muscles and the obturator internus tendon.

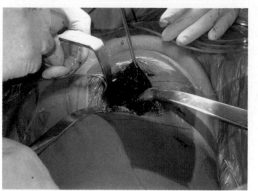

Figure 18-7
The femoral head is removed after resection of the neck.

XIII. Use a femoral neck retractor to elevate the proximal femur out of the wound.

XIX. Flex the knee to 90 degrees and internally rotate the hip so that the leg is perpendicular with the ground.

XX. Identify the lesser trochanter, and use the Bovie to mark the level of the neck cut, which is usually approximately 10 to 15 mm above the lesser trochanter. The exact level of the neck cut should be determined on preoperative templating.

XXI. Make the femoral neck cut using a reciprocating saw blade (complete cuts with an osteotome).

XXII. The neck cut can be made in two directions (transverse and vertical) to avoid cutting the greater trochanter.

XXIII. Use a sweetheart forceps to grab and remove the femoral head once the cuts are complete; use a ligamentum teres knife as needed to assist in femoral head removal (Fig. 18-7).

Acetabular Preparation

I. Position retractors onto the anterior lip of the acetabulum, under the transverse acetabular ligament, and posterosuperiorly.

II. Once the acetabulum is adequately exposed, use a long-handled knife or Bovie to remove the acetabular labrum and remnants of the ligamentum teres.

III. Use a small reamer (usually six to eight sizes less than the templated size), and ream in a medial direction until the inner table of the tear drop is exposed (Fig. 18-8).

IV. Once medialized appropriately, use increasingly larger reamers in a direction to obtain anteversion of 20 to 25 degrees and an inclination angle of 40 to 45 degrees.

V. Insert the acetabular component with the screw holes placed in the posterior-superior quadrant of the acetabulum (Fig. 18-9).

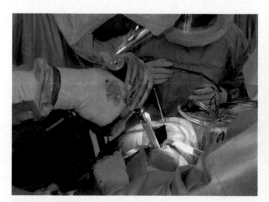

Figure 18-8
Reaming of the acetabulum is performed.

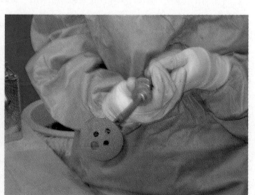

Figure 18-9
Acetabular shell with clustered screw holes.

VI. Insert optional screws if more fixation is needed. Safe screw placement can be ensured if one memorizes the four zones for acetabular screw insertion.

VII. Insert a trial liner and screw it in place and remove all retractors.

Femoral Preparation

I. Flex the hip and knee to 90 degrees and internally rotate the hip so the leg is perpendicular to the floor.

II. Use a femoral neck retractor under the proximal femur to lift it out of the wound.

III. Clear off the medial aspect of the greater trochanter with a Bovie.

IV. Use a box osteotome to open the piriformis fossa, and then use a canal finder to locate the femoral canal.

V. Use the smallest broach and mallet to advance the broach in line with the patient's natural femoral anteversion in reference to the calcar. Be sure to apply steady lateral pressure to prevent the stem being placed in a varus position.

VI. As the broaches become more difficult to advance, be sure to mallet down slowly to dissipate hoop stresses.

VII. Continue to broach until there is a tight fit between the broach and canal and rotational stability is achieved.

> Ask your attending to discuss how to determine if a stem is in varus on a radiograph.

Trial Reduction

I. Start trialing with an 0-head and a standard offset neck, or make adjustments based on preoperative templating (Fig. 18-10).

II. The assistant then reduces the hip by applying manual traction and external rotation.

III. Once reduced, check to make sure there are equal leg lengths.

IV. Check stability in extension and external rotation followed by flexion and internal rotation.

V. Make necessary adjustments until a stable hip has been reconstructed.

Wound Closure

I. Pulse irrigate the femoral canal, acetabulum, and wound.

II. Insert the final acetabular liner in the correct orientation and mallet it into place with the impactor.

III. Insert the final femoral stem, again tapping slowly to dissipate hoop stresses.

IV. Place the final femoral head onto the stem and tap gently with a mallet and head pusher.

V. Reduce the hip and pulse irrigate the wound again prior to closure.

VI. When repairing the capsule and external rotators, use a 2-0 drill bit to make two holes in the greater trochanter. Using a Hewson suture passer, pass the sutures

Figure 18-10
Head trials are applied to the stem.

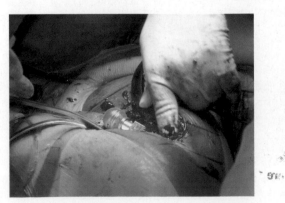

tagging the superior capsule and piriformis through the superior hole, and pass the sutures from the inferior capsule and conjoint tendon through the inferior hole. Pull the sutures to approximate the capsule and external rotators to the medial surface of the greater trochanter and tie the sutures together.

VII. Approximate the fascia, subcutaneous layer, and skin in standard fashion (see Chapter 1 for details).

VIII. Apply a sterile dressing, and place an abduction pillow between the patient's legs prior to transferring the patient from the operating room table.

POSTOPERATIVE CARE AND GENERAL REHABILITATION

I. Postoperative management includes pain control and prophylaxis against infection as well as deep venous thrombosis.

II. Common medications used for deep vein thrombosis prophylaxis include warfarin (Coumadin), low-molecular-weight heparin, aspirin, unfractionated heparin, dextran, and mechanical compression devices (e.g., stockings, Venodynes).

III. Prophylactic antibiotics can be used for up to 24 hours postoperatively. Cefazolin (Ancef), 1 g, can be given every 8 hours for 1 day to prevent surgical site infection.

IV. General rehabilitation is aimed at early mobilization to facilitate faster recovery and also aid in the prevention of deep venous thrombosis formation.

COMPLICATIONS

I. Infection

II. Nerve injury (e.g., sciatic or femoral nerve)

III. Vessel injury (e.g., external iliac vessels from screws placed in the anterior-superior quadrant of the acetabulum)

IV. Periprosthetic fracture (typically femur)

V. Early or late hip dislocation

VI. Heterotopic ossification

VII. Loss of cement fixation

VIII. Osteolysis and aseptic loosening

SUGGESTED READINGS

Berry DJ: Primary total hip arthroplasty. In Chapman MW (ed): Chapman's Orthopaedic Surgery. Philadelphia, Lippincott Williams & Wilkins, 2001.

Kusuma SK, Garino JP: Total hip arthroplasty. In Garino JP, Beredjiklian P (ed): Core Knowledge in Orthopaedics: Adult Reconstruction and Arthroplasty. Philadelphia, Mosby, 2007, pp 108–146.

McPherson EJ: Adult reconstruction. In Miller MD (ed): Review of Orthopaedics, 4th ed. Philadelphia, Saunders, 2004, pp 266–284.

Pellici PM, Tria AJ, Garvin KL: Orthopaedic Knowledge Update: Hip and Knee Reconstruction 2. Rosemont, IL, American Academy of Orthopaedic Surgeons, 2000.

Compression devices prevent venous stasis by improving blood return to the heart, and they also stimulate the release of fibrinolytic factors by endothelial cells lining the vessels.

Early postoperative infection is typically the result of direct inoculation of the operative site, whereas late infections are usually the result of hematogenous spread to the prosthetic joint from a distant site.

Hip

CHAPTER 19

Hip Fractures

J. Stuart Melvin   and   R. Bruce Heppenstall

Case Study 1

A 76-year-old female presents with left groin pain and inability to bear weight on the left lower extremity after suffering a fall from standing. She normally ambulates without assistance and denies prior hip pain. Her left lower extremity is 3 cm shorter than the right and is held in external rotation. There is marked groin pain with attempted passive hip range of motion. She denies having had a syncopal event or any loss of consciousness. The physical examination reveals the hip fracture to be an isolated injury. The motor and sensory examinations are intact and the vascular status of the limb is within normal limits. Anteroposterior (AP) and lateral radiographs of the left hip are presented for two different fracture patterns that may result from a similar mechanism of injury: a femoral neck fracture (Fig. 19-1) and an intertrochanteric hip fracture (Fig. 19-2).

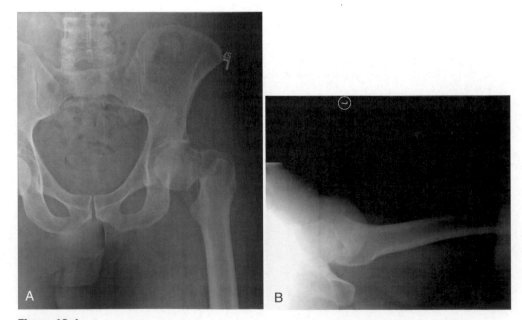

Figure 19-1
Anteroposterior (**A**) and lateral (**B**) radiographs of the left hip demonstrating a displaced femoral neck fracture.

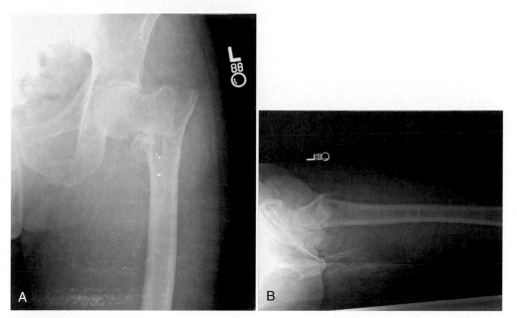

Figure 19-2
Anteroposterior (**A**) and lateral (**B**) radiographs of the left hip demonstrating an intertrochanteric fracture.

Case Study 2

A 47-year-old man presents to the trauma bay after falling 20 feet from a ladder. The patient is awake and alert and complains of left thigh pain. The left leg is shortened and there is an obvious varus deformity of the proximal thigh. The skin is intact, and the motor and sensory examinations are within normal limits. There is a palpable dorsalis pedis pulse. There was no loss of consciousness. An AP radiograph taken in the trauma bay is presented in Figure 19-3.

BACKGROUND

I. Hip fractures are common injuries most often seen in the geriatric population. These fractures have an impact that reaches far beyond the obvious orthopaedic

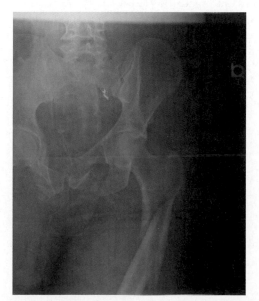

Figure 19-3
Anteroposterior view of the hip demonstrating a displaced subtrochanteric fracture.

injury and consume a large proportion of health care resources. Approximately 50% of patients who were independent prior to a hip fracture are unable to regain independence. The 1-year mortality rate for these fractures ranges from 15% to 20%.

II. The term *hip fracture* may refer to a fracture of the femoral neck, intertrochanteric femur, or subtrochanteric femur. The location of the fracture within one of these anatomic regions is important and dictates the potential treatment options.

III. In elderly patients, hip fractures are most often low-energy fractures related to osteoporosis. Thus, hip fractures are more common in women.

IV. In younger patients, hip fractures occur infrequently. When they do occur, they are most often due to high-energy trauma or are pathologic fractures secondary to a bone tumor.

V. Approximately 300,000 hip fractures occur annually in the United States. With the aging population, the number of hip fractures is expected to double by the year 2050.

VI. The major goals of treatment of hip fractures are as follows:
A. Relief of pain
B. Restoration of function
C. Early mobilization

Femoral Neck Fractures

I. **Nondisplaced or Impacted Femoral Neck Fractures**
A. Approximately 8% to 15% of nondisplaced fractures become displaced without treatment.
B. Less than 8% of nondisplaced fractures progress to osteonecrosis of the femoral head.
C. Less than 5% of non-displaced fracture progress to a nonunion.

II. **Displaced Femoral Neck Fractures**
A. Osteonecrosis occurs in 15% to 33% of cases.
B. Nonunion occurs in 10% to 30% of cases.

III. **Anatomy**
A. The femoral neck is an intracapsular structure. On average, the femoral neck and head are anteverted 10 ± 6 degrees and the neck-shaft angle is typically 130 ± 7 degrees.
B. The vascular supply to the femoral head is defined as follows (Fig. 19-4):
1. Arteries traverse the length of the femoral neck and may be disrupted in a fracture of the femoral neck, contributing to the risk of osteonecrosis or nonunion. Extracapsular hip fractures (intertrochanteric and subtrochanteric) have a negligible risk of osteonecrosis.
2. An extracapsular arterial ring is formed at the base of the femoral neck by contributions from the lateral and medial femoral circumflex arteries.

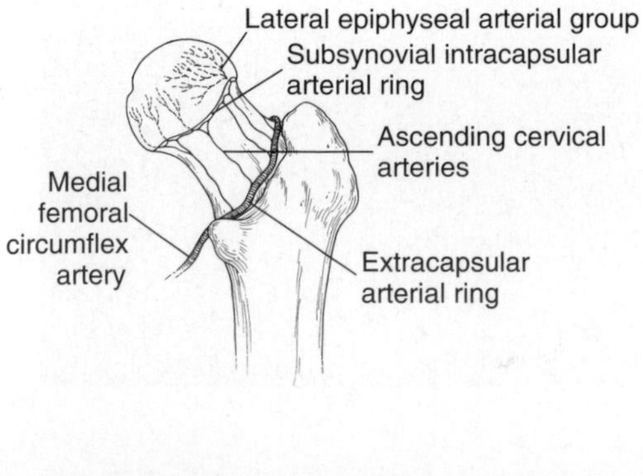

> The average femoral neck-shaft angle is 130 ± 7 degrees.

Figure 19-4
Blood supply to the femoral head. *(From Canale ST [ed]: Campbell's Operative Orthopaedics, 10th ed. Philadelphia, Mosby, 2003.)*

Lateral epiphyseal arterial group
Subsynovial intracapsular arterial ring
Ascending cervical arteries
Medial femoral circumflex artery
Extracapsular arterial ring

Ascending cervical branches from this ring pierce the capsule and run along the femoral neck as the retinacular arteries. These retinacular arteries form a subsynovial ring at the base of the femoral head and pierce the femoral head as the epiphyseal branches.

3. The lateral epiphyseal arteries from the posterior-superior ascending cervical branches arise from the medial femoral circumflex artery to supply the majority of the femoral head.

4. The artery of the ligamentum teres, a branch of the obturator artery, supplies a small portion of the femoral head in adults, although it contributes a great deal to the femoral head blood supply in children younger than 4 years of age.

IV. **Fracture Classifications**
  A. Anatomic location
    1. Subcapital
    2. Transcervical
    3. Basicervical
  B. Pauwels classification
    1. This classification is based on the angle formed by the fracture line in the femoral neck and a horizontal line.
      a. Type I: 30 degrees
      b. Type II: 50 degrees
      c. Type III: 70 degrees
    2. An increasing angle leads to higher shear forces and instability across the fracture site.
  C. Garden classification. This classification is based on the degree of fracture fragment displacement (Fig. 19-5).

> The posterior-superior ascending cervical branches from the medial femoral circumflex artery supply the majority of the femoral head.

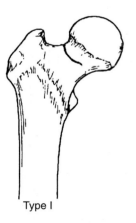

Type I

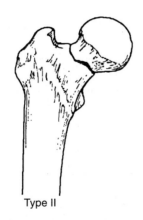

Type II

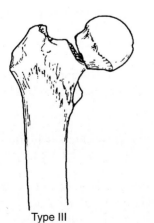

Type III

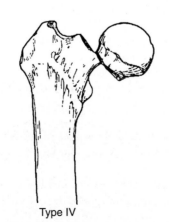

Type IV

Figure 19-5
Garden classification of femoral neck fractures. *(From Kyle RF: Fractures of the hip. In Gustilo RB, Kyle RF, Templeman DC [eds]: Fractures and Dislocations. St Louis, Mosby, 1993.)*

Hip

1. Type I: incomplete or impacted
2. Type II: complete and nondisplaced
3. Type III: complete with partial displacement
4. Type IV: completely displaced

Intertrochanteric Hip Fractures

I. Intertrochanteric (IT) fractures are the most common hip fracture in the elderly and are most often related to osteoporosis. When they occur in younger patients, they are secondary to high-energy trauma or pathologic fracture.

II. **Anatomy**

A. IT fractures occur between the greater and lesser trochanters with occasional extension into the subtrochanteric region.

B. These fractures occur through cancellous bone and thus possess great healing potential. The nonunion rate is less than 2%.

C. The calcar femorale is an area of dense cortical bone at the posterior-medial aspect of the proximal femur that acts as a strong strut to transfer load from the femoral neck to the intertrochanteric region and is critical for stability. The integrity of this region is the basis for whether a fracture is considered stable or unstable.

III. **Fracture Classifications**

A. Boyd and Griffin

1. Type I: fracture line extends along the intertrochanteric line—stable
2. Type II: fracture line extends along the intertrochanteric line with comminution and displacement—stable
3. Type III: fracture at level of the lesser trochanter with posteromedial comminution—reverse obliquity—unstable
4. Type IV: intertrochanteric fracture with subtrochanteric extension—unstable

B. Evans

1. Divided into stable and unstable fracture patterns with stability dependent on continuity of the posteromedial cortex
2. Reverse obliquity fractures—inherently unstable

C. Orthopaedic Trauma Association

Subtrochanteric Hip Fractures

I. Subtrochanteric (ST) fractures occur in a zone extending from the lesser trochanter to 5 cm distal to the lesser trochanter.

II. These fractures are notoriously difficult to treat because of the powerful muscle forces acting on the fragments as well as the tremendous stress that is normally placed through this region. The proximal fragment is typically flexed, abducted, and externally rotated while the distal fragment is typically adducted.

III. When seen in young patients, ST fractures are due to high-energy trauma or pathologic fracture. In the elderly, they are often related to osteoporosis.

IV. Fractures may also occur at the site of screw placement for a femoral neck fracture if the inferior screw is placed too low as this creates a cortical defect and results in a stress riser.

V. **Anatomy**

A. The medial and posteromedial cortices of the ST femur experience the highest compressive stresses in the body. The lateral cortex is under a high degree of tensile stress.

B. These fractures occur at the corticocancellous junction. The high composition of cortical bone and subsequently the decreased vascularity impairs the capacity

---

An intact calcar femorale or posteromedial cortex is the defining factor for classifying an intertrochanteric fracture's stability.

The proximal fragment in subtrochanteric fractures is usually flexed, abducted, and externally rotated due to the pull of the psoas, gluteus medius, and short external rotators, respectively.

Approximately 10% of subtrochanteric fractures are a result of gunshot wounds.

for healing of these fractures when compared with the abundant cancellous bone of the IT region.

VI. **Fracture Classifications**
  A. Fielding. This is an anatomic classification based on location of the fracture.
    1. Type I: at the level of the lesser trochanter
    2. Type II: less than 2.5 cm below the lesser trochanter
    3. Type III: 2.5 to 5 cm below the lesser trochanter
  B. Seinsheimer. This system incorporates factors affecting stability and offers management guidelines.
    1. Type I: nondisplaced
    2. Type II: two-part fractures. Subtypes based on fracture pattern and displacement.
    3. Type III: three-part spiral fracture. Subtypes based on type of fracture fragments.
    4. Type IV: comminuted
    5. Type V: IT extension
  C. Russell-Taylor. This classification is based on integrity of the piriformis fossa. It was designed to guide treatment of intramedullary nails using a piriformis fossa starting point.
    1. Type I: intact piriformis fossa
      a. A: lesser trochanter attached to the proximal fragment
      b. B: lesser trochanter detached from the proximal fragment
    2. Type II: fracture extending into piriformis fossa
      a. A: stable posterior-medial buttress
      b. B: comminution of lesser trochanter
  D. Orthopaedic Trauma Association

RADIOGRAPHIC ASSESSMENT

  I. For all hip fractures, an AP of the pelvis, internal rotation AP, and cross-table lateral radiographs of the affected hip should be obtained.
  II. For femoral neck fractures, magnetic resonance imaging is indicated if plain radiography fails to reveal a fracture and suspicion is high for an occult fracture or stress fracture of the femoral neck. Bone scans may also show increased uptake with occult or stress fractures of the hip.
  III. Magnetic resonance imaging may also be required for pathologic fractures to evaluate the proximal femur for soft tissue extension of an underlying bone tumor.

TREATMENT ALGORITHM

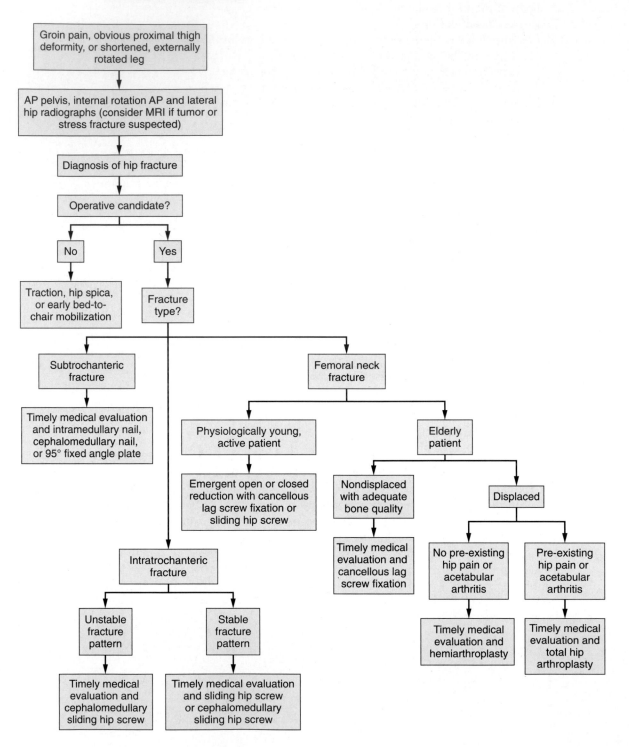

TREATMENT PROTOCOLS

I. **Treatment Considerations**
   A. Patient age
   B. Activity level prior to injury. Nonambulators may be considered nonoperative candidates.
   C. Location of fracture within the femoral neck. Low neck fractures abutting the intertrochanteric region (basic cervical) may be treated as IT fractures because of similar bone quality and vascular status.

D. Displaced femoral neck fractures. Displaced fractures have a much higher rate of nonunion and osteonecrosis, making arthroplasty (partial or total hip replacement) a more predictable treatment option.

E. Presence and severity of acetabular osteoarthritis. Preexisting acetabular osteoarthritis makes total hip arthroplasty (THA) the best treatment option.

F. Associated injuries

G. Timing of surgery. Surgery is indicated within 96 hours after injury if the patient is medically stable.

H. Overall health status. Nonoperative treatment methods may be considered if the surgical risk is excessively high secondary to patient comorbidities.

I. Fracture stability. Stability of IT and ST fractures is based on the integrity of the posteromedial cortex.

J. Fracture pattern. Reverse obliquity fracture patterns are unstable by definition and are best treated as ST fractures.

II. **Nonoperative Treatment**

A. Surgical treatment is the standard of care for all hip fractures. Nonoperative treatment is to be considered only when the risk of surgery outweighs the benefit.

B. Treatment options include skeletal traction, Buck's skin traction, application of a hip spica cast, or non–weight bearing with acceptance of the ensuing proximal femoral deformity.

C. For ST fractures, skeletal traction after closed reduction is the most common nonoperative treatment protocol. Closed reduction is performed with a distal femoral transcondylar Steinmann pin by flexing the hip to 90 degrees, correcting the external rotation deformity, and applying traction to decrease abduction. Traction is typically applied for 12 to 16 weeks.

D. Regardless of treatment modality, early bed-to-chair mobilization is paramount and should begin as soon as pain permits to prevent complications of prolonged recumbency.

> Ask the patient about preexisting hip pain because this may indicate preinjury hip osteoarthritis.

SURGICAL ALTERNATIVES, INDICATIONS, AND CONTRAINDICATIONS

Nondisplaced or Impacted Femoral Neck Fractures

I. In situ pinning with multiple cancellous lag screws

A. This is the preferred treatment for nondisplaced femoral neck fractures. Three screws are placed parallel in an inverted triangle configuration.

B. Advantages
   1. Quicker procedure
   2. Minimal soft tissue damage

C. Disadvantages
   1. Less rigid fixation
   2. Potentially creates a stress riser in the subtrochanteric region of the proximal femur

II. Sliding hip screw and side plate

A. If a sliding hip screw and side plate is used, a derotational pin may be placed parallel to the sliding screw to avoid rotation of the head fragment.

B. Advantages
   1. Greater biomechanical strength
   2. Allows for compression across fracture site with weight bearing
   3. Minimizes the creation of a stress riser in the subtrochanteric region

C. Disadvantages
   1. Requires a larger exposure
   2. Potential for rotational malalignment at time of screw placement

Displaced Femoral Neck Fractures

I. Open or closed reduction with multiple cancellous lag screws or sliding hip screw

A. Surgical stabilization with cancellous screws should be urgently performed for young patients with a high-energy injury and good bone quality.

B. This may also be performed after timely medical evaluation for highly functional elderly patients with good bone quality and minimal osteoarthritis.

II. **Hip Hemiarthroplasty** (see Chapter 18 for femoral stem insertion)

A. This involves replacement of the femoral head and neck with a femoral prosthesis and is the treatment of choice for elderly patients with lower functional demands, poor bone quality, and minimal acetabular osteoarthritis.

B. Unipolar and bipolar prosthesis are considered to have similar functional outcomes.

C. Cement to secure the prosthesis to bone should be considered for patients with osteoporosis.

D. Advantages
   1. Decreased operative time compared with THA
   2. Increased stability due to larger femoral head size
   3. Immediate weight bearing
   4. Lower rates of reoperation compared to multiple cannulated screws or sliding hip screw

E. Disadvantages
   1. May lead to erosion of acetabular cartilage
   2. Femoral stem loosening

III. **Total Hip Arthroplasty** (THA; see Chapter 18 for details)

A. THA involves the replacement of the femoral head and neck as well as the articular surface of the acetabulum. This treatment option should be considered in the following scenarios:
   1. Elderly patients with preinjury hip pain or significant radiographic evidence of osteoarthritis
   2. Rheumatoid arthritis
   3. Paget's disease involving the acetabulum
   4. Salvage procedure for failed open reduction and internal fixation or hemiarthroplasty

B. Advantages: very good and predictable long-term functional results and relief of pain

C. Disadvantages
   1. Higher dislocation rate when compared with hemiarthroplasty or primary THA for osteoarthritis
   2. Requires a longer surgical time with greater blood loss

Intertrochanteric Hip Fractures

I. **Sliding Hip Screw**

A. Historically the most common method of operative fixation

B. The plate is available in fixed angles from 130 to 150 degrees and should be matched to the native anatomy.

C. Advantages
   1. Ease of application
   2. Broad surgeon familiarity
   3. Relatively less expensive
   4. Allows compression at the fracture site with weight bearing

D. Disadvantages
   1. Greater tensile stress on the screw due to longer lever arm of a plate placed on the lateral femur
   2. Greater screw sliding, which can lead to medialization of distal fragment
   3. Failure rate of 10% for fixation, most often in unstable fractures due to errant screw placement or failure of the screw to slide in the plate

II. **Cephalomedullary Sliding Hip Screw**

A. Has become the most common method of operative fixation

B. Uses a sliding screw or helical blade placed through an intramedullary nail

C. Advantages
1. Shorter lever arm for the lag screw, which decreases tensile stress on the screw
2. Avoids excessive screw sliding, because the proximal fragment would abut the nail before it would abut a side plate
3. Placed through a limited skin incision, requiring minimal dissection and thus less tissue trauma and blood loss

D. Disadvantages
1. Early generation devices associated with a higher rate of femoral shaft fractures at the tip of the nail or interlocking screws
2. No demonstrated clinical advantage over the sliding hip screw and side plate for stable IT fracture
3. More expensive device

III. **Hip Hemiarthroplasty** (see Chapter 18 for femoral stem insertion)
A. This is not usually indicated for primary treatment of IT fractures; however, it may be indicated after failed internal fixation.
B. If using to primarily treat an IT fracture, a calcar replacing implant must be used. Consideration must also be given to reattachment of the greater trochanter to restore abductor function.

> What is your attending's preference for operative treatment of intertrochanteric fractures?

Subtrochanteric Hip Fractures

I. **Intramedullary Nail**
A. Intramedullary fixation is the preferred treatment.
B. First-generation interlocking nails (centromedullary) are indicated when both trochanters are intact.
C. Second-generation interlocking nails with a locking screw that extends into the femoral neck (cephalomedullary) offer more stable fixation and are indicated when the lesser trochanter is displaced or comminuted.
D. Advantages
1. Potential for closed treatment with preservation of fracture hematoma and blood supply to fracture fragments
2. Decreases the moment arm on the implant compared with a lateral plate and thus decreases the tensile stress on the implant
3. Reaming the canal in preparation of the implant, which provides internal bone graft
E. Disadvantages
1. Placement of an intramedullary implant, which can be technically demanding
2. Possible need for the fracture site to be opened to facilitate reduction and guide pin insertion, thus lessening benefits of closed intramedullary fixation

II. **Ninety-Five–Degree Fixed Angled Device**
A. Historically the most common device used for operative fixation
B. Has a fixed angle construct, which provides rigid fixation
C. Advantages
1. Offers a treatment option for fractures with comminution of the trochanters that may make intramedullary implant insertion difficult
2. Provides for multiple points of proximal fixation
D. Disadvantages
1. Technically very demanding
2. Extensive soft tissue dissection
3. High risk of implant failure due to tremendous stress applied to the plate laterally

III. **Sliding Hip Screw**
A. Indicated only for very proximal fractures
B. Sliding of the screw to allow medialization of the distal fragment, which reduces bending moment on fracture and implant

C. Necessity for sliding mechanism to cross the fracture site to lessen the risk of implant failure

D. Essential to reconstruct the posteromedial cortex to decrease the stress on the device

GENERAL PRINCIPLES FOR PARALLEL CANCELLOUS LAG SCREW FIXATION OF NONDISPLACED FEMORAL NECK FRACTURES

I. Typically, three screws are placed in an inverted triangle configuration. The first screw is inserted inferiorly along the calcar to control inferior displacement. The second screw is placed posterosuperiorly along the neck to prevent posterior displacement. The third screw is placed anterosuperiorly.

II. A fourth screw may be placed posteriorly for additional support in the presence of posterior comminution.

III. Lag screw threads should be in the femoral head and not remain crossing the fracture site. This impedes fracture compression.

IV. It is important to place the screws above the level of the lesser trochanter at the comparable point on the lateral femoral cortex. This prevents the formation of a stress riser along the lateral cortical-cancellous junction, which may lead to a subsequent fracture.

V. Acceptable reduction

A. Valgus angulation is more mechanically stable and can be accepted more so than varus angulation.

B. Try to avoid posterior translation of the neck while maintaining anteversion on lateral radiograph.

C. Assess for comminution posteriorly and place pins appropriately.

D. The convexity of the femoral head should form a shallow S-shaped curve with the concavity of the femoral neck on all fluoroscopic views. A C-shaped curve or sharp apex on fluoroscopic views indicates malreduction.

E. The Garden alignment index is a method of assessing adequacy of reduction. For an adequate reduction, the primary compression trabeculae of the femoral neck should form an angle of 160 to 180 degrees with the femoral shaft on both an AP and lateral radiograph (Fig. 19-6).

COMPONENTS OF THE PROCEDURE: CLOSED REDUCTION AND PARALLEL CANCELLOUS LAG SCREW FIXATION OF NONDISPLACED FEMORAL NECK FRACTURES

Positioning

I. Patient positioning is on the fracture table. See Chapter 17 for positioning on the fracture table.

Figure 19-6
Garden alignment index. *(From DeLee JC: Fractures and dislocations of the hip. In Rockwood CA Jr, Green DP [eds]: Fractures in Adults, 2nd ed. Philadelphia, JB Lippincott, 1984.)*

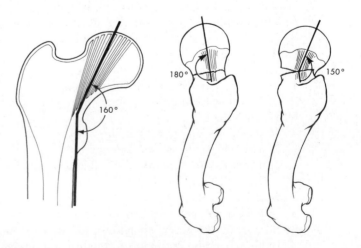

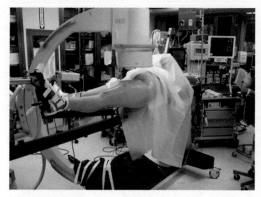
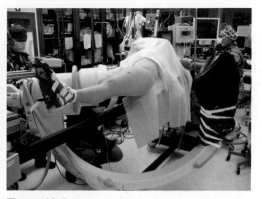

Figure 19-7
Fluoroscope positioning for anteroposterior fluoroscopy of hip.

Figure 19-8
Fluoroscope positioning for lateral fluoroscopy of hip.

II. Positioning of fluoroscope machine (Figs. 19-7 and 19-8)
   A. The fluoroscope should be positioned between the patient's legs for AP and lateral views of the hip. The lateral is obtained by swinging the fluoroscope along its axis beneath the operative leg.
   B. Ensure that adequate unobstructed AP and lateral views of the fracture can be obtained prior to draping. Mark the position of the fluoroscope for these views by placing tape on the floor.

Closed Reduction

I. Begin by disengaging the fracture, which is achieved via traction, flexion, and external rotation. These maneuvers are performed by using the traction gears or through manipulation of the position of the traction boot.
II. Next, obtain the reduction through slow extension, abduction, and internal rotation. The adequacy of the reduction should be checked with fluoroscopy using the guidelines set forth in the previous section on acceptable reduction.
III. If reduction cannot be achieved in a young patient, proceed to open reduction via an anterior-lateral approach to the hip.

Prepping and Draping

See Chapter 17 for details on prepping and draping.

Surgical Approach and Applied Anatomy

I. Begin by marking the angle of the femoral neck in the AP plane and the femoral shaft in the lateral plane on the skin. A sterile pen is used to trace a K-wire positioned appropriately in the AP and lateral plane. When making the skin marks, make sure that all screws will be superior to the lesser trochanter.
II. The incision should extend 1.5 cm superiorly and inferiorly to the point where these lines cross. Make the incision with a 15-blade and use a Bovie to incise the subcutaneous fat and fascia in line with the incision.

Screw Placement

I. Three screws should be placed parallel along the femoral neck in an inverted triangle configuration. For placement of the first screw, drive a guide pin at an angle of 130 to 135 degrees along the inferior neck on the AP fluoroscopic view and in the center of the neck on the lateral fluoroscopic view to within 1 cm of subchondral bone. Slightly more valgus may be acceptable for

> The anterolateral approach to the hip is in the intermuscular plane between the tensor fascia lata and the gluteus medius muscles. This is not an internervous plane because they are both innervated by the superior gluteal nerve.

Hip

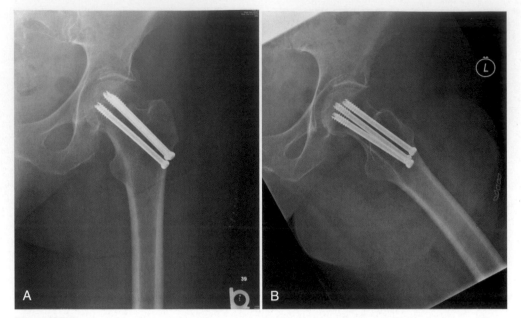

Figure 19-9
Anteroposterior (**A**) and lateral (**B**) postoperative radiographs of hip following parallel cancellous screw fixation.

valgus-impacted fractures, taking care that the entry point is above the lesser trochanter.

II. Using the inverted triangle guide, drive the second and third guide pins along the posterosuperior and anterosuperior neck, respectively. Use an army-navy retractor as needed to avoid catching the IT band and fascia in the drill.

III. Remove the pin guide and measure the screw lengths with the depth gauge. Using the screwdriver, place the appropriate length cannulated lag screws in the same order as they were drilled. Ensure that the threads of the lag screws do not cross the fracture line when fully seated, because this will prevent compression across the fracture line.

IV. Take final AP and lateral fluoroscopy images (Fig. 19-9).

V. See Chapter 18 for insertion of the femoral component only (hemiarthroplasty) and THA for treatment of displaced femoral neck fractures.

Wound Closure

I. For all procedures, the wound is copiously irrigated with sterile saline and hemostasis is achieved prior to closure.

II. The wound is closed in layers and staples are used to reapproximate the skin edges (see Chapter 1 for details).

GENERAL PRINCIPLES OF SLIDING HIP SCREWS: INTERTROCHANTERIC HIP FRACTURES

I. It is important to place the screw in the center of the femoral head on AP and lateral views and within 1 cm of subchondral bone. This position has been shown to decrease the rate of superior screw cutout and varus collapse.

II. The tip-apex distance is a method to predict screw cutout and is calculated as the sum of the distance from the tip of the lag screw to the apex of the femoral head on both the AP and lateral radiographs (Fig. 19-10).

CALCULATE THE TIP-APEX DISTANCE TO ENSURE PROPER SCREW POSITIONING.

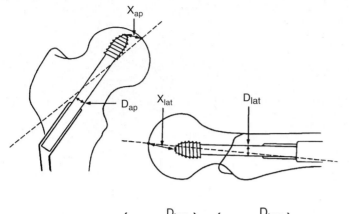

Figure 19-10

Calculation of tip-apex distance. *(From Baumgaertner MR, Curtin SL, Lindskog DM, Keggi JM: The value of the tip-apex distance in predicting failure of fixation of peritrochanteric fractures of the hip. J Bone Joint Surg 77A:1058, 1995. Reprinted with permission from The Journal of Bone and Joint Surgery, Inc.)*

$$TAD 5 \left(X_{ap} \times \frac{D_{true}}{D_{ap}} \right) + \left(X_{lat} \times \frac{D_{true}}{D_{lat}} \right)$$

III. A tip-apex distance of less than 25 mm is associated with lower rate of screw cutout.

COMPONENTS OF THE PROCEDURE: CLOSED REDUCTION AND APPLICATION OF SLIDING HIP SCREW AND SIDE PLATE

Positioning

I. Positioning on the fracture table. See Chapter 17 for patient positioning on the fracture table.
II. Positioning of the fluoroscope machine. Please see previous section on treatment of nondisplaced femoral neck fractures.

Closed Reduction

I. To obtain a closed reduction, begin by taking initial AP and lateral fluoroscopy images.
II. Begin the reduction maneuver by applying traction with the leg in external rotation. Internally rotate the leg by manipulating the position of the traction boot to achieve the reduction. Posterior sag of the distal fragment can often be corrected with placement of a crutch below the distal fragment, whereas excessive varus can often be corrected with additional traction.
III. Check the reduction with AP and lateral fluoroscopy.

Prepping and Draping

See Chapter 17 for details on prepping and draping.

Surgical Approach and Applied Anatomy

I. Under image intensification, mark the skin incision by using a guide pin placed on the skin parallel to the femoral neck on the AP view and femoral shaft on the lateral view. An incision is carried 10 cm distally along the lateral femur from the point where these lines cross.
II. Incise down through the subcutaneous tissue to the level of the fascia. Make a longitudinal incision in the fascia in line with the incision. Split the vastus lateralis between the muscle fibers and get down to bone. Stay approximately 0.5 cm from the lateral intermuscular septum to avoid perforating vessels from the profunda femoris artery. Reflect the vastus lateralis superiorly with a Bennett retractor.

> **BE CAREFUL OF PERFORATING BRANCHES OF THE PROFUNDA FEMORIS ARTERY. THESE VESSELS TYPICALLY PIERCE THE LATERAL INTERMUSCULAR SEPTUM AND CAN LEAD TO A GREAT DEAL OF BLEEDING IF THEY ARE INADVERTENTLY DISRUPTED.**

Hip

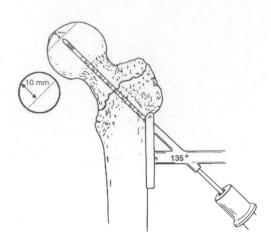

Figure 19-11
Alignment guide demonstrating proper placement of guidewire. *(From Baumgaertner MR: Compression Hip Screw Plates Technique Manual. Memphis, Smith & Nephew Richards, 1996.)*

Placement of Screw and Side-Plate

I. Using the angle guide, select the appropriate plate angle that will place a screw parallel to the femoral neck in the center of the femoral head on AP and lateral views. The 135-degree plate is the most commonly used plate. Higher angle plates increase the risk of placing the screw below the lesser trochanter, increasing the risk of fracture.

II. Under image intensification, use the wire driver and plate angle guide to drive a threaded guidewire to within 1 cm of subchondral bone in the center of the femoral head on AP and lateral views. Assess the tip-apex distance at this time and replace the guidewire if it is greater than 25 mm (Fig. 19-11).

III. Next, measure the screw length from the length of the guidewire and ream over the guidewire to the appropriate length per the specific device. Beware of guide pin advancement into the joint.

IV. Tap over the guidewire and insert the appropriate length screw over the guide-wire. Use firm continuous pressure to place the screw within 1 cm of subchondral bone. Avoid levering on the screw as it is being inserted.

V. Align the screwdriver handle parallel with the shaft of the femur when the screw is seated. This will align the key mechanism with the side plate. Most often a "keyed" system is used in which the side plate captures the lag screw and prevents rotation of the screw but allows sliding along the barrel of the plate.

VI. Place the side plate over the screw and secure it to the lateral femur.

VII. Place a clamp around the femur and sideplate to hold the plate to the femur and release traction on the leg to allow fracture impaction and sliding.

VIII. Now, insert 4.5-mm cortical screws to fill the holes of the sideplate making sure to obtain bicortical purchase. The clamp may be released after two screws have been secured. Retighten all screws prior to closure (Fig. 19-12).

BEWARE OF GUIDEWIRE ADVANCEMENT INTO THE HIP JOINT AND PELVIS WHEN REAMING OR DRILLING OVER THE GUIDEWIRE.

RELEASE TRACTION PRIOR TO PLACING FEMORAL SHAFT SCREWS TO ALLOW FOR FRACTURE IMPACTION.

Wound Closure

The wound is closed in standard fashion according to the surgical principles outlined in Chapter 1.

GENERAL PRINCIPLES OF CEPAHLOMEDULLARY SLIDING HIP SCREW PLACEMENT: INTERTROCHANTERIC AND SUBTROCHANTERIC HIP FRACTURES

I. A cephalomedullary sliding hip screw is placed typically using a greater trochanteric starting point. The starting point for ST fractures may be slightly

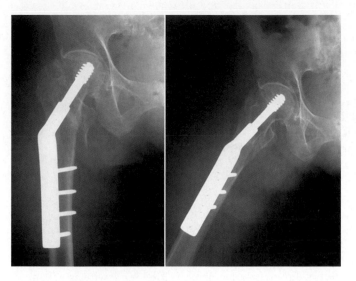

Figure 19-12
Anteroposterior and lateral view
of sliding hip screw and sideplate. *(From Canale ST [ed]:
Campbell's Operative Orthopaedics,
10th ed. Philadelphia, Mosby, 2003.)*

more medial due to the higher tendency of these fractures to fall into a varus
position.

II. A short cephalomedullary screw can be used for IT fractures, whereas a long device
must be used for ST fractures.

III. A screw and side plate can be used for standard IT fractures; however, their use
is contraindicated in reverse obliquity IT fractures and ST fractures.

IV. The proximal fragment of an ST hip fracture is likely to be in flexion, abduction,
and external rotation. A small open anterior incision may be needed to manipulate
the proximal fragment while placing the guidewire. If adequate reduction cannot
be achieved, then use an extension of the lateral incision to visualize the fracture
site.

V. Also, use the tip-apex distance with this device to minimize screw cutout in the
postoperative period.

COMPONENTS OF THE PROCEDURE: CLOSED REDUCTION AND CEPHALOMEDULLARY SLIDING HIP SCREW PLACEMENT

Positioning

I. Patient positioning is on the fracture table. See Chapter 17 for positioning on the
fracture table.

II. Positioning of the fluoroscope machine. Refer to the previous section on treatment
of nondisplaced femoral neck fractures.

Closed Reduction

I. To obtain a closed reduction, begin by taking initial AP and lateral fluoroscopy
images.

II. Begin the reduction maneuver by applying traction with the leg in external rotation. Internally rotate the leg by manipulating the position of the traction boot to
achieve the reduction. Posterior sag of the distal fragment can often be corrected
with placement of a crutch below the distal fragment, whereas excessive varus can
often be corrected with additional traction. This is especially important with
intramedullary devices because varus makes obtaining the starting point more
difficult. If excessive varus cannot be corrected, consider a sliding hip screw or
open reduction.

III. Check the reduction with AP and lateral fluoroscopy.

IV. Have the leg placed in neutral or slight adduction to facilitate access to the greater
trochanter starting point.

Hip

Prepping and Draping

See Chapter 17 for prepping and draping.

Surgical Approach

I. This section will detail the greater trochanter starting point. The appropriate starting point depends on the specific device, but usually it is at the superior tip of the greater trochanter in the AP projection and at the junction of the anterior third and posterior two thirds of the greater trochanter in the lateral projection.

II. Place a 3.2-mm K-wire percutaneously on the anticipated starting point. Use fluoroscopy to guide the insertion of the K-wire to the correct position. The starting point for percutaneous K-wire placement in obese patients is often located more proximally.

III. Make a 2-cm longitudinal incision at the K-wire skin entry point and bluntly dissect to the entry point on the greater trochanter. The guidewire is advanced from the starting point down to the level of the lesser trochanter.

Placement of the Cephalomedullary Sliding Hip Screw

I. Place a tissue protector and a conical reamer to the starting point to open the medullary canal over the guide pin. Alternatively, a curved awl under fluoroscopy may be used to locate the starting point and prepare the proximal femur.

II. Once the entry reamer has opened up the proximal femur, pass a ball-tipped guidewire down the femoral shaft; this guides the flexible reamers while reaming the femoral canal. Reaming may not be necessary in elderly individuals who have large-diameter canals.

III. See Chapter 24 for details regarding placement of an intramedullary nail. The remainder of this section will focus on placing the lag screw through an already properly placed intramedullary nail component.

IV. When positioned appropriately, insert the screw sleeve guide and incise the skin where this guide contacts the skin. Dissect down through the iliotibial band and vastus lateralis to bone. Advance the sleeve guide to bone and stabilize the screw sleeve guide to ensure that it is flush to bone. Next, drill the lateral cortex.

V. Replace the screw sleeve guide and place a K-wire sleeve guide. This centrally positions the K-wire within the hole in the lateral wall. Now, advance a 3.2-mm K-wire to subchondral bone. Check K-wire placement on AP and lateral fluoroscopy.

VI. Measure the screw depth from the K-wire and drill the screw path to within 1 cm of subchondral bone. Ensure that the K-wire does not advance into the joint. Compression at the fracture site can be achieved by selecting a screw 5 mm shorter than measured.

VII. Now insert the screw and ensure that it is free to slide. Tighten the set screw and then loosen it a quarter-turn. The set screw allows sliding but not rotation of the lag screw. Insert the end cap.

VIII. Finish by placing locking screws using the targeting guide. If a long nail is used, distal locking screws should be placed using free hand perfect circle technique (Fig. 19-13). (See Chapter 24 for perfect circles technique.)

Wound Closure

The wound is closed in standard fashion according to the surgical principles outlined in Chapter 1.

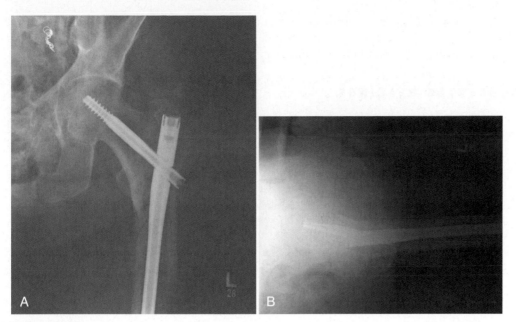

Figure 19-13
Anteroposterior (**A**) and lateral (**B**) postoperative views of cephalomedullary sliding hip screw used to treat a subtrochanteric fracture.

POSTOPERATIVE CARE AND GENERAL REHABILITATION OF HIP FRACTURES

I. Postoperative management includes pain control and prophylaxis against infection and deep venous thromboembolism.

II. Twenty-four hours of postoperative antibiotics should be administered.

III. Unless contraindicated, systemic anticoagulation with warfarin or low-molecular-weight heparin should be administered for 2 to 6 weeks.

IV. Pharmacologic treatment is augmented with compression stocking, a mechanical compression device, and early mobilization.

V. Physical therapy or out-of-bed mobilization is started on postoperative day 1.

VI. Weight-bearing status in the elderly is controversial.

A. Elderly patients with decreased upper extremity strength often have difficulty maintaining partial or non–weight-bearing protocols. Additionally, partial or non–weight-bearing protocols may generate considerable force across the hip. Thus, many believe that weight bearing as tolerated is the most appropriate recommendation to mobilize these patients early.

B. For younger patients whose fractures are often pathologic or higher energy with comminution, weight-bearing status depends on stability of fracture and internal fixation.

> Ask your attending about the patient's postoperative weight-bearing status and thromboprophylaxis.

COMPLICATIONS

I. Infection

II. Malunion

III. Nonunion

IV. Osteonecrosis (femoral neck fracture)

V. Screw cutout of the femoral head (sliding hip screw and cephalomedullary devices)

VI. Hardware failure

VII. Intra-articular screw placement

VIII. Continued pain and stiffness

IX. Subtrochanteric femur fracture (cancellous lag screws)

Hip

X. Periprosthetic fracture (short cephalomedullary sliding hip screw)
XI. Leg length discrepancy (comminuted subtrochanteric fractures)
XII. Deep vein thrombosis and pulmonary embolus

SUGGESTED READINGS

Bucholz RW, Heckman JD, Court-Brown C: Fractures in Adults, 6th ed. Philadelphia, Lippincott Williams & Wilkins, 2006, pp 1753–1844.

Canale ST (ed): Campbell's Operative Orthopaedics, 10th ed. Philadelphia, Mosby, 2003, pp 2873–2938.

Koval KJ, Zuckerman JD: Hip fractures: I. Overview and evaluation and treatment of femoral-neck fractures. J Am Acad Orthop Surg 2:141–149, 1994.

Koval KJ, Zuckerman JD: Hip fractures: II. Evaluation and treatment of intertrochanteric hip fractures. J Am Acad Orthop Surg 2:150–156, 1994.

KNEE

CHAPTER 20

Quadriceps and Patellar Tendon Repair

Karen J. Boselli, Albert O. Gee, and Craig L. Israelite

Case Study 1

A 29-year-old male recreational basketball player presents to the emergency department with a chief complaint of left knee pain. He reports that during a pick-up game, he landed "off-balance" on his left knee after a jump shot. His knee buckled, and he noticed immediate swelling. He was unable to bear weight on the knee after the injury and noted that he was unable to straighten the leg. When prompted, the patient reports a 3-month history of "jumper's knee" for which he had been using a Cho-Pat strap and anti-inflammatory medications. Physical examination reveals a grossly swollen and slightly ecchymotic left knee, with a palpable defect at the level of the patellar tendon. A lateral radiograph is presented in Figure 20-1.

Case Study 2

A 54-year-old obese man comes to the emergency department complaining of right knee pain after slipping and falling at work as a firefighter. He has since been unable to bear

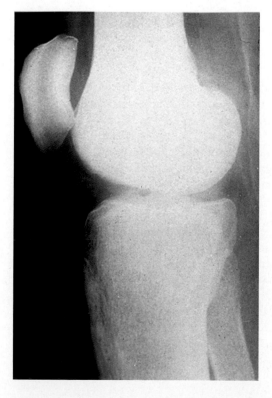

Figure 20-1
A lateral radiograph of the knee demonstrating patella alta. *(From McRae R, Esser M: Practical Fracture Treatment, 4th ed. Edinburgh, Churchill Livingstone, 2002.)*

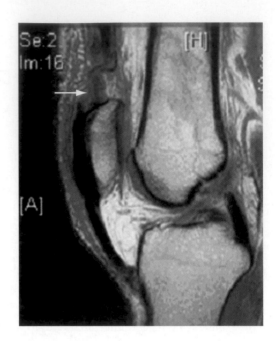

Figure 20-2
Sagittal magnetic resonance imaging scan of the
knee. The arrow is pointing to a complete rupture
of the quadriceps tendon.

weight. He recalls a tearing sensation in his knee at the time of his fall but does not recall
any direct trauma. He has a history of diabetes, for which he takes oral hypoglycemic
agents. On examination, he has a large right knee effusion and is lying in the stretcher
with his knee extended. He is able to flex his knee slightly but is unable to actively extend
it or raise his leg from the bed. There is a palpable depression over the superior aspect of
his patella, with moderate ecchymosis. A magnetic resonance image of the right knee is
presented in Figure 20-2.

BACKGROUND

    I. The most common disruption of the extensor mechanism of the knee is a trans-
verse patella fracture; this is followed in frequency by quadriceps tendon ruptures,
which are three times more common than patellar tendon ruptures.

    II. Quadriceps tendon ruptures occur most commonly in patients older than 40 years
of age, whereas patellar tendon ruptures occur more frequently in young, athletic
patients. Given an increase in activity level and athletic participation in all age
groups, however, it is not uncommon to see patellar tendon ruptures in older
patients.

    III. Quadriceps tendon ruptures usually occur transversely within 2 cm of the superior
pole of the patella, and they propagate distally and transversely into the medial
and lateral retinacula. Patellar tendon tears generally occur at the insertion site of
the tendon onto the inferior pole of the patella. They are less frequently seen as
avulsions from the tibial tubercle or as intrasubstance tears.

    IV. As a general rule, ruptures do not occur in healthy tendons; more often a rupture
occurs as the result of repetitive microtrauma. When prompted, patients often
report preexisting knee pain or tendinitis. In an athlete who does not give a history
of prior knee pain, there was likely a subclinical process contributing to degeneration and tendinopathy.

    V. Systemic medical conditions can contribute to the degeneration of the tendon and
make it more susceptible to injury. This is especially true of the quadriceps tendon.
These conditions may include lupus, gout, rheumatoid arthritis, chronic renal
failure, obesity, and diabetes mellitus. Bilateral injuries are also more common in

patients with these conditions because they are predisposed to systemic weakening of collagen.

VI. Quadriceps and patellar tendon ruptures have been associated with systemic steroid use as well as previous local steroid injections into the tendon.

VII. Mechanism of injury. Most commonly, the quadriceps or patellar tendon is ruptured by an eccentric violent contraction of the quadriceps muscles with the knee partially flexed.

    A. With a quadriceps tendon rupture, the patient may have been attempting to prevent a fall or regain balance during a fall.

    B. With a patellar tendon rupture, the injury may occur during a strenuous contraction of the quadriceps during athletic activity.

    C. Ruptures may occur during less strenuous activities in patients whose tendons are weakened by systemic illness or administration of steroids.

    D. Rarely, the quadriceps or patellar tendon can be injured by a direct penetrating trauma. Tendon disruption can also occur after total knee arthroplasty, and has been reported after anterior cruciate ligament reconstructions with patellar tendon autograft harvest.

TREATMENT ALGORITHM

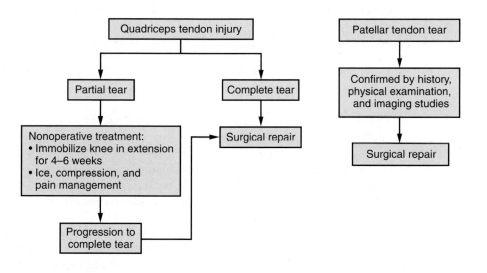

TREATMENT PROTOCOLS

I. **Treatment Considerations**

    A. Accurate diagnosis

    B. Identification of systemic medical illnesses

    C. Timing of tear—acute versus chronic rupture

    D. Extent of tear—partial versus complete rupture

II. **Initial Approach**

    A. Clinical presentation

        1. History

            a. Diagnosis of extensor mechanism ruptures can be difficult and is often delayed.

            b. With acute ruptures, patients give a history of immediate pain and inability to bear weight on the injured extremity. Some report an audible pop or tearing sensation at the time of injury.

The presence of any extension with a complete quadriceps or patellar tendon rupture indicates that the medial and lateral patellar retinacula are intact.

In the acute setting, aspiration of the knee hemarthrosis and administration of 10 mL of intra-articular lidocaine for analgesia assists in obtaining an accurate physical examination.

IT IS POSSIBLE FOR A QUADRICEPS OR PATELLAR TENDON RUPTURE TO OCCUR CONCOMITANTLY WITH OTHER LIGAMENTOUS INJURIES, WHICH CAN EASILY BE MISSED. A THOROUGH PHYSICAL EXAMINATION IS IMPORTANT, INCLUDING EXAMINATION OF THE KNEE UNDER ANESTHESIA AT THE TIME OF TENDON REPAIR.

It may be helpful to obtain a lateral radiograph of the contralateral knee for comparison.

The Insall-Salvati ratio is the ratio between patellar height and patellar tendon length; on a lateral radiograph, this ratio should be 1:1. An abnormal ratio indicates patella alta or patella baja (increased or decreased ratio, respectively).

Blumensaat's line is a line drawn along the roof of the intercondylar notch, seen on a lateral radiograph. This is an important landmark to determine the position of the patella.

---

c. A thorough past medical history should be elicited for any systemic conditions that may predispose the patient to an extensor mechanism rupture. Any history of previous knee surgeries and local steroid injection should also be documented.

d. With chronic injuries, patients may not recall a history of trauma. They may complain of weakness or instability with single-leg stance.

2. Physical examination
   a. On inspection and palpation of the knee joint, there is often a large, tense hemarthrosis. There may be ecchymosis or a painful, palpable gap in the tendon. The patella may be displaced superiorly or inferiorly.
   b. The hallmark of a complete injury is the inability to extend the knee (or maintain extension against gravity). If unable to perform a straight-leg raise against gravity due to pain, the patient may be more comfortable sitting at the edge of an examination table and attempting to extend the knee.
   c. With a partial injury, the medial and lateral retinacula may be intact, allowing some active extension. However, the patient lacks several degrees of terminal extension.
   d. If physical examination is limited by patient discomfort, consider performing an aspiration to decompress the hematoma. Local anesthetic can also be injected into the joint to facilitate a complete ligamentous examination.
   e. In chronic injuries, consolidated hematoma or scar tissue may obscure a palpable defect in the tendon, making the diagnosis more difficult.

B. Radiographic evaluation
   1. AP and lateral radiographs are most often sufficient in confirming the diagnosis of a suspected quadriceps or patellar tendon rupture.
      a. A patient with a quadriceps tendon rupture may have patella baja, and may have a small bony avulsion fragment from the superior pole of the patella.
      b. A patient with a patellar tendon rupture may have patella alta, with the patella lying superior to Blumensaat's line on a lateral radiograph with the knee flexed 30 degrees.
      c. Merchant or tunnel views can also be obtained to rule out patellar dislocations or osteochondral injuries, if suspected.
      d. Patients with chronic quadriceps tendinopathy may show a "tooth sign," or degenerative spurring at the patella.
   2. Ultrasound is highly operator-dependent but has been proven to be very accurate in the diagnosis of extensor mechanism injuries. It is also helpful for diagnosing this injury in patients with a previous total knee replacement.
   3. Magnetic resonance imaging is an excellent modality for evaluation of tendon pathology, especially if the diagnosis is in question. It can differentiate partial from complete rupture, and can also be used to estimate the size and extent of the tear. Additionally, it can be used to evaluate other intra- and extra-articular structures for concomitant injuries.
      a. Normal tendon has a homogeneous low signal with smooth margins.
      b. A ruptured tendon shows discontinuity of the fibers with wavy ends and an increased T2-signal, representing hemorrhage and edema.

TREATMENT OPTIONS

I. **Nonoperative Treatment**
   A. Conservative management is only indicated for incomplete ruptures. Complete ruptures must be managed with surgical restoration of the extensor mechanism.
   B. Nonoperative treatment should be reserved for patients who have normal or near-normal knee extension strength when compared to the uninjured knee,

and who have evidence of a small partial thickness tear on magnetic resonance imaging.

C. Treatment usually consists of immobilization with the knee in full extension for 4 to 6 weeks.

D. The patient should be closely monitored for progression to complete rupture, which requires prompt surgical treatment.

II. **Operative Treatment**

A. Operative treatment is indicated for acute complete ruptures of the quadriceps or patellar tendon.

B. Early or immediate repair (provided that the skin is in adequate condition) is recommended to restore the disrupted extensor mechanism and achieve optimal functional results. The prognosis for recovery is dependent on the time between injury and repair. Ideally, the repair should be performed within 10 to 14 days following the injury to prevent significant scar formation.

C. There are multiple techniques by which the quadriceps or patellar tendon can be surgically repaired. No studies have shown that one particular technique is superior to the others.

D. Chronic ruptures are more difficult to repair and may have less favorable outcomes than acute tears that undergo immediate repair. The remaining tendon and quadriceps muscle have often undergone degeneration and contraction, which makes apposition of the tendon back to the patella more difficult. Treatment of chronic tendon ruptures is beyond the scope of this chapter.

GENERAL PRINCIPLES OF EXTENSOR MECHANISM REPAIR

I. **Goals**

A. Successful repair of quadriceps or patellar tendon back to its bony insertion, or reapproximation of the torn ends

B. Repair of torn retinaculum

C. Restoration of active knee extension while maintaining full knee range of motion (ROM)

D. Avoiding patella alta or patella baja by tensioning the suture appropriately

E. Cerclage suture for reinforcement of patellar tendon repair as needed

II. The extensor mechanism of the knee consists of the quadriceps musculature (rectus femoris, vastus lateralis, vastus intermedius, and vastus medialis), the quadriceps tendon, the patella, the patellar tendon, the tibial tubercle, and the adjacent soft tissues.

III. The extensor mechanism originates above the hip joint at the origin of the rectus femoris muscle on the anterior inferior iliac spine. The remainder of the quadriceps muscles originate on the shaft of the femur.

IV. The individual quadriceps muscles come together distally to form the quadriceps tendon, which has three laminae, or layers.

A. The anterior (superficial) layer of the quadriceps tendon consists of the rectus femoris tendon.

B. The middle layer is composed of the vastus lateralis and vastus medialis.

C. The posterior (deepest) layer is formed by the vastus intermedius tendon.

V. The extensor mechanism has several functions. With the leg elevated, the extensor mechanism serves to extend or straighten the knee joint. With the foot planted on the ground, the extensor mechanism serves to stabilize the knee joint.

VI. The patella is the largest sesamoid bone in the body. Its purpose within the extensor mechanism is to increase the moment arm of the quadriceps femoris muscle, thereby providing a mechanical advantage in knee extension.

VII. The adjacent soft tissues about the knee are also important in knee stability and for proper knee extensor mechanism function.

A. The patellar retinaculum is a fibrous structure consisting of medial and lateral components, and it serves an important role in patellofemoral joint stability.

Knee

> When does your attending prefer to use cerclage wiring to augment the tendon repair?

B. The iliotibial band supports the extensor mechanism laterally, and it also serves as a patellofemoral joint stabilizer.

VIII. Each component of the extensor mechanism plays a critical role in the stability and function of the knee and therefore is essential to restore during surgical repair.

COMPONENTS OF THE PROCEDURE

Positioning, Prepping, and Draping

I. The patient is placed in a supine position on the operating room table. If intra-operative fluoroscopy is to be used, consider placing the patient on a radiolucent Jackson table.

II. The anesthesiologist administers general or regional (spinal/epidural) anesthesia. A femoral block may be given prior to the start of the case for postoperative pain control.

III. ROM and ligamentous examination should be performed to check for any motion deficits or concomitant ligamentous injuries.

IV. A bump should be placed under the ipsilateral hip to minimize hip external rotation, and the leg should be shaved proximal and distal to the knee.

V. A tourniquet is placed high on the proximal thigh of the operative leg, and the extremity is prepped and draped in standard fashion according to the surgical principles outlined in Chapter 1 (Fig. 20-3).

VI. The skin incision is marked over the midline of the knee anteriorly (Fig. 20-4).

A. For a quadriceps tendon, the incision should be centered from proximal to distal on the superior pole of the patella.

B. For a patellar tendon, the incision should extend from the mid-patella to the tibial tubercle.

> Ask your attending about his or her choice of incision for extensor mechanism repair.

VII. Less commonly, a transverse incision can be used. This is thought to be more cosmetic because it follows Langer's lines; however, it may make exposure more difficult.

Surgical Exposure

I. **Applied Surgical Anatomy**

A. The quadriceps femoris consists of the rectus femoris, vastus intermedius, vastus medialis, and vastus lateralis muscles.

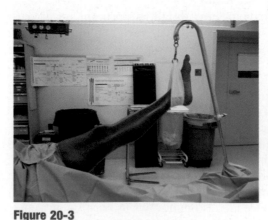

Figure 20-3
The operative extremity suspended with the candy cane. The impervious drape has been placed high on the thigh, just below the level of the tourniquet.

Figure 20-4
Skin incision for quadriceps tendon repair. The bony landmarks have been identified, including the borders of the patella and the tibial tubercle. There is significant ecchymosis due to hematoma at the site of rupture.

B. The extensor mechanism consists of the quadriceps femoris, quadriceps tendon, patella, patellar tendon, and tibial tubercle.

C. The patella is the largest sesamoid bone, lying within the expansion of the quadriceps tendon.

D. The lateral retinaculum is an expansion of the vastus lateralis muscle, attaching to the superolateral patella and proximal lateral tibia.

E. The medial retinaculum is an extension of the vastus medialis muscle, to the superomedial patella and proximal medial tibia.

F. The blood supply to the quadriceps tendon arises from the descending branches of the lateral femoral circumflex artery, branches of the descending geniculate artery, and branches of the medial and lateral superior geniculate arteries. The superficial tendon is well vascularized; however, the deep layer has a relatively avascular area that may play a role in tendon degeneration.

G. The blood supply to the patellar tendon arises from the inferior medial and inferior lateral geniculate arteries, reaching the tendon via the infrapatellar fat pad and retinacula.

H. The infrapatellar branch of the saphenous nerve exits from the adductor canal, pierces the sartorius muscle, and courses anteriorly to supply the skin at the medial and anterior knee, as well as the patellar tendon (Fig. 20-5).

II. The tourniquet is inflated prior to making the incision.

III. An incision is made with a 15-blade through the skin and superficial subcutaneous tissues. Self-retaining retractors or sharp rakes can then be placed to assist in the subcutaneous dissection.

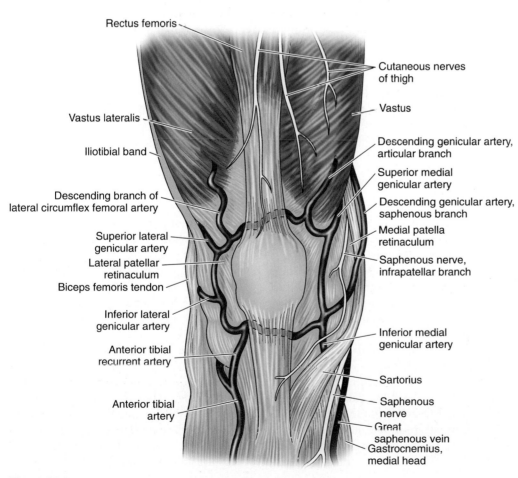

Figure 20-5
Superficial neurovascular structures of the anterior aspect of the knee. *(From Scott WN: Insall and Scott Surgery of the Knee, 4th ed. Philadelphia, Churchill Livingstone, 2006.)*

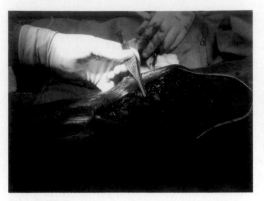

Figure 20-6

Exposure of the distal quadriceps tendon, patella, medial, and lateral retinacula. The distal pole of the patella should be exposed to facilitate passage of suture through drill holes.

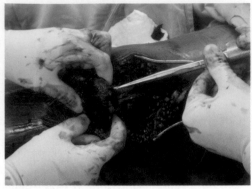

Figure 20-7

Débridement of soft tissue at the proximal pole of the patella, using a curette.

IV. Thick medial and lateral subcutaneous flaps are developed to identify the extent of the retinacular tears. This dissection can be performed sharply with a scalpel, or with the use of dissecting scissors (Fig. 20-6).

V. Once the medial and lateral extents of the retinacular tear are identified, they may be tagged with an absorbable suture for ease of later repair.

VI. There is usually a large hematoma present from the rupture, which needs to be removed with copious irrigation. This allows for exposure of the full extent of the tendon rupture; the torn ends can be identified and mobilized. The joint should also be inspected for any evidence of articular chondral injury or loose bodies.

VII. Any frayed or nonviable tissue should be débrided. Small, avulsed bony fragments that are too small for repair should be excised.

VIII. Depending on the location of the tear, the tibial tubercle, inferior pole of the patella, or superior pole of the patella are débrided of any remaining soft tissue. A rongeur, burr, or curette can be used to decorticate the bony insertion, and create a bleeding bed of bone for tendon healing (Fig. 20-7).

Tendon and Retinacular Repair

I. Once the edges of the torn tendon have been thoroughly débrided back to viable tissue, the actual repair may be performed. There are several surgical techniques available for repair; the choice of technique depends on the type of injury and surgeon preference.

II. If the rupture is in the midsubstance of the tendon, it can be repaired end-to-end using a heavy nonabsorbable suture.

III. Most often the rupture occurs at the osseotendinous junction, and it is not amenable to end-to-end repair. In this case, the tendon is reattached to its insertion using heavy suture and bone tunnels.

IV. The tendon should be realigned into its anatomic position to allow for normal patellar tracking.

V. Two heavy nonabsorbable sutures are inserted into the tendon using a running locked Krackow stitch (see Fig. 20-9). Although this is a diagram of the quadriceps tendon, a similar pattern should be used for patellar tendon repair. The suture should start from the torn tendon edge, travel approximately 2 to 3 cm until normal healthy tendon is encountered, and then turn back toward the tendon edge. One suture is placed medially within the tendon, and the other is placed laterally.

VI. Three parallel drill holes, spaced by about 1 cm, are placed along the long axis of the patella using a 2- or 3-mm drill bit. The drill holes should start at the bleeding

Ask your attending about his or her choice of suture pattern and suture material for repair.

CONFIRM THAT THE DRILL HOLES HAVE NOT VIOLATED THE ARTICULAR SURFACE BY DIRECT INSPECTION, PALPATION, OR FLUOROSCOPY.

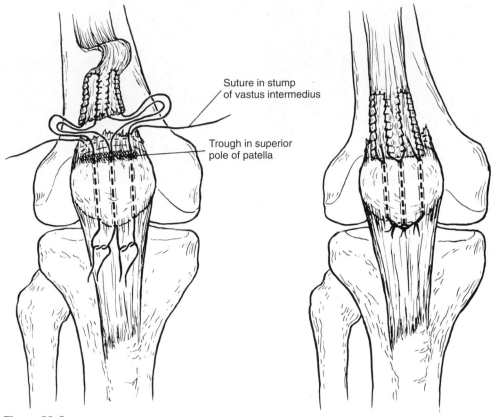

Suture in stump
of vastus intermedius

Trough in superior
pole of patella

Figure 20-8
Two depictions of the method of quadriceps tendon repair, using heavy sutures passed through intraosseous tunnels (*dotted* lines). The pattern is similar for repair of a patellar tendon rupture. (*Adapted from Azar FM: Traumatic disorders. In Canale ST [ed]: Campbell's Operative Orthopaedics, 10th ed. Philadelphia, Mosby, 2003.*)

bed of bone that was previously created and exit at the opposite pole of the patella. If the tendon has avulsed from the tibial tubercle, transverse drill holes must be placed in the tibial tubercle.

VII. The patellar tendon should be repaired adjacent to the articular surface and not to the anterior surface of the patella. If the tendon is positioned too anterior, an increase in patellofemoral contact forces results, yielding patellofemoral pain and premature arthritis.

VIII. There are four heavy suture limbs exiting at the torn tendon edge. Using a Hewson suture passer, pass these sutures through the drill holes as shown in Figure 20-8. The inner limbs pass together through the center drill hole, and the outer limbs pass through the medial and lateral drill holes, respectively.

IX. **Cerclage Suture Augmentation of Patellar Tendon Repair**
   A. If augmentation of the patellar tendon repair is required, begin by creating a transverse drill hole approximately 1 cm posterior to the tibial tubercle.
   B. Another heavy nonabsorbable suture or Mersilene tape is passed through the tunnel. The suture is then passed superiorly within the quadriceps tendon, along the superior pole of the patella, and tied. A wire can also be used, although it will require removal at a later date.

X. **Tensioning of Repair**
   A. Each pair of passed sutures is temporarily secured with a hemostat, applying gentle tension. The alignment of the patella on the distal femur should be inspected to ensure proper tracking during ROM (Fig. 20-9).
   B. During patellar tendon repair, the patellar height needs to be assessed. The knee is positioned in 30 degrees of flexion, and the patellar height is measured from the tibial tubercle to the inferior pole of the patella. This height can be

Consider augmentation of repair for midsubstance ruptures, or those in patients with systemic illnesses that have predisposed them to rupture. It should also be considered in patients who will be managed with aggressive early range of motion or those with excessive tension on the repair during intraoperative range of motion.

Knee

Excessive tensioning of the patellar tendon suture may result in patella baja.

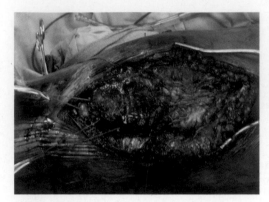

Figure 20-9
Tensioning of the quadriceps tendon repair, using hemostats. The Krackow stitch has been completed in the quadriceps tendon, and the suture limbs have been passed through drill holes through the patella.

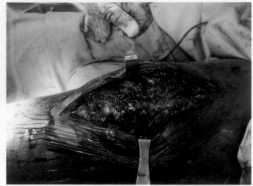

Figure 20-10
Completed quadriceps tendon repair. The knots are visible at the distal aspect of the patella (at the left of the image), and should be kept as small as possible.

> What is your attending's preferred method of estimating patellar height during suture tensioning?

compared to the unaffected extremity, and the height adjusted by increasing or decreasing tension on the cerclage suture.

C. If necessary, an intraoperative lateral radiograph can be obtained and compared with the contralateral extremity to ensure appropriate patellar position.

D. Once the correct position is obtained, the sutures are tied. The knee is flexed to determine the degree of flexion that can be tolerated without causing excessive tension on the repair.

E. Try to avoid excessively large knots, as they may be prominent beneath the skin and cause difficulty for the patient postoperatively.

F. Oversew the tendon repair with an interrupted #0 or 2-0 absorbable suture, to approximate any remaining loose ends (Fig. 20-10).

XI. **Retinacular Repair**

A. The medial and lateral retinacula are repaired using absorbable sutures in an interrupted fashion. Start at the most medial or lateral extent of the tear, using the tag sutures that were previously placed.

B. The retinacula should be repaired with the knee held in 30 degrees of flexion, to prevent limiting postoperative ROM.

Wound Closure

I. If exposed, the patellar paratenon should be closed first using a 2-0 or 3-0 absorbable suture.

II. Based on surgeon preference, the tourniquet may be released prior to closure or once the dressings have been secured. A closed suction drain can be used in the wound if necessary.

III. The subcutaneous layer and skin are closed in standard fashion (see Chapter 1 for details). After staples are placed to approximate the skin edges, a sterile dressing is applied and an Ace wrap is used to wrap the entire extremity.

IV. A knee immobilizer or locked hinge brace is placed on the extremity. Make sure that the brace is secure prior to the patient awaking from anesthesia.

POSTOPERATIVE CARE AND REHABILITATION

I. Perioperative antibiotics are continued for 24 hours, or until the Hemovac drain is removed.

II. Pain should initially be managed with patient-controlled analgesia and later controlled with oral narcotic mediation.

III. Deep vein thrombosis prophylaxis is based on the preference of the attending physician; warfarin (Coumadin), aspirin, or low-molecular-weight heparin

(Lovenox) are common choices. Sequential lower extremity compression devices should also be used routinely.

IV. If drains were placed, they are usually discontinued within the first two postoperative days, when the output is sufficiently low.

V. The knee immobilizer is kept in place until postoperative day 2, when the dressings are changed and the wound is inspected to assess appropriate healing.

VI. After the first wound check, a cylinder cast can be placed with the knee in full extension. Alternately, a reliable patient can be maintained in a locked hinged knee brace or immobilizer.

VII. Patients are allowed to bear weight as tolerated using crutches for assistance with ambulation. A physical therapy consult is obtained during the patient's hospital stay.

VIII. The remainder of rehabilitation is largely dependent on surgeon preference. For a quadriceps tendon repair, straight-leg-raise exercises may begin at 3 to 6 weeks, and the ROM exercises may start at 6 to 12 weeks. For a patellar tendon repair, isometric quadriceps strengthening may begin immediately, and ROM exercises may start as early as 2 weeks postoperatively.

IX. With the use of a hinged knee brace, motion may be increased by 10 to 15 degrees each week for a quadriceps tendon repair and 30 degrees each week for a patellar tendon repair. Full return to strenuous activity should be delayed until 4 to 6 months, when ROM has been restored and quadriceps strength has returned to nearly the strength of the contralateral extremity.

> What is your attending's rehabilitation protocol following extensor mechanism repair?

COMPLICATIONS

I. Loss of knee motion is the most common complication after extensor mechanism repair. Specifically, full knee flexion is most commonly affected.

II. Extensor weakness is usually secondary to quadriceps atrophy and is more common after patellar tendon repair.

III. Other complications may include:

A. Wound infection

B. Wound dehiscence, usually related to superficial location of the large nonabsorbable sutures

C. Patellar incongruity with patellofemoral degenerative changes, anterior knee pain, and arthritis

D. Rerupture of the repaired tendon, requiring revision repair surgery

SUGGESTED READINGS

Azar FM: Traumatic disorders. In Canale ST (ed): Campbell's Operative Orthopaedics, 10th ed., vol. 3. Philadelphia, Mosby, 2003.

Beynnon BD, Johnson RJ, Coughlin KM: Knee. In DeLee JC (ed): DeLee and Drez's Orthopaedic Sports Medicine, 2nd ed., vol. 2. Philadelphia, Saunders, 2003.

Ilan DI, Tejwani N, et al: Quadriceps tendon rupture. J Am Acad Ortho Surg 11:192–200, 2003.

Matava MJ: Patellar tendon ruptures. J Am Acad Ortho Surg 4:287–296, 1996.

Siwek CW, Rao JP: Ruptures of the extensor mechanism of the knee joint. J Bone Joint Surg Am 63:932–937, 1981.

Knee

CHAPTER 21

Arthroscopic Meniscectomy

Andrea L. Bowers and Brian J. Sennett

Case Study

A 55-year-old male presents with right knee pain and swelling. Six months ago, he stepped awkwardly off a curb and noted immediate pain on the inside of his knee. His pain is intermittent but is much worse with weight bearing, changing directions while walking, and especially with squatting or pivoting. Sometimes his knee "catches" or feels as if it is going to give out on him; occasionally it swells. His symptoms have not improved despite use of nonsteroidal anti-inflammatory medications, icing, and a course of physical therapy prescribed by his primary physician. Plain radiographs of the knee are unremarkable. Sagittal and coronal magnetic resonance images of the knee are presented in Figure 21-1.

BACKGROUND

I. The medial and lateral menisci are located within the knee joint between the femoral condyles and the tibial plateau. The menisci comprise type I collagen and serve to increase contact area, distribute load, and absorb shock with weight bearing. Menisci are largely insensate and have a limited blood supply. The peripheral third of the meniscus (the "red-red" zone) has greater perfusion than

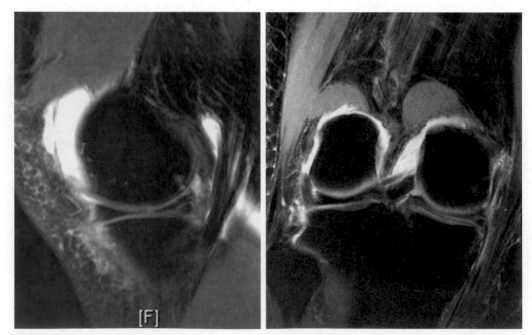

Figure 21-1
Sagittal and coronal T2 magnetic resonance imaging scans demonstrating a medial meniscus tear.

the middle ("red-white") and central ("white-white") zones. The color of the zones is based on the vascularity in that region of the meniscus.

II. The knee contains a semicircular lateral meniscus and a larger, oblong medial meniscus. Both are triangular in cross section. The menisci typically attach via bony attachments anteriorly and posteriorly. In addition, the medial meniscus is adherent to the deep portion of the medial collateral ligament and may attach to the lateral meniscus via the transverse intermeniscal ligament. The lateral meniscus occasionally attaches posteriorly by the ligaments of Humphry and Wrisberg to the femur (see Fig. 23-14).

III. The medial meniscus has less excursion than the lateral meniscus (5 mm vs. 11 mm, respectively) because the knee flexes from an extended position, and the medial meniscus is three times more likely to tear than the lateral meniscus.

IV. Tears of the meniscus are generally seen in two different patient populations. One is the young athlete who sustains a twisting injury and tears an otherwise healthy meniscus. Such tears may also be seen in the setting of a tear of the cruciate or collateral ligaments, and in limited instances, these tears may be amenable to repair. Tears are also seen in the middle-aged or older individual with underlying degenerative changes in the meniscus that render it susceptible to tearing with low-energy injury mechanisms.

V. Because of the poor vascular supply in the older patient, the underlying tissue is often incapable of healing, and tears of the meniscus are commonly excised rather than repaired. Historically, the meniscus was removed entirely; however, follow-up revealed an alarming incidence of degenerative arthritis after complete meniscectomy. Current standard of care is the arthroscopic partial meniscectomy, in which the tear and degenerative area are trimmed to a smooth peripheral rim, preserving as much meniscus as is possible.

VI. **Goals.** The major goals of arthroscopic meniscectomy are as follows:
   A. Relief of pain
   B. Removal of any mechanical block to motion
   C. Débridement to a stable rim of remaining meniscus
   D. Preservation of as much uninjured meniscus as possible
   E. Documentation of concomitant injury/degeneration of intra-articular structures

> An actual tear of the meniscus is distinguished from degenerative changes on a magnetic resonance imaging scan by communication of the intra-substance signal with the edge of the meniscus.

TREATMENT ALGORITHM

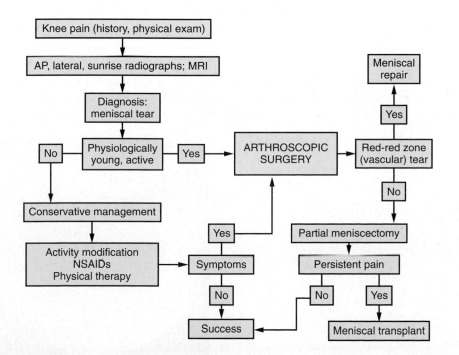

TREATMENT PROTOCOLS

Asymptomatic, partial-thickness tears less than 5 to 10 mm in length that are stable to probing may be treated nonoperatively, although there is a theoretical risk of tear propagation.

I. **Treatment Considerations**
   A. Patient age
   B. Concomitant injury (cruciate or collateral ligament tear)
   C. Symptomatology
   D. Size of tear
   E. Location of tear
   F. Orientation of tear
   G. Stability of tear
   H. Quality of meniscal tissue

II. **Nonoperative Treatment Options**
   A. Activity modification
   B. Nonsteroidal anti-inflammatory drugs
   C. Cryotherapy (icing)
   D. Physical therapy

SURGICAL ALTERNATIVES TO ARTHROSCOPIC MENISCECTOMY

I. **Open Meniscectomy:** fallen out of favor due to well-known association between complete meniscectomy and late osteoarthritis

II. **Meniscal Repair**
   A. Reserved for acute, peripheral tears (outer "red-red" zone) in a non-degenerative meniscus
   B. Ideal candidate: presents with a 1- to 2-cm acute, longitudinal peripheral (vascular) tear with concomitant anterior cruciate ligament reconstruction
   C. Techniques
      1. Open repair
      2. *Inside-out (gold standard)*
      3. Outside-in
      4. All-inside (e.g., sutures, arrows, darts)

III. **Meniscal Transplantation:** for young symptomatic patients after near-total or total meniscectomy with minimal degenerative changes in either the medial or lateral compartments

SURGICAL INDICATIONS FOR ARTHROSCOPIC MENISCECTOMY

I. Symptomatic radial or longitudinal tears in active individuals
II. Meniscal tears that have failed nonoperative management, such as physical therapy or injections
III. Displaced bucket-handle tears: a longitudinal tear of the central or posterior horn in which the inner one third, which is still attached to the edges of the periphery like a handle on a bucket, can displace into the notch (Fig. 21-2)

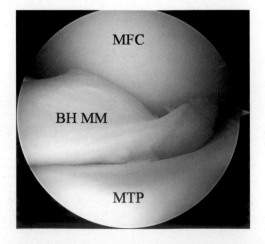

Figure 21-2
Bucket-handle tear of the medial meniscus (BH MM). The torn rim of the meniscus displaces toward the notch between the medial femoral condyle (MFC) and medial tibial plateau (MTP).

IV. Tears creating a mechanical block to knee range of motion

V. The symptomatic discoid lateral meniscus, with or without a tear

RELATIVE CONTRAINDICATIONS FOR ARTHROSCOPIC MENISCECTOMY

I. Significant comorbidities compromising the safety of a surgical candidate

II. Asymptomatic meniscus tear, particularly when stable (<5 mm, partial thickness, and displaceable <3 mm)

III. End-stage degenerative joint disease: these patients may be better served with total knee replacement (see Chapter 23)

GENERAL PRINCIPLES OF ARTHROSCOPIC MENISCECTOMY

I. Arthroscopy involves evaluation of the joint with a small arthroscopic camera ("scope") with a fiberoptic light source. The scope itself comes in different diameters and viewing angles. A 30-degree scope is the most frequently used scope in knee arthroscopy. The 70-degree scope is occasionally used to visualize the posterior joint.

II. The scope is inserted through a small 0.5- to 1-cm portal that penetrates the skin, subcutaneous tissues, and capsule. The capsule is distended with pressurized sterile irrigant (saline or lactated Ringer's) passed through the inflow cannula (which may be separate or a component of the scope).

III. The internal image is displayed on a screen positioned so the surgeon can comfortably view it while examining or manipulating the knee. Still photographs or video can be taken by the camera to document findings and treatment.

IV. Through a separate portal, a series of probes, shavers, and biters can be introduced into the joint to treat intra articular pathology. Care must be taken to avoid iatrogenic injury to the articular cartilage or other structures when inserting the scope or other instruments into the joint (Fig. 21-3).

V. Multiple portals can be made about the knee joint as needed to obtain the correct approach to the meniscus. In general, the medial and lateral parapatellar portals are the workhorses of arthroscopic meniscectomy.

VI. The following compartments of the joint should be inspected (Fig. 21-4).

A. Medial compartment

B. Lateral compartment

C. Notch (the central space occupied by the cruciate ligaments)

D. Patellofemoral articulation

E. Suprapatellar pouch

F. Medial gutter

G. Lateral gutter

VII. The order of examination does not necessarily matter, but a systematic, repeatable examination sequence can ensure that the entire joint is always thoroughly assessed.

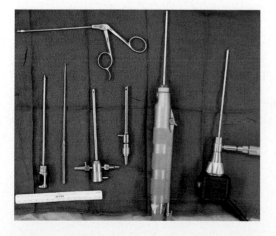

Figure 21-3

Arthroscopic instruments: blunt, probe, cannulae, biter, shaver, and 30-degree scope.

Knee

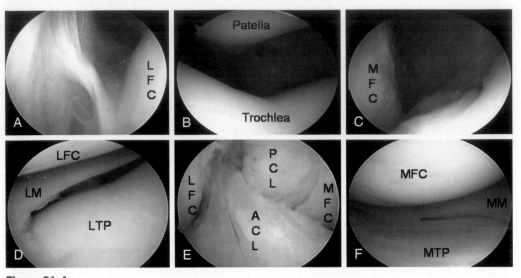

Figure 21-4

Arthroscopic images of the knee. **A,** Lateral gutter. **B,** Patellofemoral joint. **C,** Medial gutter. **D,** Medial hemijoint. **E,** Intercondylar. **F,** Lateral hemijoint. ACL, anterior cruciate ligament; LFC, lateral femoral condyle; LM, lateral meniscus; LTP, lateral tibial plateau; MFC, medial femoral condyle; MM, medial meniscus; MTP, medial tibial plateau; PCL, posterior cruciate ligament.

Documentation of concomitant or incidental findings is a critical element of the arthroscopic examination.

VIII. Periodically throughout the procedure, the joint may need to be irrigated through the outflow cannula to provide egress of accumulated intra-articular blood or debris and maintain a clear view.

IX. A meniscal tear that meets surgical criteria is either repaired or trimmed with a series of shavers and biters to a smooth, stable peripheral rim of remaining healthy meniscus.

> What sequence does your attending use to examine and treat the knee compartments, and why?

COMPONENTS OF THE PROCEDURE

Positioning, Prepping, and Draping

> What is your attending's preferred anesthetic for a straightforward partial meniscectomy?

I. The procedure can be performed under general endotracheal anesthesia, epidural or spinal, peripheral block, or intra-articular injection with sedation.

II. The patient is positioned supine on a standard operating table. To improve visualization, a valgus (lateral) post or knee holder is utilized. A valgus post is positioned approximately three fingerbreadths proximal to the knee flexion crease when the knee is flexed 90 degrees over the side of the table. When the post is up and a lateral force is applied to the distal extremity, the patient's thigh presses against the post and creates a valgus stress on the knee to open the medial hemijoint (Fig. 21-5). A leg holder allows the knee to flex off the end of the table and allows valgus and varus forces to be applied to improve visualization.

III. The extremity should be shaved to approximately 6 inches above and below the knee.

> Does your attending routinely apply or inflate a tourniquet for partial meniscectomy?

IV. Some surgeons apply a tourniquet to the proximal thigh, which may or may not be inflated. A nonsterile 34-inch tourniquet is usually sufficient and is secured over Webril padding.

V. Prepping and draping are performed according to the general principles outlined in Chapter 1. Ask the attending surgeon about his or her preferences.

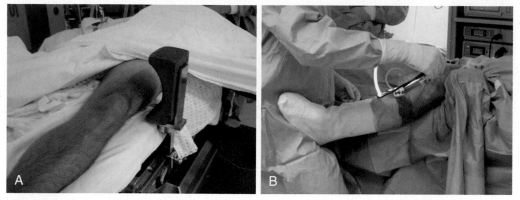

Figure 21-5
Lateral post. **A,** The lateral post is positioned proximal to the knee joint. **B,** During surgery the arthroscopist uses his or her own leg to stress the patient's leg against the draped valgus post and open the medial hemijoint.

Surgical Approach and Applied Anatomy

I. The leg is positioned in an extended position on the table. The knee is examined for an effusion, and the joint capsule is injected with approximately 40 mL of fluid (either saline or local anesthetic with epinephrine, depending on the type of anesthesia).

II. The knee is flexed over the side of the table.

III. The surface anatomy of the knee, including the patella, medial and lateral edges of the patellar tendon, and medial and lateral tibial plateau are palpated and marked with a marking pen. The lateral and medial parapatellar portal sites are positioned approximately 1 and 1.5 cm, respectively, away from the patellar tendon halfway between the distance from the patella to the tibial plateau (Fig. 21-6).

IV. The projected portal sites can be injected with local anesthetic with epinephrine before the incision is made, to reduce capsular bleeding.

V. An 11-blade is used to create the first portal, first through skin and then through subcutaneous tissues into the capsule. The incision can be dilated with a hemostat. The blunt trocar for the scope is introduced and positioned within the joint.

> **BE CAREFUL NOT TO TRANSECT THE MENISCUS ITSELF WHEN MAKING YOUR PORTALS WITH AN 11-BLADE.**

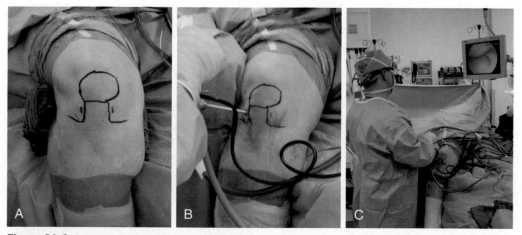

Figure 21-6
A, Surface landmarks are marked on a prepped and draped knee. **B,** An arthroscope is introduced via a portal. **C,** The surgeon visualizes the internal joint on a viewing screen.

Knee

VI. The blunt trocar is removed and the camera is inserted. An inflow cannula is established, either connected to the scope itself or through a separate portal.

VII. A second portal is created to allow instruments to be introduced into the joint. This portal can be created under direct visualization by the camera inserted in the original portal. This can minimize the risk of iatrogenic injury to the articular surfaces introduced with blind or forceful portal entry.

Diagnostic Arthroscopy

I. A diagnostic arthroscopy is performed, in which the aforementioned compartments of the knee are systematically inspected and probed. Photographs are taken of each compartment and any pathology encountered. The order of the examination varies by surgeon preference, and the following is an example of one technique.

II. The medial compartment examination is facilitated by applying a valgus force against the lateral post. The knee can be flexed or extended gently to better visualize specific areas within the compartment. Typically the scope is inserted through the lateral portal and the probe through the medial portal. The articular surfaces and the medial meniscus are examined.

III. The modified Gillquist technique can facilitate visualization of the posterior medial hemijoint. The knee is flexed to 90 degrees, and a varus force is applied to the tibia. The camera is passed from the lateral portal medial to the posterior cruciate ligament, levering against the posterior cruciate ligament and away from condyle, to observe the posterior horn of the medial meniscus and the posteromedial aspect of the knee.

IV. The camera is carefully withdrawn from the medial compartment into the notch. The anterior and posterior cruciate ligaments are probed to assess their integrity.

V. The lateral hemijoint is entered. A varus force or figure-of-four positioning allows access to the lateral compartment (Fig. 21-7). Again, the articular cartilage and meniscus are examined. The popliteus tendon can be visualized coursing behind the posterolateral aspect of the lateral meniscus. The popliteal hiatus is evaluated for the presence of loose bodies.

VI. The camera is pulled back toward the notch, and then it is advanced up and forward along the trochlea as the knee is slowly extended. The patellofemoral joint and suprapatellar pouch can be examined from this position.

VII. Finally, the medial and lateral gutters can be examined by positioning the camera around and down the sides of the femoral condyles.

VIII. Easy passage of the scope may be restricted by plica, which are remnants from embryonic joint development. Such plica are typically benign, although the medial patellar plica in particular can become enlarged and cause pain in the region of the medial femoral condyle.

Figure 21-7

The figure-of-four position facilitates access to the lateral compartment.

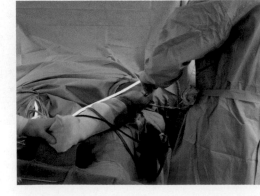

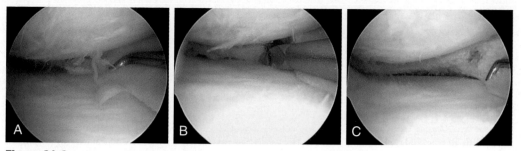

Figure 21-8
A, Medial meniscus tear. **B,** Débridement of tear. **C,** Trimmed meniscus.

Partial Meniscectomy

I. Attention is turned to the meniscal tear. The entire length of the meniscus is probed and the margin of the tear is assessed for stability. An attempt should be made to reduce any portions of the meniscus that are displaced (e.g., parrot-beak or bucket-handle tears).

II. As a general rule, for the posterior half of the meniscal body and the posterior horn, the probe/shaver/biter should enter on the ipsilateral side of the knee (i.e., medial meniscus, the shaver should enter from the medial portal). For tears that are located in the anterior horn and anterior half of the meniscal body, access to the tear may be enhanced if the shaver is inserted from the contralateral portal.

III. A motorized shaver is used to débride wispy, irregular edges. A biter is used repeatedly to trim jagged edges. Biters are available with variable-angled necks to achieve access to all parts of the tear.

IV. The shaver and biters are alternated as needed to excise the torn portion of meniscus and débride to a smooth, stable rim of remaining tissue. Care must be taken to débride enough meniscus to create an even edge without excising too much and destabilizing remaining tissue.

V. The trimmed meniscus is probed again to verify stability of the remaining segment (Fig. 21-8).

Wound Closure

I. The instrument and camera are withdrawn. The inflow is closed and the outflow portal opened to allow drainage of the remaining irrigation.

II. Some surgeons may choose to instill intra-articular anesthetic at closure. Sterile dressings are applied per surgeon's preference.

POSTOPERATIVE CARE AND GENERAL REHABILITATION

I. Arthroscopic meniscectomy is commonly performed on an outpatient basis, and the patient is sent home the same day.

II. Oral narcotic medicines are prescribed for management of postoperative pain.

III. Cryotherapy can enhance postoperative analgesia and minimize effusion.

IV. Sterile dressings are not removed until a few days postoperatively.

V. In general, patients can bear weight as tolerated immediately on the operative lower extremity. Early range of motion is encouraged. Physical therapy may be necessary.

COMMON COMPLICATIONS

I. Iatrogenic intra-articular injury
II. Hemarthrosis

> INTRODUCE INSTRUMENTS INTO THE JOINT WITH SHARP EDGES ANGLED AWAY FROM THE ARTICULAR CARTILAGE TO AVOID IATROGENIC INJURY TO THE ARTICULAR CARTILAGE ABOVE AND BELOW THE MENISCUS.

> OVERLY AGGRESSIVE DÉBRIDEMENT CAN DESTABILIZE THE REMAINING MENISCAL TISSUE.

> All components of the diagnostic arthroscopy and partial meniscectomy should be documented with photographic images taken with the arthroscope.

> Does your attending typically instill anesthetic or analgesics into the joint at the end of the case?

Knee

III. Destabilization of the remaining meniscus
IV. Sensory deficit over lateral proximal tibia (infrapatellar branch of the saphenous nerve)
V. Fluid extravasation into the calf or thigh
VI. Focal osteonecrosis from laser-assisted chondroplasty

SUGGESTED READINGS

Greis PE, Bardana DD, Holmstrom MC, Burks RT: Meniscal injury: I. Basic science and evaluation. J Am Acad Orthop Surg 10:168–176, 2002.

Greis PE, Holmstrom MC, Bardana DD, Burks RT: Meniscal injury: II. Management. J Am Acad Orthop Surg 10:177–187, 2002.

McCarty EC, Spindler KP, Bartz R: Meniscal injury. In Vaccaro AR: Orthopaedic Knowledge, Update 8. Rosemont, IL, American Academy of Orthopaedic Surgeons, 2005, pp 449–451.

Miller MD, Cooper DE, Warner JJP: Review of Sports Medicine and Arthroscopy, 2nd ed. Philadelphia, Elsevier, 2002.

CHAPTER 22

Anterior Cruciate Ligament Reconstruction

J. Todd R. Lawrence   and   Brian J. Sennett

Case Study

A 20-year-old female collegiate athlete presents with complaints of left knee pain, swelling, and a feeling of instability after a twisting injury to her knee that she sustained while she was playing soccer about 7 weeks ago. She reports hearing and sensing a "pop" at the time of injury. Her knee became swollen over the course of the next few hours and has been swollen since that time. Aspiration of her knee by her team physician the next day revealed a hemarthrosis. She is currently able to ambulate with minimal pain but notes that her knee feels unstable, as if "the bones are moving places they are not supposed to," especially while performing cutting and jumping activities. She denies any locking, catching, or clicking in the left knee. Physical examination is notable for a mild effusion and positive Lachman, anterior drawer, and pivot shift tests. No examination findings are suggestive of patellar pathology, meniscal tears, or other ligamentous injuries about the knee. A magnetic resonance image of the knee and an intraoperative arthroscopic view of the ruptured anterior cruciate ligament (ACL) are presented in Figures 22-1 and 22-2.

BACKGROUND

I. Anatomy/biomechanics. The ACL is an intra-articular extrasynovial ligament of the knee. In the notch of the knee, it courses obliquely from the medial aspect of the lateral femoral condyle to insert just anterior to and between the intercondylar eminences of the tibia. In total, it is approximately 33 mm long and 11 mm in diameter and can resist a load of approximately 2200 newtons. It is thought to have two functional bundles. The anteromedial bundle is tighter in flexion and

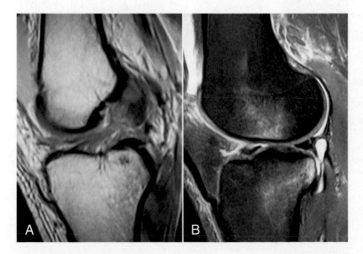

Figure 22-1

Magnetic resonance imaging scans demonstrating an anterior cruciate ligament (ACL) tear. **A,** A sagittal, T1-weighted image through the notch demonstrates a complete tear of the ACL. **B,** A sagittal, T2-weighted image through the lateral tibiofemoral joint demonstrates edema in the distal femur and posterior one third of the tibial plateau, a characteristic "bone bruise" pattern of ACL tears.

237

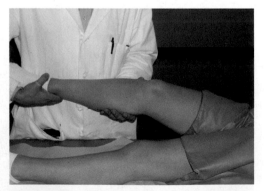

Figure 22-2
Intraoperative view demonstrating an ACL tear. An arthroscopic view of the notch demonstrating a tear of the ACL from the femoral insertion site. Note the empty medial wall of the lateral femoral condyle.

resists anterior translation of the tibia on the femur. The posterolateral bundle is tighter in extension and is more responsible for countering rotational forces. The primary blood supply is the middle geniculate artery.

II. The most common mechanism of injury responsible for ACL rupture is a non-contact pivoting injury with the foot firmly planted on the ground. Most patients report hearing or sensing a "pop" and experience swelling of the knee that occurs within 6 hours of the injury. If this effusion is aspirated, it typically reveals bloody fluid referred to as a *hemarthrosis*.

III. The Lachman test is the most sensitive physical examination maneuver for detecting an ACL tear. The pivot shift test is also useful for assessing rotational instability; however, it typically requires general anesthesia in the acute setting because the patients guard against the test (Figs. 22-3 and 22-4).

IV. Female athletes have a two- to eightfold increased risk of ACL tear compared with male athletes. The etiology of this is not known but may be due to differences in neuromuscular control.

V. Chronic ACL deficiency results in a higher incidence of cartilage damage and meniscal tears compared with ACL-intact knees. Despite this fact, the develop-

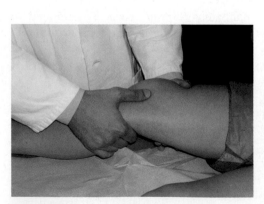

Figure 22-3
Lachman test. The Lachman test is the most sensitive physical examination test for anterior cruciate ligament tears. The knee is held at 30 degrees of flexion, and an anteriorly directed force is applied to the proximal tibia while the femur is held stationary. The amount of translation and the nature of the endpoint are assessed.

Figure 22-4
Pivot shift test. The pivot shift test is useful for assessing rotational instability. The extremity is held by the lower leg with the knee in extension, and a valgus force is applied to the knee. In this position, in an anterior cruciate ligament–deficient knee, the tibia is subluxated anteriorly. The knee is slowly flexed by the examiner and at about 20 to 30 degrees of knee flexion, the knee "shifts" or reduces as the iliotibial band slips posterior to the axis of rotation of the knee. Tibial internal rotation can be used to accentuate this effect.